OCCUPATIONAL EPIDEMIOLOGY

OCCUPATIONAL EPIDEMIOLOGY

Proceedings of the Seventh International Symposium on Epidemiology in Occupational Health, Tokyo, Japan, 11–13 October 1989

Editors:

Haruhiko Sakurai
Department of Preventive Medicine and Public Health
Keio University, School of Medicine
Tokyo, Japan

Isao Okazaki
Department of Preventive Medicine and Public Health
Keio University, School of Medicine
Tokyo, Japan

Kazuyuki Omae
Department of Preventive Medicine and Public Health
Keio University, School of Medicine
Tokyo, Japan

1990

EXCERPTA MEDICA, Amsterdam – New York – Oxford

International Congress Series No. 889
ISBN 0 444 81337 3

This book is printed on acid-free paper.

Published by:
Elsevier Science Publishers B.V.
(Biomedical Division)
P.O. Box 211
1000 AE Amsterdam
The Netherlands

Sole distributors for the USA and Canada:
Elsevier Science Publishing Company Inc.
655 Avenue of the Americas
New York, NY 10010
USA

Printed in The Netherlands

Preface

This Proceedings volume is composed of papers presented at the Seventh Symposium of the Scientific Committee on Epidemiology in Occupational Health of the International Commission on Occupational Health. The Symposium was held at the Meiji Kinenkan, Minato-ku, Tokyo, October 11–13, 1989.

The International Commission on Occupational Health (ICOH) holds regular meetings called the International Congress on Occupational Health every three years. The activities within the ICOH are organized into a number of scientific committees. The Scientific Committee on Epidemiology in Occupational Health was formed in 1980 and its 29 members represent 17 countries from around the globe. A Symposium is held every year, except for the year of the ICOH triennial congress, for the purpose of bringing together active research workers in occupational epidemiology to discuss methodology, findings, and applications of their work. It has become an important forum of exchange in the field of occupational epidemiology. Previous symposiums have been held in Helsinki, Finland (1980); Montreal, Canada (1982); Singapore (1983); Como, Italy (1985); Los Angeles, U.S.A. (1986); and Stockholm, Sweden (1988).

The 1989 Symposium was organized by the Department of Preventive Medicine and Public Health, School of Medicine, Keio University in Tokyo, Japan. The Symposium Organizing Committee consisted of myself, Haruhiko Sakurai (Chairman), Professor, Keio University; Professor Hideyasu Aoyama, Okayama University; Professor Shunichi Araki, University of Tokyo; Professor Masayuki Ikeda, University of Kyoto; Professor Noburu Ishinishi, Kyushu University; Professor Ken-ichi Nakamura, Showa University; Professor Kuniomi Nakamura, National Institute of Industrial Health; Professor Kazuo Nomiyama, Jichi Medical School; Professor Toshiteru Okubo, Universty of Occupational and Environmental Health; Professor Kazuo Saito, Hokkaido University; Professor Tsuguyoshi Suzuki, University of Tokyo. An Evaluation Committee consisting of Professor J. Malcolm Harrington, University of Birmingham, Birmingham, United Kingdom; Professor Christer Hogstedt, National Institute of Occupational Health, Solna, Sweden; Professor Okubo, Professor Araki, and myself were responsible for the review of all originally submitted abstracts.

I would like to express my sincere gratitude to the Advisory Board, to Dr. Hiroshi Nakajima (Director-General, WHO), to the invited lecturers, to the chairpersons of the various sessions, and especially to all the participants whose research, paper presentations, and discussions provided this Seventh International Symposium on Epidemiology in Occupational Health with many scientifically stimulating sessions. Their contributions made this Symposium a success, both scientifically with the many topics of provocative and meticulous research and work that were presented as well as socially with the warmth of meeting fellow researchers in the field. I would also like to express my appreciation to the Ministry of Labor, Japan Medical Association, Japan Association of Industrial Health, Japan Industrial Safety and Health Association, Occupational Health Promotion Foundation, Japan World Exposition Commemorative Fund, Uehara Memorial Foundation, The Cooperative Foundation Against Environmental Pollution, as well as various industrial associations and private corporations without whose financial support and encouragement, we would have not been able to bring this Symposium to fruition. Finally, I am indebted to all the authors who undertook the work of preparing manuscripts for this proceedings volume, thereby contributing to a broad overview of current occupational epidemiology research. It is hoped that this will further stimulate future interest in occupational epidemiology.

All authors, whose abstracts were accepted for presentation at the Symposium, were invited to prepare manuscripts for this Proceedings volume. For the purpose of rapid publication, these manuscripts have undergone no editing. The papers are grouped into the different themes of the Symposium and ordered alphabetically, by the first author, within each theme.

Haruhiko Sakurai, M.D.
Chairman, ISEOH-89

CONTENTS

INVITED LECTURES

METHODS AND EXPOSURE ASSESSMENT

OCCUPATIONAL CANCER

INVITED LECTURES

Occupational Epidemiology. H. Sakurai et al., editors

OCCUPATIONAL EPIDEMIOLOGY AND ITS APPLICATION TO HEALTH CARE WORKERS

J M HARRINGTON
Institute of Occupational Health University of Birmingham University Road West PO Box 363 BIRMINGHAM B15 2TT United Kingdom

INTRODUCTION

The science (and art) of epidemiology is usually applied to occupational health problems as they arise but irrespective of the industry. Rarely does one consider an entire industry as a challenge to occupational epidemiology. In this review the health care industry is highlighted as a suitable case for epidemiological concern.

THE SIGNIFICANCE OF HEALTH CARE WORKERS AS AN OCCUPATIONAL GROUP

The health care industry has a number of features which warrant special attention. These are its size, the multiplicity of its occupational hazards, the patchy attention it has received from investigators thus far, its unique culture and the opportunities it affords for advancing knowledge on occupational health problems which would be applicable elsewhere.

Size

The health care industry employs a large sector of the workforce in most countries. In the United States of America in 1984., there were seven million health care workers (HCW) and this figure is estimated to rise to 11 million by 1990.[1] In the United Kingdom, the current figure is one million which makes the Department of Health the largest employer of labour in Western Europe. In many countries the HCW population is about 5% of the total workforce, though most work outside the hospital environment.[2]

Multiplicity of Occupational Hazards

The range of hazards to which the HCW may be exposed is vast. It covers a wide range of physical agents - fires, explosions, gassings, electrocutions, radiation, noise etc, many chemical hazards including carcinogens, allergens, mutagens and narcotics, mechanical and ergonomic issues as well as psychological problems such as work patterns and job stress. Theoretically all the microbiological hazards are possible.

An underinvestigated population

Given the range and complexity of the health care industry, the published literature does not accurately reflect these occupational health risks and hazards. Much of the early literature was anecdotal until the advent of non-communicable disease epidemiology. Even thereafter the populations studied have been either those where tracing procedures were relatively easy or those for which the researchers had a particular - perhaps egocentric - interest[3]. The surfeit of studies of physicians epitomises this patchy coverage. On the other hand, there is some evidence that the level of accidents [4,5,6,7,8] and sickness absence[9] is extremely high among HCW's but little systematic work has been undertaken to follow up these important observations.

A unique culture

Attitudes to health and safety are modified by the culture within which a group of employees work. Emmett & Baetz[4] have summarised these features for HCW's. They include a concern with a curative rather than a preventive approach in their own professional dealings combined with a low personal concern for their own well being. Both these features are closely related to the role of caring for the health of others. Many employees are resident at the site of work. On the other hand, few health industry managements have established high quality occupational health services. Indeed, management attitude to occupational health is frequently primeval compared with their counterparts in major industries.

Epidemiology Opportunities

The health care industry affords potential exposure to some uniquely interesting agents. In particular, infectious agents; occupational, rather than therapeutic, exposure to chemotherapeutic agents and pockets of workers exposed to chemicals of current concern such as ethylene oxide, glutaraldehyde and formaldehyde. Furthermore, the professional associations which represent many of the sub-groups of the workforce - physicians, nurses, radiographers, physiotherapists - have a membership which remains stable throughout their working life.

CURRENT OCCUPATIONAL HEALTH CONCERNS

There are many, but perhaps some predominate. They are:

INFECTIONS	STRESS
ALLERGENS	ADDICTION
TERATOGENS	MANUAL HANDLING
CARCINOGENS.	

All of these hazards have been studied in one or more of the main sub-groups of HCW's but as Table 1 shows, the coverage is patchy. Physicians and nurses predominate as the occupational groups which have been studied the most, whilst cancer is clearly the health issue of greatest concern - though not necessarily of greatest importance.

THE EPIDEMIOLOGICAL METHOD AND HEALTH CARE POPULATIONS

Perhaps one way of reviewing the epidemiological difficulties of studying HCW's is to develop a matrix of HCW sub-groups by the steps necessary to complete an adequate epidemiological study (Table 2). The logical steps in any epidemiological study are to assemble an adequate study population, determine the exposure status, select comparison groups, measure health outcome, limit non-response and establish effective follow up.[10] A review of these steps for the major HCW sub-groups perhaps demonstrates why some groups have been studied more extensively than others.

Physicians clearly provide more fertile ground for study as there are excellent prospects for the successful completion of each step in the epidemiological method with possible exception of deciding on an appropriate comparison group. By contrast, technical and support staff in health care facilities score poorly for most steps. Nevertheless, they are one of the largest sub-groups with some of the greatest exposures to hazards of interest. Assembling adequate study populations, limiting non-response and monitoring effective follow up clearly are the major methodological constraints.

EXAMPLES OF POPULATIONS STUDIED AND PROBLEMS REVIEWED

The following sections are concerned with reviewing studies of sub-groups of HCW's in order to highlight some of these difficulties. The selection of the sub-groups demonstrates an unashamed bias as it is easier to discuss research with which one is most familiar. Such a bias also limits the desire inherent in all epidemiologists to criticise other people's work. One's own work, is after all, so much more valuable than that of any one else! A further restriction imposed was to concentrate on more recent work as a number of reviews[11,12,13,14] have been published in the last few years.

Hospital staff in general

Studies of hospital staff as a group have tended to concentrate on infectious disease risks[8] or have attempted to review accidents[5] or sickness absence.[9] Recent interest has been generated in the risks to various HCW groups from hepatitis B and human immunodeficiency viruses. Despite the publicity surrounding the theoretical occupational risk of acquiring HIV infection, hepatitis B virus (HBV) is a much more serious threat to health.[15] The epidemiology of HBV is also much more clearly delineated. The advent of effective and safe vaccines against HBV should eliminate this occupational risk which was significant (10-30% seroconversion rate in HCW's with a 2% mortality). The epidemiology of HIV transmission is less clearcut. Few good quality longitudinal studies have been published but from the meagre evidence available, it appears that seroconversion rates following needlestick injuries with infected blood are less than 0.5%.[15] Nevertheless, needlestick injuries are grossly underreported.[16] One unpublished report from a medical student in my university suggested that medical students

Table 1

STUDIES OF THE HEALTH RISKS OF HEALTH CARE WORKERS

	INFECTION	PREG OUTCOME	CANCER	ALLERGY	ERGONOMICS	TOXIC	STRESS
PHYSICIANS	✓		✓			✓	
ANAESTHETISTS		✓	✓			✓	
ONCOLOGY STAFF			✓			✓	
LABORATORY STAFF	✓		✓	✓			
RADIOLOGY STAFF		✓	✓			✓	
DENTISTS					✓		
NURSES			✓	✓	✓		✓
PHARMACEUTICAL WORKERS			✓	✓		✓	
MAINTAINANCE STAFF							
DOMESTIC STAFF			FEW STUDIES				

Table 2

THE EPIDEMIOLOGICAL METHOD & HEALTH CARE POPULATIONS

	PHYSICIANS	NURSES	TECH STAFF	MAINT/DOM	PHARM WORKERS
ASSEMBLE ADEQUATE STUDY POPULATION	••••	•••	••	•	•
DETERMINE EXPOSURE STATUS	••••	••	••	••	••
SELECT COMPARISON GROUPS	••	•	•••	•••	•••
MEASURE HEALTH OUTCOME	••••	••	••	••	••
LIMIT NON-RESPONSE	••••	•	•	•	••
EFFECTIVE FOLLOW UP/TRACE RATE	••••	•	•	•	••

•••• Excellent
••• Good
•• Fair
• Poor

experience between 600 and 1000 injuries from needles or during surgery per 1000 person years. Injuries whilst assisting in the operating theatre contributed 36% of all reported injuries. If these figures are a closer estimate of injury, then the seroconversion rate for HIV is perhaps an order of magnitude lower than that reported.

By contrast, tuberculosis was traditionally an occupational infection of HCW's. In the 1950's in Britain, medical laboratory staff were noted to have a ninefold excess risk of acquiring the disease,[17] whereas two decades later the excess risk was still fivefold.[18] A recent survey of UK health service employees[19] suggests that although the risk is now comparable to UK national rates, mortuary attendants remain a high risk group.

Physicians

As stated earlier, physicians have received more attention from epidemiologists than other groups of HCW's. Indeed, Doll's early work on cigarette smoking and lung cancer made use of this very stable and eminently traceable group. As a group such tracing is easy in most countries and recent studies from Japan[20] and Finland[21] have emphasised their exceptionally low SMR's for many disease groupings - particularly for cancer. By contrast, increasing attention is being devoted to their mental state - a much more difficult subject for epidemiological study. There is no doubt that sick doctors are a problem to themselves and for their patients. Psychiatric illness in doctors may interfere with their competence as practitioners. In the UK, doctors do have greater likelihood of dying from suicide, accidents and cirrhosis than the general population even after allowing for social class influences.[22] When morbidity is taken into account as well as mortality it may be concluded that physicians have better physical health but poorer mental health than others.[23] Stressors identified as being particularly important were job demands and patient expectations, interference with family life, constant interuptions and the administration of the practice.[24] These stressors seem to start at the most junior levels in hospital[25] and as alcoholism is one coping strategy, excess drinking seems to be a problem even at medical school.[26] Many of these studies, however, lack a good epidemiological basis and the response rates for the attitudinal studies rarely exceed 50%.

Long hours of work are blamed for much of the ills and complaints of junior doctors. We recently reviewed the literature on the subject[27] and discovered that little work had been done to study the effects of such fatigue on doctors and even less on developing appropriate performance tests for sleep-deprived doctors.

Pathologists and pathology staff

Whilst we have published mortality studies of pathologists suggesting an excess of lymphoma[8] or brain tumours[28], less work has been published on other laboratory staff. Such studies are difficult to mount for the reasons outlined earlier but a recent doctoral thesis in my department has attempted to study one particular group which, a priori, might be assumed to be at high risk of occupational disease - namely the post mortem room workers.[29] The study plan was a simple one: to see if post mortem room workers had a poorer health record than comparable groups (who is a comparable group?) and to study whether the working environment of the post mortem room was as hazardous as it appears. Surprisingly, although these workers frequently puncture their gloves and injure themselves, they do not have a high incidence of infections which could be ascribed to contact with autopsy material. Interestingly, a follow up study of our cohort of pathologists suggest that the brain tumour excess, although modest, is still present after a further decade of surveillance.

Anaesthetists

Workers in the anaesthetic room have been studied extensively both for mortality and pregnancy outcome. Reviews of these studies have been published from time to time but critical reviews of the literature are few and far between. Again, expressing a personal bias, the conclusions drawn by one of my staff[30] after such a critical review in 1986 perhaps summarises the present state of knowledge and highlights many of the problems inherent in studying even a well delineated group of HCW's

> "In the interpretation of epidemiological studies, attention must be paid to both the *quality* and the *quantity* of the data. If quantity alone were important, we could conclude that occupational exposure to anaesthetic gases does indeed present serious reproductive hazards, and possibly a number of other health effects. On closer examination, however, many of the studies present considerably flawed data, subject to strong confounding and reporting biases which severely limit the conclusions which may be drawn from their findings.
>
> First, none of the surveys considered here appears to have solved the problem of finding a suitable control group, and, secondly, no epidemiological study specifically implicates anaesthetic gases alone as a factor in disease causation."

Studies of the working environment of anaesthetists have started to appear more frequently of late.[31,32] If anaesthetic gases are the cause of abnormal pregnancy outcome and other adverse health effects in this popultion and if these hygiene studies are valid, then much remains to be done to clean up the operating theatre as a workplace.

Oncology staff

Although the clinical toxicology of anti neoplastic drugs is well documented so far as patients are concerned, little information exists on the risks to health of those who adminster these drugs.[33] Out of 28 specific chemicals listed by IARC as Group 1 Carcinogens, eight are chemo therapeutic agents. Indeed, it has been known for a decade[34] that oncology nurses can and do absorb enough of these agents to produce increased mutagenicity in their urine. Measureable amounts of cyclophosphamide or platinum have also been noted in their urine. Nevertheless, studies showing adverse health effects such as on pregnancy outcome[35] or neoplasia are exceedingly difficult to mount given the small numbers of workers in any hospital, the wide variety of agents handled and the long latency induction required for neoplastic change. (Pregnancy outcome studies are a methodological problem of the first order in any case.)

Nurses

One might imagine that nurses would be a relatively easy group to study. The numbers are large and many follow no other profession during their working lives. However, most are female, they marry, change their names, leave work to raise children and may not return to work thereafter. They rotate on a variety of specialist services. Epidemiological studies of nurses are few and far between - even mortality studies are a rare commodity for this group. One recent study from Wisconsin[36] relied on a proportional morality analysis but found little of note apart from an excess risk of suicide. Certainly nurses seem to experience high abseenteeism.[37] Much of this abseenteeism has been construed as a withdrawal from a physically and psychologically demanding job but there is no doubt either that lung and skin allergies cause some fof the absences (with particular interest of late concentrated on glutaraldehyde[38]). Nurses are, however, the prime group exposed to anti neoplastic drugs as well. High on any list of causes of absence among nurses comes back disorders of one sort or other. There are many epidemiological difficulties in studying back pain, given that 80% of the population will experience this symptom at some stage in their lives. Furthermore, as lifting patients seems to be a major hazard in this context for nurses, it is difficult to design a mechanical procedure to cope with such loads given the wide variety of circumstances in which a nurse will have to move or lift a patient. Nevertheless, work practice approaches to the problem are likely to be more successful in limiting the injuries than pre-employment evaluations.[39]

Pharmaceutical workers

This group of workers has held a particular fascination since we investigated a population of oral contraceptive formulators in Puerto Rico in 1978.[40] This study was more straightforward than most because the plant was new, employed a previously unexposed population of workers, handled only two therapeutically active materials and had a high incidence of health effects.

For most pharmaceutical plants, the workers rotate around the jobs, the work is "campaign driven" - that is, one drug may be formulated for only a few weeks before a switch to another - and there is good occupational hygiene control. Nevertheless the workplace contains agents which, by definition, are biologically active and frequently so at concentrations orders of magnitude lower than more common agents in chemical plants. Furthermore, the pharmacodynamics of these therapeutic agents are well known for the oral or parenteral routes but frequenly little is known concerning the "effective dose" for inhalation. The potential health effects from occupational exposure are thus legion.[41]

Several recent papers have addressed the issue of airborne exposure limits in general terms,[42, 43] but following a study by one of my staff on occupational exposure to an animal growth promoter[43], we reviewed the problems inherent in arriving at a justifiable approach to establishing numerical standards for airborne concentrations.[45] For this occupational group, the problems are as difficult as they are fascinating.

Maintenance and support staff

These HCW's are the most difficult to identify for epidemiological studies and yet their occupational exposures to chemicals, sterilants and, hospital waste, as well as physical factors such as heat and radiation render them a particularly vulnerable group. They are also the least well served by health services and provide a low profile but vital service to the industry. Dermatoses have been identified as a particular problem for hospital cleaning women[46] with as many as 40% developing a skin problem at some stage during their employment. They have been described as the forgotten majority[47] - though in fact in most hospital environments they constitute about a quarter of the workforce and are thus the second largest group after the nurses. It is safe to say that the working conditions of this group would not be tolerated in most factories, yet in hospitals with less interest in their wellbeing and virtually no environmental monitoring, their workplaces are rarely good and often are frankly hazardous. Epidemiological studies of maintenance and support staff are long overdue in order to highlight their problems and quantify the risks.

CONCLUSIONS AND FUTURE CONSIDERATIONS

This review makes no attempt to cover the field of health care work in any exhaustive way. The object was to highlight certain areas of concern to occupational physicians and to emphasise certain problems faced by occupational epidemiologists wishing to study sub-groups of this population. Clearly there are many interesting questions requiring answers not only to quantify health effects, but also to measure - often for the first time - the exposure characteristics of different work situations in the health service. The population employed in this industry is large and disparate. What risks have been identified are either life-threatening - such as neoplasia or expensive - such as back pain or dermatitis. Yet there are major methodological difficulties in studying some of the more important sub-groups of HCW's.

Thus some new study initiatives are required. So far as small scattered workforces are concerned, collaborative exercises are needed to investigate occupational exposures to such agents as ethylene oxide or perchlorethylene. Neurosurgeons would be a suitable group to study in relation to their intimate exposure to brain tissue and their possible links with slow virus and central nervous system disorders including neoplasia. Such a study might even have to be international in order to acquire a large enough population.

Exposure registers is one way forward here and consideration should be given to exposure to agents known to be animal carcinogens but for whom human data are lacking. The natural history of back disorders could be studied by following a cohort of trainee nurses. The effective dose of chemo therapeutic agents or other pharmaceutical preparations necessary to produce a human health effect could be determined by studying populations of nurses or pharmaceutical company workers. But, effort and collaboration would be needed to achieve a scientifically valid outcome.

Much remains to be done. If there is one message from this presentation it is this: the health care industry is a large one which has received scant attention from epidemiologists to date. Yet the occupational exposures these workers face could answer many of the questions which face the broader kirk of occupational health today. That is the challenge we face as epidemiologists. It is for us to take up that challenge but to do so we must collaborate with each other. That surely is one of the main purposes of the very existence of ICOH.

REFERENCES

1 Ommen GS, Morris SL (1984) Occupational hazards to health care workers: report of a conference. Am J Indust Med 6:129-137

2 US Public Health Service (1988) Guidelines for protecting the safety and health of health care workers US Govt Printing Office Washington DC

3 Harrington JM (1981) The health industry In: McDonald JC (ed) Recent Advances in Occupational Health - 1. Churchill Livingstone, Edinburgh, pp 75-84

4 Emmett, EA Baetz J (1987) Health in the health care industry? In: Emmett EA (ed) State of the Art Reviews: Occupatioanal Medicine. Hanley & Belfus, Philadelphia, pp ix-xv

5 Pines A, Skulkeo K, Pollak E, Peritz E, Steif J (1985) Rates of sickness absenteeism among employees of a modern hospital: the role of demographic and occupational factors. Brit J Indust Med 42:326-335

6 Lunn JA (1975) The health of staff in hospitals. Heineman Medical Books, London

7 Harrington JM (1976) MD Thesis, University of London

8 Gestal JJ (1987) Occupational hazards in hospitals: accidents, radiation, exposure to noxious chemicals, drug addiction and psychic problems, and assault. Brit J Indust Med 42:510-520

9 Pines A, Cleghorn, de Rohrmoser DC, Pollak E (1985) Occupational accidents in a hospital setting: an epidemiological analysis. J Occup Accidents 7:195-215

10 Kelsey JL, Thompson WD, Evans AS (1986) Methods in observational analysis. Monographs in Epidemiology and Biostatistics Vol 10. Oxford University Press, Oxford

11 Murray RM (1979) The health of doctors: a review. J Roy Coll Phys 12:403-415

12 Harrington JM (1983) Cancer and the health industry. J Soc Occup Med 33:114-118

13 Gestal JJ (1987) Occupational hazards in hospitals: risk of infection. Brit J Indust Med 44:435-442

14 Emmett EA (1987) Health problems of health care workers. (ed) State of the Art Reviews: Occupational Medicine Vol 2, No 3. Hanley & Belfus, Philadelphia

15 US Public Health Service (1989) Guidelines for prevention of transmission of human immunodeficiency virus and hepatitis B virus to health care workers and public safety workers - a response to PL 100-607. US Dept of Health & Human Services, Washington DC

16 Hamory BH (1983) Underreporting of needlestick injuries in a university hospital. Amer J Infect Control 11:174-177

17 Reid DD (1957) Incidence of tuberculosis among workers in medical laboratories. Brit Med J 2:1-14

18 Harrington JM, Shannon HS (1976) Incidence of tuberculosis, hepatitis, brucellosis and shigeillosis in British medical laboratory workers. Brit Med J 1:759-762

19 Lunn JA, Mayho GV (1989) Incidence of pulmonary tuberculosis by occupation of hospital employees in the National Health Service in England & Wales 1980-1984. J Soc Occ Med 39:30-32

20 Araki S, Muraia K, Kumagai K, Nagasu M (1986) Mortality of medical practitioners in Japan: social class and the "healthy worker effect". Amer J Indust Med 10:91-99

21 Nurminen M, Rimpela A, Pukkala E (1988) Exceptionally low cancer incidence in doctors. Lancet 1:190-191

22 Murray RM (1983) The sick doctor. Medicine International:1582-1584

23 Pilowski L, O'Sullivan G (1989) Mental illness in doctors. Brit Med J 298:269-270

24 Cooper CL, Rout V, Faragher B (1989) Mental health, job satisfaction, and job stress among general practitioners. Brit Med J 298:366-370

25 Firth-Cozens J (1987) Emotional distress in junior hospital officers. Brit Med J 295:533-536

26 Collier DJ, Beales ILP (1989) Drinking among medical students: a questionnaire survey. Brit Med J 299:19-22

27 Spurgeon A, Harrington JM (1989) Work performance and the health of junior hospital doctors - a review of the literature. Work & Stress 3:117-128

28 Harrington JM, Oakes D (1984) Mortality study of British pathologists 1974-1980. Brit J Indust Med 41:188-191

29 Hall AJ (1989) PhD Thesis, University of Birmingham

30 Shackleton S, Harrington JM (1986) The pollution controversy. In: Lunn JN (ed) Epidemiology in Anaesthesia. Edward Arnold, London, pp 93-122

31 Rajhans GG, Brown DA, Whaley D, Wong L, Guirguis SS (1989) Hygiene aspects of occupational exposure to waste anaesthetic gases in Ontario hospitals. Ann Occup Hyg 33:27-45

32 Gardner RJ (1989) Inhalational anaesthetics - exposure and control: a statistical comparison of personal exposures in operating theatres with and without anaesthetic gas scavenging. Ann Occup Hyg 33: 159-173

33 Vainio H (1982) Inhalation anaesthetics, anti cancer drugs and sterilants as chemical hazards in hospital. Scand J Work Environ Health 8:94-107

34 Falck K, Grohn P, Sorsa M, Vainio H, Heinonen E, Holsti LR (1979) Mutagenicity in urine of nurses handling cytostatic drugs. Lancet 1:1250-1251

35 Selevan S, Lindbohm ML, Hornung RW, Hemminki K (1985) A study of occupational exposure to anti neoplastic drugs and fetal loss in nurses. N Eng J Med 313:1173-1178

36 Katz RM (1983) Causes of death among registered nurses. J Occup Med 25:760-762

37 Redfern SJ (1978) Absence and wastage of trained nurses: a selective review of the literature. J Adv Nurs 3:231-249

38 Norback D (1988) Skin and respiratory symptoms from exposure to alkaline glutaraldehyde in medical services. Scand J Work Environ Health 14:366-371

39 Agnew JE (1987) Back pain in hospital workers. In: Emmett EA (ed) Health Problems of Health Care Workers, Hanley & Belfus, Philadelphia. Vol 2, No 3, 609-616

40 Harrington JM, Stein GF, Rivera RO, de Morales AV (1978) The occupational hazards of formulating oral contraceptives - a survey of plant employees. Arch Environ Health 33:12-15

41 Teichman RF, Fallow LF, Brandt-Rauf PW (1988) Health effects of workers in the pharmaceutical industry: a review. J Soc Occup Med 38:55-57

42 Sargent EV, Kirk GD (1988) Establishing airborne exposure control limits in the pharmaceutical industry. Am Indust Hyg Assoc J 49:309-313

43 Rackham M, McHattie GV, Teasdale EL (1989) Occupational hygiene assesment strategy in the pharmaceutical industry. J Soc Occ Med 39:15-18

44 Aw TC, Smith AB, Stephenson RL, Glueck CJ (1989) Occupational exposure to zeranol, an animal growth promoter. Brit J Indust Med 46:341-346

45 Aw TC, Harrington JM (1989) Occupational exposure standards for pharmaceutical agents. Asia-Pacific J of Public Health (in press)

46 Hansen KS (1983) Occupational dermatoses in hospital cleaning women. Contact Dermatitis 9:343-351

47 Clever LH (1983) The forgotten majority: health hazards in hospital support service personnel. Occ Health Nursing April:20-30

Occupational Epidemiology. H. Sakurai et al., editors

RISK ASSESSMENT OF A-BOMB RADIATION

HIROO KATO

Department of Epidemiology, Radiation Effects Research Foundation,
Hiroshima JAPAN 732

INTRODUCTION

Atomic bombs were dropped on Hiroshima and Nagasaki in August 1945. The number of acute deaths due to the atomic bomb radiation, burns and/or mechanical injuries as of the end of 1945 is estimated to be somewhere between 90,000 and 120,000 out of population of approximately 330,000 in Hiroshima. The corresponding figures in Nagasaki would be between 60,000 and 80,000 out of around 250,000[1].

As acute radiation effects, nausea and vomiting and successive diarrhoea and stools contained mucus and blood were observed within 2-3 days after bombing. Epilation and purpula began to appear 2-3 weeks after bombing.

The Atomic Bomb Casualty Commission (ABCC) was established in the two cities by the United States government in 1947 to initiate follow-up studies on the late health effects of atomic bomb radiation. ABCC was soon joined in its studies by a branch laboratory of the Japanese National Institute of Health (JNIH). Under a reorganization in 1975, responsibility for the research performed by ABCC and JNIH was assumed by the Radiation Effects Research Foundation (RERF), an independent binational institution equally funded by the governments of Japan and the United States.

SAMPLE FOR THE STUDY AND METHOD OF FOLLOW-UP SURVEY

A nation-wide survey of atomic bomb survivors was first conducted in 1950, enumerating a total of 285,000 survivors throughout the country. A cohort of about 120,000 subjects was thus selected from among these survivors, both radiation exposed and non-exposed controls, who were resident in Hiroshima and Nagasaki at the time of this survey.

Mortality in this cohort has been under study since 1950, and autopsies have also been performed on 20-30% of the individuals who have died. Ascertainment of survival status and causes of death: a family registration system was established in Japan about 100 years ago, under which all vital events which affect a family composition such as birth, death and marriage are registered at the legal address (Honseki) of the family. Therefore, it is possible to easily and accurately ascertain the survival status of a study subject by checking his or her Koseki (Honseki) regardless of the actual residence of the person. Ascertainment of death is almost 100% complete because the Koseki of the study subjects are checked periodically. Upon knowing the fact of death and the address of the deceased as a result of Koseki check, the cause of death has been obtained from the vital statistics death schedule kept at the Health Center in which the deceased's address is covered. The vital statistics death schedules are prepared, of course, from death certificates, and thus the accuracy of the cause of death is a problem. The accuracy of the cause classification on death certificates as revealed by autopsy findings for those individuals who came to autopsy[2] in terms of confirmation rate and detection rate. Confirmation rates differ according to the cause of death: the rate is high for cancers such as leukemia, lung cancer and stomach cancer, being 70-80%, but the accuracy is poor for cancers such as those of the pancreas and liver where the confirmation rate is less than 50%. In studying a cause of death having low accuracy, it is possible to restrict the study to only those were that have been histologically confirmed either through autopsy or surgical pathology report. The underlying cause of death is classified according to the International Classification of Diseases (ICD).

Since 1958, detailed biennial medical examinations have been carried out with 75-85% participation rates on a subsample comprising about 1/5 of this cohort. A separate cohort of 2,800 in-utero exposed children and their non-exposed controls has been followed for mortality after birth and for morbidity.

In addition, a large scale genetic study was conducted based on the pregnancy registration in both Hiroshima and Nagasaki City in 1948-1953. Furthermore, a cohort consisting of 70,000 children whose parents were either exposed or not exposed was set up in 1958 for mortality follow-up and cytogenetic and biochemical genetic studies.

There is a record linkage with the tumor registry, from which incidences of cancers (i.e., breast and thyroid cancers) have been determined in relation to radiation exposure.

Radiation dose (shielding kerma dose) received by individuals was estimated by air dose and shielding condition (Japanese house, concrete building and so on) under the revised dose system in 1986 (DS86). Organ dose for specific organs was further estimated.

Information on other carcinogenic etiological factors is obtained from the cohort through interviews, mail surveys, and record linkage with census data. Information is obtained on the following: smoking, occupation, history of mental illness, family history, dietary habits, exposure to medical X-rays.

EXPOSURE ASSESSMENT

The atomic bombs dropped on Hiroshima and Nagasaki were of different design and content. A uranium bomb with an explosive yield equivalent of 15 kilotons of TNT was used in Hiroshima and a plutonium bomb with that of 21 kilotons of TNT in Nagasaki. Whereas the radiation generated was almost entirely gamma rays in Nagasaki, neutrons made a some contribution to the total dose received by survivors in Hiroshima in the tentatively estimated dose system in 1965 (T65D).

However, as a result of reassessment of A-bomb dosimetry, the new Dosimetry System was introduced in 1986 (DS86). Briefly, the difference between the new (DS86) and the old (T65D)[3] could be summarized as follows: 1) Under DS86, neutron air dose decreases greatly in both cities, to about 10% of T65D value in Hiroshima and 30% in Nagasaki. 2) The transmission factor for gamma ray in wooden Japanese structure is smaller around 50%, but the transmission factors for organs are higher as compared with that of T65D. Thus, the change in the transmission factor of gamma rays from house shielding and organs tend to cancel each other. As a result, mean organ-absorbed doses do not change significantly between the two dose system.

LATE HEALTH EFFECTS

Brief summary

The late health effects of atomic bomb radiation which have been studied based on the afore-mentioned various research programs are summarized in Table 1. These effects can be divided into the following three types: (1) effects for which a definite relationship to atomic bomb exposure has been established; (2) effects for which there is a borderline or suggestive relationship; and (3) effects for which no relationship has been shown.

Radiation effects are limited to an increase in some sites of malignant tumors as well as an excess of cataracts, chromosomal aberrations, small head size and mental retardation in the in-utero exposed, and a delay in growth and development which occurred shortly after bombing.

So far, we failed to observe significant radiation-related acceleration of nonspecific aging, suppression of immune response and fertility, or genetic effects. However, these negative findings can not be considered as establishing that such effects do not exist. They may mean that sample sizes were not adequate or the indices of radiation effects employed were not sufficiently sensitive.

Table 1. Summary of Findings on Late Effects of Atomic Bomb Radiation

I. Established Increase in:
1. Malignant tumors (leukemia, thyroid, breast, lung, stomach, multiple myeloma)
2. Cataracts
3. Lymphocyte chromosomal aberrations
4. Small head size and mental retardation in the in-utero exposed
5. Delay in growth and development

II. Suggestive Increase in:
1. Malignant tumors (esophagus, colon, ovary, salivary glands, urinary tract, malignant lymphoma)
2. Certain changes of humoral and cell-mediated immunity

III. No Demonstrable Increase in:
1. Malignant tumors (chronic lymphatic leukemia, osteosarcoma)
2. Mortality from other than malignant tumors
3. Accelerated aging
4. Infertility
5. Birth defects or mortality in F_1 generation

Radiation-induced cancer

The most recent findings regarding cancer mortality[4] and incidence can be briefly summarized as follows: 1) An increase in leukemia mortality among A-bomb survivors peaked 5-6 years after the bombing and has decreased with time thereafter. In addition to leukemia, the incidence of cancer of the lung, breast, esophagus, stomach, colon, thyroid, ovary, urinary tract, and multiple myeloma increases with dose. At present, there is no indication of an increase in cancer of the rectum or uterus among A-bomb survivors. In general, radiation-induced solid cancers begin to appear after the age at which they are normally prone to develop, and have continued to increase with time in proportion to the natural increase in mortality of the control group. 2) There are factors which modify the effects of radiation, such as age at the time of bombing (ATB) and sex. Sensitivity to radiation, in terms of cancer induction, is higher for persons who were young ATB in general, than for those who were older ATB. 3) There was no increase in childhood cancer among those exposed while in utero, but there is a recent indication of an increase in cancer incidence among these persons as they age.[5] 4) There seems to be no interaction in a multiplicative way between radiation and smoking and lung cancer induction.

As an index of the magnitude of the radiation effect, the proportion of cancer deaths among 42,000 A-bomb survivors exposed with 0.01 Gy and over (average 0.30 Gy) in the cohort which are radiation induced has been estimated for the period 1950-85 on the assumption that the dose-response curve is linear. Although radiation-induced leukemia accounts for 55.4% of the total leukemia deaths occurring in the cohort, 7.9% of the total deaths from malignant tumors other than leukemia are estimated to have been radiation induced. By site, the proportion of radiation-related cancers ranges from 6.3% for stomach cancer, to 32.5% for multiple myeloma.

Effects on growth and development

Radiation exposure while in utero have had profound effects on growth and development. The most striking findings has been the increased occurrence of small head size with mental retardation. It was revealed that 8-15 weeks of gestation is the most sensitive stage of pregnancy for mental retardation caused by radiation. There was no increase of risk before 8 weeks of gestation.[6]

Genetic effects

Perhaps the most important studies for which the results have been negative are those relating to the genetic effects of A-bomb exposure. No significant effects of parental exposure to the A-bombs were observed on the occurrence of stillbirths, birth defects, infant mortality, or alterations in birth weight in 70,000 pregnancy terminations during the period 1948-1953. Subsequent studies have failed to demonstrate any relationship between parental exposure and mortality of children.

The fact that no untoward medical effects have been detected in the F_1 generation does not prove that genetic effects do not exist. It may reflect only that the effect is too small to be detected by the study methods employed or that the methodology is not appropriate. An awareness of this was the reason for extension of the cytogenetics studies to the F_1 individuals and development of the Biochemical Genetics Program to search for the possible increased occurrence of radiation-induced mutations at the molecular level.

These studies, which use electrophoresis and enzyme activity measurement to search for mutations occurring in serum and red blood cell protein systems, are under way. Results obtained thus far have not shown any relationship to parents exposure status and an intensive study using, more advanced techniques such as DNA analysis is under way.

REFERENCES

1. Ohkita T (1984) In: Effects of Naclear War on Health and Health and Heatlh services. World Health Organization Geneva, Annex 4, pp 101-115
2. Yamamoto T, Moriyama IM, Asano M, and Guralnich L (1978) Radiation Effects Research Foundation Technical Report 18-78
3. Shimizu Y, Kato H, Schull WJ, Preston DL, Fujita S and Pierce DA (1989) Radiat Res 118: 502-24
4. Shimizu Y, Kato H, Schull WJ (1988) Radiation Effects Research Foundation Techinical Report 5-88
5. Yoshimoto Y, Kato H, and Schull WJ (1988) Lancet ii:665-9
6. Otake M, Yoshimaru H, Schull WJ (1987) Radiation Effects Research Foundation Technical Report 16-87

Occupational Epidemiology. H. Sakurai et al., editors

THE POLICIES AND STRATEGIES OF WHO ON OCCUPATIONAL HEALTH AND EPIDEMIOLOGY

Hiroshi Nakajima

Director-General, World Health Organization
CH-1211 Geneva 27, Switzerland.

The Scientific Committee on Epidemiology in Occupational Health of the International Commission on Occupational Health has been in official relations with WHO since 1961. I would like to take this opportunity to explain WHO's policies and strategies in the field of Occupational Health.

Ever since it came into existence in 1948, WHO has paid special attention to workers' health. In fact, the subject of "industrial hygiene" was placed by the First World Health Assembly under "Public health administration", a topic that was accorded high priority. It was pointed out at the time that a broad interpretation should be given to the term "industrial", and that it might be replaced by the term "occupational". The Assembly recommended the establishment of a small joint committee with the ILO on this subject.

The first meeting of this joint committee was held two years later, in 1950, and advised that the term "occupational health" should in fact be used instead of "industrial hygiene". Furthermore, it produced a statement on the aims of occupational health, and this has since become the definition quoted in almost every textbook in the field. I do not therefore see any need to repeat it here, but as 40 years have now elapsed, it seems necessary to revise the definition, and I hope that an up-to-date definition can be developed by the next Joint ILO/WHO Committee on Occupational Health.

So far, 10 such committees have been convened, on a wide range of topics. Examples are: the notification of occupational diseases, in 1952; medical causes of absenteeism, in 1957; occupational health problems in agriculture, in 1962; occupational health and safety of migrant workers, in 1975; education and training in occupational health, safety, and ergonomics, in 1981; and recognition and control of adverse psychosocial factors at work, in 1984. At the last meeting, held in 1987, the topic was the epidemiology of work-related diseases and accidents. I shall return to the report of that meeting later on.

In WHO, we use a six-yearly planning cycle, and prepare a biennial programme budget. Our Eighth General Programme of Work covering the period 1990-1995 is ready for implementation while in May of this year, the World Health Assembly approved our programme budget for the 1990-1991 biennium.

The Workers' Health Programme is one of the five programmes in the group known as the Programme for Protection and Promotion of the Health of Specific Population Groups.

The specific objectives of the Workers' Health Programme during the period 1990-1995 are: 1) to cooperate with Member States in developing or strengthening national workers' health programmes, designed to achieve the full coverage of people at work; 2) to support the development of infrastructures for workers' health in national health systems, based on the primary health care approach; and 3) to stimulate and support the continuous development and adaptation of the technology and approaches to implement national workers' health programmes, giving priority to workers at high risk.

The WHO Office of Occupational Health in Geneva monitors

changes in the health problems of workers associated with the introduction of new materials and technologies, and supports countries in dealing with new work-related health problems, together with existing problems in the field of occupational health that vary from place to place in the present-day world. I believe that in this area, the Scientific Committee on Epidemiology in Occupational Health of the ICOH could provide very substantial support to WHO's Workers' Health Programme.

In 1990-1991, only 0.48% of our regular budget is allocated to the Workers' Health Programme. I would however like to emphasize that WHO's contribution to the health of working populations is by no means restricted to this particular Programme. Many other programmes also contribute to varying extents. Let me explain. First, I should mention our Programme on Health Risk Assessment of Potentially Toxic Chemicals. This Programme is implemented by WHO as its contribution to the International Programme on Chemical Safety, which is jointly operated by WHO, the International Labour Organisation, and the United Nations Environment Programme. It compiles, evaluates, and disseminates, in a manner that is suitable for all our Member States, information on the health and environmental risks associated with priority chemicals of global significance. It promotes the development of improved methods, including epidemiological methods, for assessing the risk to health and the environment of chemicals, and for their testing. It also develops guidelines on how to detect and control human diseases of chemical etiology; how to respond to accidents involving chemicals, including the diagnosis and treatment of poisoning; how to identify and quantify health problems related to the safe use of chemicals locally; how to formulate corresponding national programmes, including enabling legislation; how to maintain vigilance over toxic chemicals; and how to prevent and control poisoning.

Next, come the group of programmes within the Division of Noncommunicable Diseases. These include the programmes on cardiovascular diseases, cancer, and other noncommunicable diseases. Our Programme on Tobacco or Health also works closely with the Workers' Health Programme.

Programmes relating to the protection and promotion of mental health, together with and including ever-increasing drug and alcohol-related problems, are closely related to workers' health, as are programmes dealing with rehabilitation, prevention of blindness and deafness, and accident prevention. This latter programme has recently been transferred from the Regional Office for Europe to headquarters, in order to ensure better coordination and collaboration.

The list goes on to include the programmes on health situation and trend assessment, health legislation, organization of health systems based on primary health care, development of human resources for health, public information and education for health, etc.

The catalytic role of the WHO Workers' Health Programme is greatly enhanced by its network of 40 collaborating centres and its advisory panel consisting of 120 experts around the world. Cooperation with nongovernmental organizations, such as the International Commission on Occupational Health, and with other United Nations agencies, particularly the ILO, greatly enhances the output and impact of WHO's contribution to the health of working populations.

So much for occupational health, and let me now move to epidemiology. I shall begin with general epidemiology, followed by occupational epidemiology. In November 1988, a Meeting on Uses of Epidemiology in Support of Health for All Strategies was held in Geneva. That meeting pointed out that the main challenge for epidemiology today was to serve as an effective instrument in the design and evaluation of health policies and plans. It identified the basic scope of epidemiological methods as providing the ability to measure health problems and risks, to compare them over time and between groups, and to assess the impact of interventions. It was pointed out that epidemiological methodologies had a number of uses, including the following: 1) identifying and measuring the importance of health problems elucidating the causes of these problems, and describing high-risk groups; 2) undertaking disease surveillance and control; 3) planning, distributing, monitoring, and evaluating health resources and their use; and 4) formulating and evaluating health policies and interventions (social, behavioural, economic, and by health services).

It was emphasized that the capacities for applying these methods should be developed and supported within countries.

The discussions at the meeting led to recommendations in the following areas: 1) the uses of epidemiology as a fundamental science in public health and in Health-for-All policies; 2) development within countries of a set of essential capacities for an epidemiological approach; 3) research, especially to support or integrate health systems research; 4) training; and 5) the future work of WHO in this field.

I would like to inform you that the full report of the

meeting is in active preparation and should shortly be available.

After examining the summary report of the meeting in January this year, the WHO Executive Board discussed the role of epidemiology in attaining Health for All. Stress was laid on the need to develop capabilities for the local collection, analysis, and use of epidemiological data in association with sciences such as economics and health planning; it was emphasized that training and appropriate research should form an integral part of the process, and that nongovernmental organizations should be closely involved. It was also proposed that appropriate mechanisms should be set up in the Secretariat and a plan of action formulated, with suitable resources, including the strengthening of WHO's epidemiological capabilities.

As a matter of fact, epidemiological capabilities already exist in all WHO technical programmes and the Workers' Health Programme is no exception. In 1987, it formed the joint Secretariat with the ILO's Occupational Safety and Health Branch for the Tenth Joint ILO/WHO Committee on Occupational Health to discuss the epidemiology of work-related diseases and accidents. I note that the International Commission on Occupational health, was deeply involved in this meeting. The Chairman, Professor S. Hernberg, was, I understand, President of the International Commission on Occupational Health and the first Chairman of the Scientific Committee on Epidemiology in Occupational Health.

That meeting was convened for a number of reasons. Its main objectives were to review the causes of work-related diseases, accidents, and injuries, to propose epidemiological approaches for research, and to make appropriate recommendations. In fact there were 14 recommendations in the report, which has been published in our Technical Report Series. At the international level, the meeting recommended that WHO and the ILO should consider cooperating with national governments, at their request, to undertake research and training and to develop educational materials, standard reporting models, and guidelines for the identification and prevention of work-related diseases and accidents. As a priority, WHO and the ILO should consider developing a programme addressing the issue of standardized systems for reporting work-related diseases and accidents.

At its session in May of this year, our Executive Board commented favourably on this report and suggested certain lines of action, particularly with reference to developing countries. It further recommended that WHO should promote the exchange of experience in various countries in the world on the application of epidemiology in occupational health.

In my humble opinion, this recommendation is entirely consistent with the objectives of this Symposium, in other words to bring active research workers together to discuss methodologies, findings, and applications in occupational epidemiology. This is why I have endeavoured to explain to you today our Organization's policies and strategy in regard to occupational health and epidemiology. And this is why I have come to seek your support for this very important field of work of the World Health Organization.

© 1990 Elsevier Science Publishers B.V. (Biomedical Division)
Occupational Epidemiology. H. Sakurai et al., editors

THE IMPACT OF EPIDEMIOLOGY ON THE PREVENTION OF OCCUPATIONAL DISEASE

DAVID H. WEGMAN, MD

Work Environment Department, College of Engineering, University of Lowell, Lowell, MA 01854, (USA)

The products of epidemiologic studies provide the foundation upon which to design and build disease prevention activities. Hernberg considers it a science limited to studying the occurrence of illness, not health or social behavior, while Terris calls for its extension to health. Regardless, the science can be directed to descriptive, etiologic or intervention studies. In seeking opportunities to prevent occupational disease it is essential that this discipline be plumbed for all its potential. Descriptive studies provide data for occupational health care and provide hypotheses for new occupational risks. Etiologic studies generally seek evidence of causality for work environment agents. To provide a bridge from etiologic studies to prevention, there is increasing need that such studies define exposure-effect relationships in a manner useful to intervention. Intervention studies seek evidence that the reduction of work-related risk factors results in disease reduction or improves health of the workforce. There has been an excessive emphasis in modern epidemiology on the second of these three types of studies. Epidemiologic studies of etiology should remain prominent, but these have achieved an importance and legitimacy among young energetic public health scientists almost to the exclusion of attention to the essential role of the other two study types.

<u>Descriptive Epidemiology</u>: The history of epidemiology begins with descriptive efforts; first and foremost, the excitement created by John Graunt when he searched the Bills of Mortality in Great Britain and found uses for previously unexplored data such as: for civic planning,

assessing major health problems, and geographic differences in population health. A more recent example of such an exploration was Richard Schilling's examination of these same records to generate hypotheses about cotton dust related disease. The etiologic research which has followed still derives instruction from these original observations. More important, the original descriptive epidemiology was the source of major changes in industrial practice and substantial reduction in cotton related disease in factory workers in Great Britain.

Surveillance, is a form of descriptive epidemiology first used simply to identify infectious disease cases in order that they be isolated from the community. Surveillance systems where then developed to seek secular, age and sex related patterns of infectious disease to permit preventive interventions such as immunization or to alert the medical community to impending new demands as was the case during the early poliomyelitis epidemics. The successes in surveillance of communicable disease have not been matched by parallels in occupational disease. Those which have occurred appear restricted to occupational diseases with relatively short latency, commonly recognized diagnostic features and reasonably high incidence rates. Patterns of lead palsy in painters, hepatitis B in hospital workers, acute silicosis in hard rock miners and asthma among bakery workers are examples of risks revealed in surveillance study. Intervention efforts have been focused and substantial reduction in exposure risks have ensued. New approaches to occupational disease surveillance are being explored. These are directed at the many conditions which are not uniquely caused by work environments but need presumptive rules to permit reporting, analysis and action. A parallel effort has been initiated in hazard surveillance. Based on accepted exposure-disease relationships, hazard surveillance has served as the basis for setting priorities and developing controls in most modern industrial environments. Hazard surveillance generally is based on environmental sampling schemes which search for sentinel events, e.g. excess exposures which are then treated as indicators for corrective action. Recent efforts to provide more systematic hazard surveillance data should result in more coherent and comprehensive industrial hygiene control efforts. These improved data can also contribute to population risk estimates, regional occupational health care planning, and compliance strategies for regulatory agencies. Even now, in the United States, these efforts have called attention to the need for innovative approaches to the elimination of such well known, but still prevalent problems, as lead and silica overexposure.

Etiologic Epidemiology: Etiologic epidemiology continues to provide important knowledge for preventing occupational disease. The majority of exposure-disease relationships accepted as guides for occupational disease control efforts rely on human epidemiology. The power of these studies suggests they may be necessary before serious control efforts can be mandated by the society. To the contrary, however, with the possible exception of carcinogens, the demand for epidemiologic studies has too often delayed attention to control. It is not for the epidemiologist, alone, to correct these possibly distorted demands. But the undue demand for conclusive epidemiologic evidence before taking public health actions places an important burden on each epidemiologist to take a role in proposing public health action in the face of scientific uncertainty. They are the best equipped to bridge the gap between the knowledge which exists, the knowledge which is needed and the public health context in which decisions must be made.

Developments in etiologic epidemiology and their impact can be seen in studies of acute and chronic respiratory disease. For example, well planned epidemiology studies have been used to extend and expand our understanding of the full range of effects of isocyanate exposures. These studies have succeeded in directing control efforts by focusing on the need to control risks related to: isocyanate asthma; non-specific pulmonary effects of exposures; and other exposure risks of those removed from isocyanates (through the study of the natural history of this particular asthma). A second example comes from new studies of respiratory irritants. Identification of the epidemiologic pattern of responses to acute irritants may guide efforts to prevent progression of related, less evident, chronic effects of exposure. Using new survey approaches and prospective studies both the short and long term impact of irritant exposures are being examined. Problems being addressed include unpredictable exposure patterns, the reversible nature of acute effects, and the need for objective as well as subjective measures. A final example is the importance of coupling epidemiology and toxicology to improve the nature and specificity of exposure-response relationships, (for example for silicon carbide). Refinement in these relationships can be expected to provide better guidance to setting and complying with voluntary and mandatory exposure standards.

The evolution of new methods to dissect the occupational component from other risk factors in the etiology of respiratory disease, cancer, neurologic disease, and musculoskeletal disease, among others, has played an important role in focusing attention on preventable aspects of these diseases. In this regard the World Health Organization's recent attention to the distinction between work-related and occupational disease is particularly important.

Intervention Epidemiology: Epidemiologic studies of intervention can provide further evidence related to the epidemiologic hypothesis upon which intervention is based. They also contribute to determining the success and judging the magnitude of intervention programs, thus providing the evidence necessary to extend or alter prevention efforts.

Studies of the epidemiology of silicosis in Vermont in the 1940s had a dramatic impact on prevention efforts. Years later epidemiologic studies of the same work sites provided excellent evidence on the eradication of silicosis in these occupations verifying the initial hypothesis about the exposure-disease relationship as well as the value of the controls. These studies, however, also led to a better understanding of the subtler effects of silica, effects which have since received renewed attention.

Intervention epidemiologic studies of the impact of occupational controls in industrializing nations are particularly valuable. Scarce resources are vigorously competed for, therefore requiring special attention to document and understand the use of control technology. Studies of the impact of ventilation control to reduce carbon disulfide exposures and dust suppression to reduce silica exposures in Chinese work settings are effective examples of these contributions of epidemiology.

The opportunity to use exposure-disease relationships to guide prevention efforts, however, calls attention to the need that such research continue to seek forms which ultimately can have meaning for the industrial hygienist, in the factory setting. For example, the wide range of slopes which describe lung cancer-asbestos exposure relationships, even within fiber type, suggests that the proper exposure estimator has not yet been found. An epidemiologist asked to measure the risk of disease in a manner relevant to the design of controls may need to seek models of disease risk, and measures of exposure different from those originally chosen to document etiology.

The future calls for need to carry out research on early markers of disease directed at the needs of control strategies as well as needs related to investigating disease etiology. For example, is a reduction in sister chromatid exchange in peripheral blood in exposed workers following introduction of a control an acceptable indicator of control effectiveness? How long before and after the change should the measurements be made? In general, epidemiologic evaluations of control effectiveness will involve small numbers of workers. Much more research is needed on intensive monitoring strategies which seek to partially compensate for small numbers of subjects by repeated observations on the few exposed individuals. Consideration has to be given to the problems of evaluating reduced health effects in a mobile work force when those exposed a year post-controls may be a substantially different group from those experiencing the pre-control environment. Finally, guidelines are needed to help decide when biological monitoring of exposed workers instead of, or in addition to exposure monitoring is ethically acceptable.

METHODS AND EXPOSURE ASSESSMENT

Occupational Epidemiology. H. Sakurai et al., editors

EFFECTS OF MAILING STRATEGIES ON THE RESPONSE RATE AND RESPONSE TIME IN A QUESTIONNAIRE STUDY AMONG NURSES

B.C.K. CHOI[1)], A.W.P. PAK[2)], J.T. PURDHAM[1)]

1) Occupational and Environmental Health Unit, Faculty of Medicine, University of Toronto, Toronto, Ontario, CANADA M5S 1A8
2) Department of Psychology, Brock University, St. Catharines, Ontario, CANADA L2S 3A1

This was a pilot study to determine the most efficient mailing strategy for a postal questionnaire study among nurses in Ontario. Five mailing strategies involving types of stamps on the return envelopes were considered: Business reply stamp (B), Metered stamp (M), Small regular stamp (S), Large uncommon stamp (L), No stamp (N).

From a list of all current mailing addresses of members of the Ontario Nursing Association, 400 nurses were randomly allocated to each of the 5 study groups. On Day 1, a package containing a covering letter, a one-page questionnaire, and a return envelope was sent to each of the 2,000 nurses. All of the packages were identical except for the return envelope which was treated in one of the five ways described above. The study was terminated on Day 92 (i.e. 3 months).

Response rates of the five groups were found to be: L = 43%, S = 40%, M = 37%, B = 33%, N = 26%. Financial and psychological factors, such as "no cost to the subject", "cost to the investigator", and "personal touch", which might have affected the response rates were investigated. Statistical tests based on binomial probabilities indicated that the response rate for no stamp was significantly different from those for large, small and metered stamps at the 0.05 level. Business reply stamp was significantly different from large stamp in response rate.

Response time (time from sending out to receiving questionnaires, in days) was found to follow a log normal distribution. Geometric mean response times of the five groups were: L = 14.4 days, S = 14.6 days, B = 15.5 days, N = 16.8 days, M = 16.9 days. Statistical tests based on log normal distribution did not reveal any statistically significant differences.

Total costs to send out and receive responses were: L = $438/173 responses, S = $438/159 responses, M = $431/149 responses, B = $331/132 responses, N = $278/104 responses. Costs per response received were: L = $2.53, S = $2.75, M = $2.89, B = $2.51, N = $2.68.

Therefore, if the response rate is of major concern in a postal study, paper stamps, especially large and uncommon stamps, should be used. If overall cost is of major concern, business reply stamps should be used. Response time seems little affected by mailing strategies.

Occupational Epidemiology. H. Sakurai et al., editors

A QUESTIONNAIRE FOR THE ASSESSMENT OF PHYSICAL ACTIVITY IN WORKERS

FUMIO KOBAYASHI[1], TAKEMASA WATANABE[1], KATSUHIRO SUMI[1], HIKARI FURUI[1], TOSHIKAZU TANAKA[1], MASATOSHI NAKATA[2], SHIGEO NIWA[2]

1 Department of Hygiene, Aichi Medical University, Aichi, Japan
2 Institute of Physical Fitness, Sports Medicine and Rehabilitation, Aichi Medical University, Aichi, Japan

INTRODUCTION

The exact evaluation of physical activity in daily life is important 1) for obtaining epidemiologic findings in preventive medicine and 2) for performing health education for individuals, such as improvement in dietary life, practice of proper exercises and so on. Although various questionnaires have so far been proposed for the assessment of physical activity, we developed a questionnaire to ascertain the time spent in usual daily living including work and leisure time. According to the times spent, physical activity score was calculated and daily energy expenditure was estimated.

METHODS

Subjects were 300 volunteers from the personnel, students and their families of Aichi Medical University(135 males and 165 females, mean age 32.0±11.1 and 29.0±10.2 years, respectively). Thirteen male workers (mean age 41.0±13.5 years) of an office, who came to our hospital for check-up examination were also subjected to preliminary test-retest examination. None of these subjects had any disease restrictive of physical activities. All subjects were made to fill up the questionnaire before one week and were checked up and made up for omissions by interviewers at the time of recovery. In the test-retest examination, similar examination was made twice at an interval of about 6 months.

Table1 shows the contents of the questionnaire, in which subjects are instructed to enter the respective times(minutes) spent in 21 living activities of usual life. The right column of the Table indicates codes representative of each living activity.

According to the intensity, these 21 living activities were

resumed into 8 kinds of activity (A1-A8) as follows and were calculated for the sum (T1-T8) of the times spent for each kind activity: A1 (code 1,60), A2 (code 11,15,23,24,35,36,40), A3(code 12,31,34), A4 (code 13,21,22,51), A5 (code 52), A6 (code 14,53), A7 (code 32) and A8(code 33). With reference to mean relative metabolic rate (RMR) for each of these 8 kinds of activity, the following scores (S1-S8) were given them each : S1=0, S2=0.3, S3=0.7 (T3<240), 1.1 (T3>=240), S4=1.4, S5=1.8, S6=3.1, S7=0.7, S8=1.1.

TABLE 1
LIST OF LIVING ACTIVITIES IN DAILY LIFE

Division of Life	Contents of Activities	Code
Sleep	Sleep	01
	Sitting	11
	Standing	12
Work	Walking	13
	Heavy Muscle work	14
	Driving Cars	15
Attending the office	on Foot	21
or	by Bicycle	22
Go to Market	by Car or Motorcycle	23
	by Bus or Electric Car	24
	Care of Oneself	31
	House Keeping	32
Home	Care of Children or Others	33
	Bath	34
	TV, Reading, Conversation	35
	Amusements	36
Meal	including Tea or Drinking	40
	Light(Walking, Gardening)	51
Exercise	Moderate(Golf, Baseball)	52
	Vigorous(Jogging, Swimming)	53
Rest	Lying in Bed or on the Floor	60

Physical activity score (PAS) was calculated according to the following formula; $PAS= \ (S*T/60)$. Individual daily energy expended (EN) was calculated according to the following formula;

$E1=\{PAS/((1440-T1)/60)+1.2\}*(1440-T1)*BW*BM$,

$E2=1.2*\text{rest time(code 60)}*BW*BM/60$,

E3=0.9*sleeping time(code1)*BW*BM/60,
EN=E1+E2+E3,
BW:body weight(Kg), BM:basal metabolic rate(Kcal/Kg/min).
For basal metabolic rate, Japanese nutritive requirement values were used according to sex, age and intensity division of living activities. Intensity division were set as follows:
division1 (light) : PAS < 12.5,
division2 (moderate) : 12.5 ≤ PAS <20.0
division3 (slight heavy) : 20.0≤ PAS < 25.0
division4 (heavy) : 25.0≤ PAS.

RESULTS

PAS obtained twice in the test-retest examination showed high correlation (R=0.86), confirming high reproducibility of the present questionnaire.

Table2 shows physical activity score (PAS) and kilocalory of energy expended (EN). PAS is also shown in Fig.1. PAS and EN proved to be considerably different according to the kind of job. PAS seemed to show an appropriate distribution.

TABLE 2
PHYSICAL ACTIVITY SCORE (PAS) AND KILOCALORY OF ENERGY EXPENDED(EN)

	n	Age		PAS		EN(Kcal)	
Male		Mean	SD	Mean	SD	Mean	SD
Office Worker	11	29.9	6.1	6.8	1.2	2103	309
Managerial Class	22	51.0	9.7	7.3	3.0	2212	502
Research Worker	7	38.0	4.3	9.4	4.0	2413	489
Clinician	15	33.5	5.8	10.2	3.7	2463	396
Technician	13	25.3	4.3	10.7	2.7	2252	338
Roentogenologist	13	28.5	4.5	12.9	4.4	2459	413
Engineer	5	24.6	6.3	14.4	2.2	2641	605
Medical Student	33	24.1	3.3	8.4	3.9	2297	477
	n	Age		PAS		EN(Kcal)	
Female		Mean	SD	Mean	SD	Mean	SD
Office Worker	18	29.2	8.0	9.6	2.6	1660	241
House Wife	10	42.6	10.1	10.0	1.5	1720	198
Medical Student	12	21.3	2.4	9.0	3.0	1684	215
Assistant of Nurse	17	42.9	10.9	14.7	4.0	1943	363
Nurse	43	25.4	4.9	15.3	3.9	2081	324
Obstetrical Nurse	5	26.6	2.6	14.6	2.6	1925	247
Roentogenologist	7	25.0	2.6	18.7	4.4	2173	200
Cook	4	21.3	1.0	20.9	7.6	2322	205

Table3 shows the relationship of daily energy expended (EN) and individual requirement obtained from "Japanese nutritive requirement". Mean values were almost similar, and the results of high overall correlation (R=0.73) were obtained.

TABLE 3

THE RELATION OF DAILY ENERGY EXPENDED(EN) AND INDIVIDUAL REQUIREMENT OBTAINED FROM "JAPANESE NUTRITIVE REQUIREMENT"

	Male	Female	Total
n	133	157	290
Energy Expended (Kcal)	2311±445	1886±358	2081±452
Requirement (Kcal)	2259±219	1915±247	2073±290
Correlation Coefficient	0.589**	0.699**	0.731**

** P<0.01

DISCUSSION

With our questionnaire, in which activities at work and at leisure time are scored without distinction, this PAS seems to express distinctly the difference in physical activity mainly at work. How to evaluate various physical activities at leisure time remains to be examined. The use of PAS as the index of dividing the intensity of living activities is useful in making good use of "Japanese nutritive requirement", one of the important reference for health promotion and health education. However, how to make a cut point of the score in dividing needs further examination from the viewpoint of its relationship with other physiological indexes. Although the presumption of individual daily energy expended from PAS seemed to be valid, its further verification by dietary survey is thought to be necessary with reference to energy intake.

REFERENCES

1. Shapiro S,Weinblatt E,Frank CW(1965)J Chr Dis 18:527-558
2. Wessel JA,et.al(1965)Am J Public Health 55:1430-1436
3. Reiff GG,Montoye HJ,et.al(1967)J Sport Med Phys Fit 7:135-142
4. Epstein L,Miller GW,et.al(1976)Br Heart J 38:403-409
5. Taylor HL,Jacobs DR,et.al(1978)J Chr Dis 31:741-755
6. Paffenbarger RS,Wing AL,et.al(1978)Am J Epidemiol 108:161-175
7. Kannel WB,Sorlie P(1979)Arch Intern Med 139:857-861
8. Magnus K,Matroos A,Strackee J(1979)Am J Epidemiol 110:724-733
9. Haskall WL,Taylor HL,et.al(1980)Circulation 62 suppl 5:53-61
10. Salonen JT,Puska P,et.al(1982)Am J Epidemiol 115:526-537
11. Berkman LF,Bleslow L,Wingard D(1983)Oxford Univ Press 61-112
12. Sallis JF,Haskell,WL,et.al(1985)Am J Epidemiol 121:91-106

Occupational Epidemiology. H. Sakurai et al., editors

COMPARISON OF THE PERFORMANCE OF TWO GENERAL JOB-EXPOSURE MATRICES USING THE SAME SET OF DATA

HANS KROMHOUT[1], DICK HEEDERIK[2]

[1]Department of Air Pollution, [2]Department of Environmental Health, Agricultural University Wageningen. P.O. Box 8129, 6700 EV The Netherlands

Introduction

Since the introduction of general job-exposure matrices (JEM) in the beginning of the 1980's, expectations of their performance have been rather high. Hoar et al. (1980) claimed that the NCI JEM enhanced the value of information on occupation, by placing subjects from different industries and with different occupations in the same exposure category based on similar chemical and physical exposures. They indirectly validated their job-exposure matrix by re-analyzing a case-control study of bladder cancer. The relative risk estimated for persons with heavy exposure to aromatic amines was higher than the relative risk found for any industrial category. Pannett et al. (1985) stated that although the exposure estimates from their MRC JEM were less accurate, the results of their study did not improve very much when exposure estimates inferred directly from individual job histories were used. They concluded that for occupational data elicited by means of a postal questionnaire, direct exposure estimates offer little advantage over those provided at lower cost by the JEM.

In contrast to this Hinds et al. (1985) showed in a case-control study of lung cancer that useful application of the NCI JEM is limited due to its low sensitivity. Coggon et al. (1984) also failed to identify an association of lung cancer risk with well known carcinogens like arsenic and chromium.

Material and methods

In a study using the 1960 data of a general population cohort from the small industrial town of Zutphen, the performance of two general job-exposure matrices was compared. The 1960 jobs of 796 men aged 40-59 in 1960 were coded according to the job-exposure matrices of the NCI (Hoar 1980) and the MRC (Coggon et al. 1984). The exposure of the cohort members to 22 different agents assigned by both matrices was compared after merging the 5 exposure categories of NCI JEM and the 4 categories of the MRC JEM into two categories. The exposure estimates were merged in two different ways resulting in a dichotomy of exposed versus non-exposed (**A**) and high exposed versus low & non-exposed (**B**). The agreement between the two matrices in exposure classification was assessed by calculating Cohen's Kappa (Fleiss 1981) as a measure of agreement.

The exposure information generated by both matrices was subsequently used in an analysis of the follow-up data of the cohort. The relationship between the exposure and Chronic Non-Specific Lung Disease (CNSLD) morbidity incidence was analyzed in a proportional hazard analysis (Cox 1972), allowing for smoking habits and age. This was also applied to lung cancer incidence as the outcome variable.

Results

The agreement between the 22 agents generated for the population by both matrices is summarized in table 1. Except for chromium, styrene, wood dust and cold the agreement was very poor. Classifying only high exposed cases as exposed (**B**) made the agreement even worse with the exception of the exposure to wood dust, which reached almost perfect agreement.

Table 1. Agreement (Cohen's Kappa) for 22 agents generated by two job-exposure matrices for the Zutphen cohort (796 men).

Agent	A[1]	B[2]	Agent	A	B
acrylonitrile	0.18	.	formaldehyde	-0.02	0.00
arsenic	0.15	-0.00	**styrene**	**0.57**	0.00
asbestos	0.18	0.09	carbon tetrachl.	0.36	0.00
benzene	0.28	0.02	paints	0.02	0.00
beryllium	0.01	.	waxes	-0.07	0.00
cadmium	0.08	.	**wood dust**	**0.69**	**0.95**
chromium	**0.40**	-0.03	**cold**	**0.63**	0.00
mercury	0.01	.	uv-light	-0.00	0.10
lead	0.23	0.02	pcb	0.26	.
epoxy resins	0.08	0.00	aromatic amines	0.08	0.01
ethylene oxide	-0.01	.	chlorophenols	-0.00	.

1 both high and low exposed classified as exposed
2 only high exposed classified as exposed

The MRC matrix appeared to be more conservative in attributing high exposures to arsenic, asbestos, benzene, chromium, lead, waxes, uv-light and aromatic amines than the NCI matrix. On the other hand high exposures to epoxy resins, formaldehyde, styrene, carbon tetrachloride, paints and cold were more frequently assigned by the MRC matrix.

In table 2 occupations are shown which were classified as having a high exposure to arsenic, asbestos and wood dust by one or both matrices. Most differences in classification are due to differences in assigning a specific exposure to a certain occupation.

However from table 2 it is also evident that differences occur because of differences in level of specification of the job-axis. For instance all 11 trench diggers have a high exposure to asbestos according to the MRC JEM.

Table 2. Occupations and number of persons with a high exposure to arsenic, asbestos and wood dust generated by the NCI JEM and the MRC JEM.

Exposure (n)	**NCI only** occupation (n)	**MRC only** occupation (n)	**Both** occupation (n)
Arsenic (29)	farmers (12) plant gardeners (7) exterminator (1) agric. serv. (1) food processing (6) fuel processing (1)	tanner (1)	-
Asbestos (49)	locomotive oper.(14) switchman (7) gas distribution (7)	trench digger (8) reinforced con-crete worker (6) brick layers (4)	trench digger gas distr. (3)
Wood dust (32)	-	packaging (3)	woodworkers (4) carpenters (19) cabinetmakers(6)

On the other hand, the NCI job-axis divides the 11 trench diggers over different industries and attributes a high asbestos exposure only to 3 trench diggers in gas distribution.

Table 3. Relative risk of different exposures[1] with CNSLD incidence allowed for age and smoking habits in a multivariate proportional hazard analysis of 796 men of the Zutphen cohort.

Agent	RR_{mrc}	RR_{nci}	**Agent**	RR_{mrc}	RR_{nci}
acrylonitrile	2.03	3.27	formaldehyde	1.24	1.09
arsenic	1.23	1.11	styrene	0.73	1.22
asbestos	1.27	1.60	carbo.tetrachl.	1.07	1.07
benzene	1.04	1.38*	paints	1.08	1.39
beryllium	-	1.18	waxes	1.06	1.29
cadmium	1.48	1.12	wood dust	1.30	1.25
chromium	1.68***	1.59***	cold	1.39*	1.49*
mercury	2.01*	1.05	uv-light	1.25	1.34*
lead	1.14	1.24	pcb	0.86	1.44
epoxy resins	0.90	1.03	arom. amines	1.08	1.15
ethylene oxide	1.03	2.09*	chlorophenols	1.39	-

[1] both high and low exposed classified as exposed
* $p<0.05$ *** $p<0.001$

The estimated relative risks for the exposures with CNSLD incidence (adjusted for age and smoking habits) did not differ much and were in general close to unity when the exposure categories **A** were used (table 3). Probably the low specificity of both matrices led to a negative bias and therefore to small differences in risk estimates. When only the cohort members with a high exposure according to the matrices were assumed exposed (**B**), most of the risk estimates increased. However also the differences in risk estimates for the two matrices became larger (table 4).

Table 4. Relative risk of different exposures[1] with CNSLD incidence allowed for age and smoking habits in a multivariate proportional hazard analysis of 796 men of the Zutphen cohort.

Agent	RR_{mrc}	RR_{nci}	Agent	RR_{mrc}	RR_{nci}
acrylonitrile	-	-	formaldehyde	2.25*	-
arsenic	4.80	0.83	styrene	2.13	-
asbestos	2.00	0.97	carbo.tetrachl.	2.81	-
benzene	1.02	1.61*	paints	0.91	-
beryllium	-	-	waxes	-	1.34
cadmium	-	-	wood dust	1.37	1.57
chromium	2.69**	1.54*	cold	1.26	-
mercury	-	-	uv-light	3.20*	1.12
lead	1.03	1.80*	pcb	-	-
epoxy resins	0.37	-	arom. amines	0.81	1.60*
ethylene oxide	-	-	chlorophenols	-	-

[1] only high exposed classified as exposed
* $p<0.05$ ** $p<0.01$

Although less clear than with CNSLD, the analyses with the lung cancer incidence data (not presented) showed similar results. Relative risks appeared to be close to unity, when all exposed men were assumed exposed. Larger differences between the risk estimates were present when only high exposed men were assumed exposed.

Discussion

From these results it is obvious that the two job-exposure matrices show dramatic differences in assigning exposures to occupations for most of the 22 agents. This leads to varying estimates of relative risks, which were in general lower than the relative risks found with job titles as exposure variables. More specific analyses with a reference method (for instance case by case assessment of exposure by occupational hygienists) might give further insight in reasons for poor agreement. At this moment, a definite answer regarding the usefulness of general JEM's is premature, but it is obvious from our results that they need a sound validation.

Acknowledgements
The authors are indebted to Prof. Dr. D. Kromhout National Institute of Public Health and Environmental Protection for the data of the Zutphen cohort.

References

Hoar S.K, Morrison A.S, Cole P, Silverman D.T. (1980) J Occup Med 22:722-726
Pannett B, Coggon D, Acheson E.D. (1985) Br J Ind Med 42:777-783
Hinds M.W, Kolonel L.N, Lee J. (1985) J Ntl Canc Inst 75:193-197
Coggon D, Pannett B, Acheson E.D. (1984) J Ntl Canc Inst 72:61-65
Fleiss J.L. (1981) J. Wiley & Sons 212-236
Cox D.R. (1972) J. Roy Statist Soc B 34:187-202

Occupational Epidemiology. H. Sakurai et al., editors

STABILITY AND COMPARABILITY OF RELATIVE RISK UNDER EXPOSURES TO MULTIPLE RISK FACTORS OF A DISEASE

R.SAKAI

Department of Epidemiology, School of Health Sciences, Ryukyu University, Uehara 207, Nishihara-cho, Okinawa (Japan)

INTRODUCTION

In the last century, Dr. John Snow succeeded in estimating the etiology of a cholera outbreak in London by simply pinpointing the address of each cholera victim on a city map, without the aid of any investigative methods used in microbiology. Nowadays, a central theory in epidemiology is based on relative risk calculation. There are, however, several important and difficult problems.

At first, it is required the assumption that the risk factors are measurable so that we could not calculate any relative risk if the risk factors remain undetectable and/or unmeasurable to morphological, biochemical or other analytical investigations. Second, most chronic diseases can epidemiologically have any number of risk factors that causes them to develop. To cite an example, some recognized risk factors that provoke coronary heart disease are smoking, obesity, an abnormally high blood pressure and/or cholesterol count, and too strenuous or too little exercise (1,2).

Thus, to epidemiologically analyze a particular risk or risks, we must take into account these other risk factors, apart from the suspected risk factors that are the focuses of our attention. These other risk factors compose of two elements: a "confounder" or "multiple confounders" that should have some connection with the suspected risk factors (3); and, other likely independent factors that may have cause the disease.

When the multiple risk factors are detectable and/or measurable, we can analyze these data by using any of the following methods: a multiple cross tabling (4), a stratified analysis (3), a log-linear formula, a logistic regression, or Miettinen's (5) confounder summarization or by any number of other mathematical methods. When the confounders are not measurable, Schlesslman (6) has demonstrated a simple formula based on functional relationships that assess the effect of confounders.

If the other risk factors, apart from the suspected, detectable risk factors and confounders, are neither detectable nor measurable, the influence of these unmeasurable multiple risk factors are behind the suspected, measurable risk factors. Thus, let us therm them "background risk factors" or "backgrounders".

Cornfield et al (7) demonstrated that the odds ratio observed in a case/control study will be mathematically less than the true ratio, given the existence of such a backgrounder. Therefore, relative risk is suggested to also change and be unstable under exectance of a backgrounder, but no impact from backgrounders were mathematically evident. Thus, the intent of this paper is to inspect mathematically the effect of a backgrounder exposure on the relative risk.

THE TIME-DIFFERENCE APPROACH OF A BACKGROUNDER

Unfortunately, the estimation procedure with regard to a backgrounder exposure in a cohort has not been fully elucidated. One possible approach to elucidate the effects on such an exposure may be time-differential prospective observations of the incidence of a chronic disease on a fixed cohort in which the exposure level to a backgrounder shows a change.

The above speculation with regard to a chronic disease supposes that the general human population may have multiple backgrounders apart from the suspected risk factors. To formulate this supposition mathematically, let us then assign the variable transformations of the probabilities of multiple backgrounders, i.e., (pr(BG1),pr(BG2)<....,pr(BGk)), into a composite variable Pr(BG0), for instance:

$$Pr(BG0) = \sum pr(BGi).$$

Therefore, we can summarize the total effects of the multiple backgroungers on a disease occurrence by using the effect of this composite variable. For simplification, we now shall analyze step by step the exposure to a single backgrounder (BG).

Figure 1 diagrams the relationships among four subgroups of a cohort, who may or may not be exposed to a suspected risk factor (RF) and/or to BG, and who may or may not be affected by a chronic disease. Figure 1 a and b present cohorts at the first observation, and Figure 1 c and d are at the second observation. Figure 1 a and c are the ideal diagrams and Figure 1 b and d are at the practical ones. Should the exposure level to BG be found to have changed at the second observation (see figure 1-c), the disease occurrence probability usually will have changed, too.

From Figure 1 a or b, d1 and D1 are defined to represent the case

Fig.1. Diagrams of four subgroups in a fixed cohort during the different times.

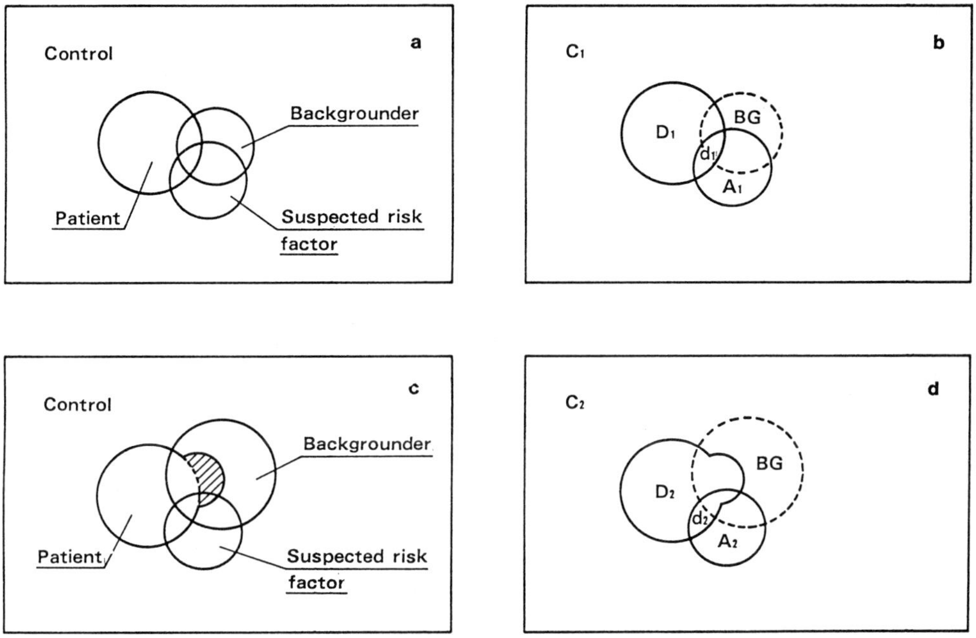

numbers with or without RF, respectively at the first obserbation. A1 and C1 also represent the number of subjects free from a disease of interest with and without RF, each other at the same time. Then, d2, D2, A2 and C2 correspond with d1, D1, A1 and C1, respectively at the second observation. Thus, we can mathematically determine the relative risk (RR1) of RF per the following formula:

$$RR1=(d1/(d1/+A1))/(D1/(D1+C1)),$$

$$RR2=(d2/(d2/+A2))/(D2/(D2+C2)),$$

wherein $C1+D1+d1+A1=C2+D2+d2+A2;$

$$d2=d1+d; \quad D2=D1+D; \quad C1=C2+D; \text{ and } A1=A2+d.$$

We can achieve the following transformations of these formulas;

$$RR2/RR1=(d2xD1x(D2+C2)x(D1+A1))/(d1xD2x(D1+C1)x(d2+A2))$$

$$=(d2xD1)/(d1xD2)=((d1+d)/d1)x(D1/(D1+D)).$$

Should the ratio be large than 1, then;

$$((d1+d)/d1)>((D1+D)/D1), \text{ and}$$

finally, $(d/d1)>(D/D1)$.

From the above, certain relations become evident. If we assume that the increase rate of cases due to combination exposure to RF and BG is greater than the increase rate of cases due to the expo-sure to only BG, then there is a new greater RR of RF, and vice versa.

DISCUSSION

Thus, it is clear that relative risk of a single risk factor is not stable, if there is a backgrounder which changes through a follow-up. It is also obvious that relative risk of a risk factor does not always coincide with that in the different population, when there is another RF of same disease. Therefore, RR is not always comparable.

On that account, if there is a backgrounder, we cannot easily accepted a result of no significant relative risk. It means that we should match an exposure level to a backgrounder, likely in the case of confounders.

However, as defined the above, a backgrounder is not measurable. So we need to devise a procedure to detect a unmeasurable back-grounder. For example, I proposes a ratio of two relative risks at the different times in a fixed cohort as an indicator to estimate a change of a backgrounder exposure level. But this method contains several limits as below.

1) If the exposure level did not change during the follow-up period, we were unable to estimate a backgrounder's existence.
2) We cannot distingush how many kinds of backgrounders exist.
3) The method is not well-adapted to a disease with a long latent priod.
4) This model could not identfy what is a backgrounder. It offers only extimation of the existance.

As shown in the above, we need to develop more suitable method to detect a backgrounder which is of course unmeasurable.

REFERENCES

1. Hammond EC (1969) Arch Environ Health 19:395-402
2. Weiss NS, Liff JM (1983) Am J Epidemiol 117:14-18
3. Sclesselman JJ, Stolley PD (1982) Case-control studies. Oxford University Press, New York
4. Cornfield J, Haenszel W (1960) J Chronic Dis 11:523-534
5. Miettinen OS (1976) Am J Epidemiol 104:609-620
6. Schlesselman JJ (1978) Am J Epidemiol 108:3-8
7. Cornfield J, Haenszel W, Hammond C et al (1959) J Natl Cancer Inst 22:173-203

© 1990 Elsevier Science Publishers B.V. (Biomedical Division)
Occupational Epidemiology. H. Sakurai et al., editors

RETROSPECTIVE EXPOSURE ASSESSMENT FOR EPIDEMIOLOGY: VAPOR EXPOSURES OF GASOLINE TRANSPORTATION WORKERS

THOMAS J. SMITH, MARILYN HALLOCK, AND S. KATHARINE HAMMOND
Environmental Health Sciences Program, Department of Family and Community Medicine, University of Massachusetts Medical School, 55 Lake Ave. North, Worcester, MA, 01655, U.S.A.

INTRODUCTION

Retrospective estimation of occupational exposures for is difficult for several reasons: quantitative exposure data are usually only available for recent times; available data are usually limited to "high" exposure jobs; and industrial operations rarely remain constant across time because of changes in job definitions, raw materials, process parameters and equipment, and other factors. The objective is to estimate each subject's time profile of exposure for all agents that might be associated with the disease of interest. Our approach is to assess exposures associated with each job and then use each subject's job history (a listing of the job titles by date kept by the company) to make a personal profile of exposure that can be used to calculate dose indices. Two simple models of exposure were used to identify the workplace factors determining the composition and intensity of exposure, and to relate them to job descriptions so that the effects of historical changes could be extrapolated.

The application of this approach will be illustrated with an example taken from an exposure assessment being performed for a U.S. cohort of workers drawn from several hundred work sites where gasoline was handled. This is part of an epidemiologic study of long-term gasoline exposures and risk of various cancers, particularly kidney cancer.

EXPOSURE EXTRAPOLATION RATIONALE

Source-Receptor Model

The source-receptor model is a concept borrowed from air pollution modeling, which describes the atmospheric transport of an air contaminant from an emission source to a receptor, eg. an exposed population (1). In our application, the industrial operation and its raw materials and products will define the sources, output strength, and composition of airborne emissions (potential agents of effects). The intensity of exposure is determined by source output strength, air movements which will transport and dilute the contaminants, and the worker's proximity to the source which is defined by his work task. Information about historical changes in materials, process, or work site configuration can be used in the model to evaluate historical changes in exposure.

Time-Weighted-Average Model

The average exposure in a job is the time-weighted-average (TWA) of exposures in its composite tasks (TWA = sum over all tasks of average exposure times fraction of time in the task). Usually historical industrial hygiene data are focussed on the high exposure tasks and job titles. The TWA model enables the use of all available data in extrapolation of exposures. Effects of historical changes in job definitions, which modify tasks included in the job or time spent at high exposure tasks, can be evaluated with the model.

APPLICATION TO GASOLINE TRANSPORTATION EXPOSURES

Gasoline Source-Receptor Model

Workers moving gasoline in the United States distribution system are primarily exposed to the inhalation of vapors displaced from headspace above liquids when transport or storage tanks are filled, and to the vapors from spills. Gasoline is a mixture of over 200 compounds. Vapor components in headspace above gasoline are represented in proportion to their mole fraction in the liquid and their intrinsic vapor pressures (2). The most volatile and abundant compounds predominate in the vapors; n-butane, isobutane, n-pentane and isopentane account for 60-80% of the vapors, but are only about 25% of the liquid (3-6). Nonhydrocarbon additives in gasoline are present at low concentrations, and are unlikely to be present in contaminated air at significant levels (5). Other common products handled by gasoline distribution workers have generally lower vapor pressures (gasoline is 150-510 mmHg (22°C) while diesel fuel and heating oil are < 1 mmHg), so tank filling with these emits much lower levels of total hydrocarbons.

The agents (if any) in gasoline vapors that may cause human kidney cancer have not been identified, so intensities of exposure to causal agents could not be directly estimated. Total hydrocarbon concentration (THC) was used as an exposure index for gasoline vapor. This was done with the assumption that each component is on average a fixed percentage of the total (7).

The configuration of equipment used in distribution has changed historically. Configuration determines the quantities of vapor emitted. Industrial hygiene data show significant differences in exposure for these configuration factors: top or bottom filling; fill pipe submerged vs. "splash loading" (fill pipe above the surface of the liquid); open vs. closed hatch (remote vent); and use of vapor recovery systems (3-5,8,9). At delivery sites, similar considerations apply. Thus historical changes in configuration of facilities at the work sites (loading area or delivery site) can be used to define past exposures.

Transportation Workers Time-Weighted-Average Exposure Model

The job title of Truck Driver will be used to illustrate the approach. This "generic" job title will be assigned to all equivalent job titles in the workers' job histories (many variants are found). These assignments are determined by long-term employees, who also provide data on historical changes in job definitions and facilities configurations at work sites.

The Truck Driver job has four component tasks: loading, driving, delivery, and other (low exposure activities, such as paper work). Published and company industrial hygiene data are available on personal exposures during loading and delivery tasks. For example, submerged filling of trucks by open hatch, top loading had an average exposure of 150 ppm THC, and delivery to large underground tanks with remote venting showed 20 ppm THC (8). Simulations of older high exposure operations, such as splash loading, were performed to provide data on tasks with configurations that were no longer in use. These limited exposure data, for tasks using various configurations of facilities can be coupled with historical data on changes in work site facilities, and time spent on tasks, to extrapolate past TWA exposures. Only the low exposures, such as driving, must be estimated indirectly based on analogy with other measured activities. A similar approach can be used with other generic job titles to make assignments of exposure for all jobs in job histories.

Error Assessment

There are many potential sources of error in this exposure assessment. Some of these may be addressed, or quantified, and others may not. Misclassification will result if exposures to causal agents do not correlate with the THC levels. Job definitions and assignments and work site facility histories should be checked within and across companies to insure consistency. Errors in TWAs can be assessed by examining contributions of component tasks. The fraction of unknown job titles and work sites can be determined; the most common generic jobs and site types can be assigned to unknowns. Company data collected in cross-sectional surveys of benzene exposures can be used to check limited THC data for representativeness. The variability across sites and workers in the same job can be determined through an analysis of variance, and the misclassification effects assessed.

REFERENCES

1. Benarie MM (1980) Urban Air Pollution Modelling. MIT Press, Cambridge, MA, USA, pp 17-18

2. Maynard JB, Sanders WN (1969) J Air Poll Control Assoc 19:505-510

3. Halder CA, Van Gorp GS, Hatoum NS, Warne TM (1986) Am Ind Hyg J 47:164-172

4. MacFarland HN, Ulrich CE, Holdsworth CE, Kitchen DN, Halliwell WH, Blum SC (1984) J Am Coll Toxicol 3:231-248

5. McDermott HJ, Killiany Jr SE (1978) Am Ind Hyg Assoc J 39:110-117

6. Runion HE (1975) Am Ind Hyg J 36:338-350

7. Rappaport SM, Selvin S, Waters MA (1987) Appl Ind Hyg 2:148-154

8. Phillips CF, Jones RK (1975) Am Ind Hyg Assoc J 39:118-128

9. Irving Jr. WS, Grumbles TG (1979) Am Ind Hyg Assoc J 40:468-473

Occupational Epidemiology. H. Sakurai et al., editors

NONPARAMETRIC ANALYSIS OF DOSE-RESPONSE RELATIONSHIPS

KURT ULM
Institute for Medical Statistics and Epidemiology, Technical University Munich,
Ismaninger Straße 22, 8000 Munich 80, Federal Republic of Germany

INTRODUCTION

The standardized mortality (or morbidity) ratio (= SMR) is a common measure used in the analysis of occupational cohort-studies. The mortality rate in a cohort of exposed workers is compared to national or regional rates, where the general population is used as reference group. The SMR is the ratio of the observed number of deaths in the cohort divided by the expected number based on the person-years at risk in the cohort and the mortality-rates in the reference population. But one has to be very cautious in drawing conclusions from a single SMR. The SMR is suspected to be biased, especially to the so-called healthy-worker-effect (HWE).

The proof of a dose-response relationship is an important criterion on the way to establish causality. The usual proceeding to proof this relationship is to divide the cohort into various subgroups according to the exposure-level or some other variables related with the exposure, like time since first exposure, length of exposure or age at onset of exposure and to calculate the SMR´s in these subgroups. If there is an association between the agent under consideration and the morality-rates, the SMR has to increase with higher exposure-levels.

The methods described in the literature to analyze the dose-response relationship are the test on trend[1] or POISSON regression models[1,2]. In these methods it is necessary to quantify the exposure in the subgroups. In the regression models it is also needed to specify the form of the relationship.

But in occupational epidemiology it is uncommon to have measurements about the exposure in the past. The result of the various methods are depending on the definition of the exposure levels, which are more or less arbitrary. For some definitions the result can be statistically significant for others not.

To show such a result the data of table 3.3 from the monograph of Breslow and Day[1] are analyzed (s. table 1). The test on trend using the values x_j to quantify the exposure leads to $X^2 = 4.43$ (statistically significant with $p < 0.05$), using the values y_j to $X^2 = 3.72$ (statistically not significant with $p > 0.05$).

One can chose the specification of the exposure level depending which result is wanted. The some is true for the analysis with regression models. A situation which is unsatisfactory.

Therefore I want to present a nonparametric method, the isotonic regression, to analyze an exposure-response relationship, the isotonic regression, which is independent of these definitions. Robertson et al.[3] provide an excellent description of this approach. There are some applications in epidemiological research [4,5], but not in analyzing SMR's.

TABLE 1:
RESPIRATORY CANCER DEATHS AMONG MONTANA SMELTER WORKERS
(Workers employed 1925 or later, from Breslow and Day[1])

subgroup (= j)	cumulative years of exposure	definition of the exposure-level x_j	y_j	Observed (=O)	Expected (=E)	SMR = O/E
1	0-0.9	0.5	0.5	100	74.12	1.35
2	1.0-4.9	3.0	3.0	38	13.84	2.75
3	5.0-14.9	10.0	10.0	15	6.83	2.20
4	15+	20.0	25.0	8	3.66	2.19
Σ				161	98.46	1.64

METHOD

Estimation-procedure

The total cohort is divided into J subgroups with increasing exposure-level. Subgroup 1 has the lowest level, subgroup J the highest one. The idea of the isotonic repression is to provide maximum-likelihood-estimates of the SMR in each of the subgroups under the constraints of monotonicity. This means, the SMR's have to fulfill the following relationship:

$$H_1: \quad SMR_1 \leq SMR_2 \leq ... \leq SMR_J \qquad (1)$$

The second step is to test, whether this result is significantly different from the null-hypothesis, all SMR's are equal:

$$H_0: \quad SMR_1 = SMR_2 = ... = SMR_J = SMR \qquad (2)$$

In the first step the crude SMR_j (= O_j/E_j) in each subgroup j (j = 1,...,J) are calculated. If for these crude SMR_j relation (1) holds, then these SMR_j´s are already the estimates of the isotonic regression. Otherwise if relation (1) is failed at pair (k, k+1) both subgroups are pooled together to:

$$SMR_k = SMR_{k+1} = \frac{O_k + O_{k+1}}{E_k + E_{k+1}} = \frac{E_k \cdot SMR_k + E_{k+1} \cdot SMR_{k+1}}{E_k + E_{k+1}} \qquad (3)$$

Then one has to go backwards to proof whether relation (1) still holds for $1 \leq j < k$. If this is true, one can move upwards, otherwise more subgroups have to be pooled together. Some algorithms are described in the monograph of Robertson et al.[3], also a program is available[6].

Test-procedure

The observed number of deaths (= Oj) is assumed to be POISSON-distributed with mean E_j [1]. A test-procedure is described for normally distributed variables with known variances[3]. The likelihood ratio statistics $R = 2 * [\ln L(H_1) - \ln L(H_0)]$ is used, which holds under H_0 the following important relation:

$$\Pr\{R > c\} = \sum_{k=2}^{J} P(k,J,w) \cdot \Pr\{\chi^2_{k-1} > c\} \quad \text{for } c > 0 \qquad (4)$$

$$\Pr\{R = 0\} = P(1,J,w)$$

$\Pr\{R > c\}$ denotes the probability that R exceeds under H_0 some constant c ($c > 0$). P(k,J,w) are the probabilities that given J different subgroups with weights $w = (w_1,..,w_J)$ the isotonic regression finishes under H_0 with k ($1 \leq k \leq J$) different estimates and $\Pr\{\chi^2_{k-1} > c\}$ lastly is the probability that a χ^2-distributed variable with k-1 degrees of freedom exceeds c ($k \geq 2$).

The reason is, if the isotonic regression finishes with k different values, the log-likelihood-ratio R is χ^2-distributed with k-1 degrees of freedom. The probability to observe such a result under H_0 is P(k,J,w). $\Pr\{R > c\}$ is the sum over all possible outcomes weighted with the corresponding probabilities. If the variable for the isotonic regression is normally distributed with known variances, relation (4) holds exactly otherwise approximately.

The log-likelihood ratio statistics R for POISSON-distributed variables turns out to be:

$$R = 2 \cdot \sum_{j=1}^{J} O_j \cdot \ln(SMR_j/SMR) \qquad (5)$$

with SMR the overall SMR and SMR_j the estimated SMR in subgroup j of the isotonic regression fulfilling relation (1).

To calculate the probability that R exceeds some constant c, the probabilities P(k,J,w) are necessary. The weights w_j are the expected number of events (= E_j) used for pooling the SMR (s. relation (3)). The probabilities P(k,J,w) are tabulated only, if all the weights are equal (s. table A10 in Robertson et al.[3]). A program is available to compute P(k,J,w) for $J \leq 5$ and any given set of weights for normally distributed variables[7], which can be used as an approximation for POISSON-distributed variables. But the differences between P(k,J) and P(k,J,w) are fairly small and have in many situations negligible effect on the significance level [3].

Independent of the probabilities P(k,J,w), the result $\Pr\{R > c\}$ can be approximated considering two facts:

a) $\Pr\{\chi^2_k > c\} > \Pr\{\chi^2_{k-1} > c\}$

b) $\sum_{k=2}^{J} \Pr\{k,J,w\} < 1$

$\Pr\{R > c\}$ has therefore the following boundaries:

$$\Pr\{\chi^2_{J-1} > c\} > \Pr\{R > c\} > \Pr\{\chi^2_1 > c\} \qquad (6)$$

R is statistically not significant at a level of α if less then $\chi^2_{1,\alpha}$ and significant if greater than $\chi^2_{J-1,\alpha}$. For values between, the exact probabilities have to be calculated to accept or reject H_0.

APPLICATION

The data of table 1 are analyzed by the isotonic regression. Relation (1) is failed between subgroup 2 and 3. Pooling these both groups together leads to:

$$SMR_2 = SMR_3 = (38 + 15)/(13.84 + 6.83) = 2.57$$

SMR_1 is still less than SMR_2. Going upwards it is to be seen that SMR_4 is less then SMR_3, which is equal to SMR_2. Subgroups 2 to 4 are pooled together. This amalgamation leads to (s. also fig.1):

$$SMR_2 = SMR_3 = SMR_4 = (38 + 15 + 8)/(13.84 + 6.83 + 3.66) = 2.51$$

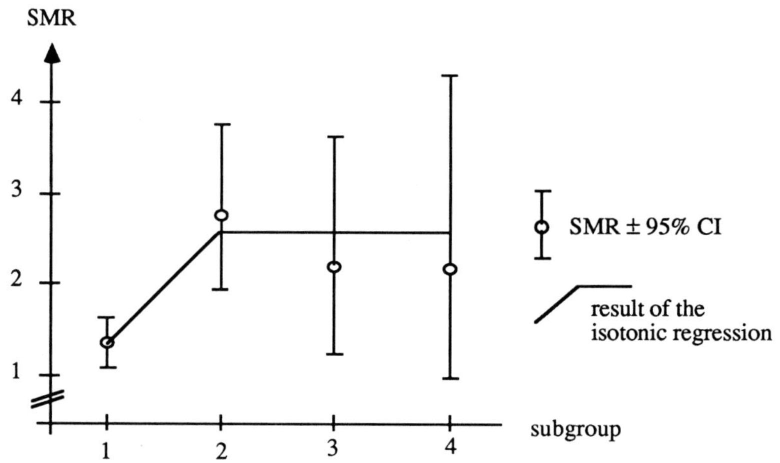

Fig. 1: Result of the isotonic regression applied to the data of table 1

The likelihood ratio statistics yields to R = 13.66. According to relation (6) the relationship is statistically significant with $p< 0.005$ ($\chi^2_{3,0.005} = 12.838$). The same result is obtained using the critical value for equal weights $Pr\{R > 12.831 | H_0\} = 0.005$ (s. table A.5 in ref.3). The exact probability $Pr\{R > c\}$ with values P(j,4,w) is $Pr\{R > 13.66 | H_0\} = 0.002$. Using equal weights the exact value will be p = 0.004. The difference between the p value using P(k,4) instead of P(k,4,w) is small.

DISCUSSION

In this paper a nonparametric approach, the isotonic regression, is described for the analysis of an exposure-SMR relationship which gives more information instead of analyzing only the overall SMR. The only assumption of this approach is monotonicity. This means, with increasing exposure the SMR cannot decrease. The application of this method frees one from all the limitations necessary to apply the test on trend or a parametric model. It is unnecessary to quantify the exposure-levels in the various subgroups, normally not available nor to specify the form of the relationship in a POISSON-regression model .

Sometimes a job-exposure matrix can be established, where the different jobs are classified into qualitative exposure groups, like low, medium or high. This can be done for different calender-periods, considered the decreasing exposure-levels with continuing time. All information can be accumulated by scoring the exposure-categories with different weights. In this situation which is common in occupational medicine the total cohort can be divided into several subgroups with respect to the exposure. In this situation the isotonic regression, a nonparametric approach, for analyzing the dose-response relationship is superior to other methods.

All calculations can be performed very easy only in using a pocket-calculator. A quick check, whether R is statistically significant can be done also easily in using relation (6) or table A5 from Robertson et al [3].

The method is presented in the context of the SMR, but it can also be applied if the risk is measured at another scale, e.g. the excess-risk or the incidence directly without use of a reference population. The extension will be to proof a dose-response relationship without use of a reference population. Then the age has to be taken into account which leads to a two dimensional isotonic regression. An algorithm for estimating the isotonic regression is available[8], but the distribution of the test value R under H_0 is unknown.

REFERENCES:

1. Breslow NE, Day NE (1987) Statistical Methods in Cancer Research Vol. II. The Design and Analysis of Cohort Studies. IARC Scientific Publications Nr. 82, Oxford Press

2. Hanley J, Liddell D (1985) J.Occup.Med. 27: 555-560

3. Robertson T, Wright F, Dykstra RL (1988) Order Restricted Statistical Influence. John Wiley & Sons, New York

4. Thomas DC (1983) Biometrics 39: 263-268

5. Ulm K (1986) Mathematical Modelling 7: 777-783

6. Cran GW (1980) Appl.Stat. 29: 209-211

7. Cran GW (1981) Appl.Stat. 30: 85-91

8. Bril G. et al (1984) Appl. Stat. 33: 85-91

OCCUPATIONAL CANCER

Occupational Epidemiology. H. Sakurai et al., editors

ETIOLOGICAL FACTORS IN LIP CANCER: A CASE-REFERENT STUDY

GIORGIO ASSENNATO[1], ANTONIO PORRO[1], LUIGI DARDANONI[2], MARIA ARDITO[1], PASQUALE F. CICCARELLI[1].

[1]Institute of Occupational Health, University of Bari, Piazza G. Cesare, 70124 Bari, Italy.
[2]Institute of Hygiene, University of Palermo, Palermo, Italy.

ABSTRACT

A case-control study has been carried out to evaluate the association between several factors (genetic, behavioral, occupational and skin-related) and lip cancer. Information on color of hair, eyes and skin, sun sensitivity, skin lesions, smoking habits, outdoor work, socio-economic status and occupation was obtained from 76 male incident cases of lip cancer, drawn from the population-based Ragusa Cancer Registry, Italy, and compared with that of 152 controls matched for sex, age, residence and hospital where cases were observed. Statistical analysis showed strong associations between genetic factors (blond hair, blue eyes, fair skin complexion, sun sensitivity), skin lesions (hyperkeratosis), occupational factors (outdoor work), low socio-economic status and lip cancer, while clerical work appeared to be a protective factor. After adjustment for genetic factors, skin lesions and occupational factors, tobacco smoking showed no significant influence on risk.

INTRODUCTION

Several epidemiological studies[1-7] on etiological factors in lip cancer have identified the following potential risk factors: genetic factors such as race, sex, skin complexion, colour of hair and eyes, and sun sensitivity; skin viral infections and non-specific skin lesions, behaviours such as exposure to tobacco smoke and alcohol; and occupationally related conditions, such as high solar radiation exposure (outdoor work, particularly in agriculture). The present study shows the results of a case-referent study analysis of lip cancer from Ragusa Cancer Registry (Sicily), Italy. An earlier study of a group of 53 cases from this registry was reported by Dardanoni, et al.[1], but it was not based on a multivariate analysis.

METHODS

Cases for the present analysis include 76 males whose lip cancer was reported to the population-based Cancer Registry in Ragusa, Sicily, Italy between January 1, 1980 and December 31, 1984. Each case was matched on sex, age (+- 2 years) and municipality of residence with two controls. Controls were selected from patients admitted to Medicine or Surgery Departments of the hospital where cases were observed, without neoplastic disease, from acute and chronic conditions, such as heart, eye or kidney diseases, trauma. Two cases and four controls were recruited in the Outpatient Department. Demographic and exposure information was collected by means of a structured questionnaire by two interviewers. The following risk factors were recorded: (1) colour of hair and eyes, complexion of unexposed skin; (2) sensitivity to solar erythema; (3) socio-economic status (SES) assessed by means of a code scoring based on education, occupation, personal hygiene, domicile; (4) outdoor work (working at least 6 hours a day outdoors); (5) occupation (before retirement): only current occupation was recorded; (6) presence of minor non-specific skin lesions (hyperkeratosis) on head, neck or hands; (7) smoking habits (cigarettes, pipe) in the previous twenty years. A two-stage data analysis process was performed. First, the association between risk factors and lip cancer was evaluated according to the matching procedures. Second, conditional logistic regression models were developed and tested in order to assess the contribution of each risk factor to lip cancer adjusted for the effects of the other variables.

RESULT

The average age was 65.30 (+- 9.31) for the cases and 64.84 (+- 9.28) for the controls.

TABLE I illustrates the relationship between genetic, skin-related, occupational and behavioral factors and lip cancer in a matched analysis. Among the most significant risk factors are: low socio-economic status, working in greenhouse, presence of skin lesions, fair complexion, blond hair and blue eyes. Working in agriculture and in greenhouse is strongly associated with lip

TABLE I

Mantel-Haenszel Relative Risk Estimates (RR-MH) and 95% Confidence Intervals (95% CI) of Lip Cancer - Matched Analysis

	Cases	Referents	RR-MH	95% CI
Hair Colour:				
Blond	9	4	4.50	1.67-14.22
Blond, Red or Brown	57	85	2.61	1.48- 4.61
Eye Colour:				
Blue	28	13	6.37	3.15-13.54
Blue, Hazel or Green	39	47	2.48	1.49- 4.18
Skin Complexion:				
Fair	53	34	8.20	4.39-16.47
Fair or Intermediate	71	116	4.25	1.71-10.25
Sun Sensitivity	39	47	2.41	1.51- 4.23
Skin Lesions				
(Hyperkeratosis)	51	24	8.80	5.31-21.44
Tobacco Smoke	58	97	1.68	1.05- 3.01
Low SES	51	16	18.20	8.00-46.55
Ourdoor Work	60	82	3.37	1.90- 6.06
Agricultural Work	44	52	3.12	1.83- 5.69
Individual Occupations:				
Farmer	39	51	2.69	1.51- 4.97
Greenhouse	5	1	10.00	1.65-93.94
Construction	9	23	0.76	0.38- 1.40
Clerk	5	31	0.25	0.11- 0.51
Sales	5	8	1.29	0.48- 3.22
Professional	0	2	----	--
Fisherman	1	4	0.50	0.08- 1.81
Various	12	32	0.67	0.33- 1.20

cancer, while clerical occupation appears to be a protective factor. TABLE II contains the results of a conditional logistic regression model of lip cancer on eight risk factors coded dichotomously. Given the previous analysis, it was decided to focus attention here only on the most extreme genetic factors. The regression analysis shows that certain phenotypic characteristics of skin complexion and eye colour, in particular blue eyes and fair skin and the presence of skin lesions are the most important risk factors for lip cancer. Hair colour seems to be less important as outdoor work and agricultural work are. Tobacco smoking and sensitivity to solar erythema were not statistically associated with lip cancer after adjustment for the effects of other risk factors.

DISCUSSION

The present analysis based on 76 cases and 152 controls supports earlier findings reported by Dardanoni, et al.[1]. The

TABLE II

Logistic Regression Model of Lip Cancer on Individual Risk Factor: Raw Coefficients, Odds Ratio and 95% Confidence Intervals

	Raw Coefficient	O.R.	95% Confidence Intervals
Blond Hair	0.72	2.06	0.28- 14.91
Blue Eyes	3.05	21.08	4.30-103.32
Fair Skin	3.01	20.37	3.88-106.85
Sun Sensitivity	0.31	1.37	0.45- 4.11
Skin Lesions	2.38	10.76	3.10- 37.37
Tobacco Smoke	0.78	2.19	0.72- 6.63
Outdoor Work	1.68	5.37	1.23- 23.43
Agricultural Work	1.75	5.74	1.04- 31.66

matched analysis confirmed the role of certain factors such as low socio-economic status, working outdoors (particularly in agriculture), presence of skin lesions, being of fair complexion, having blond hair and blue eyes. Information for socio-economic status was available only as a total score, therefore analysis for each of its components (education, occupation, domicile, personal hygiene) was impossible.

The conditional logistic regression analysis clearly shows the importance of genetic characteristics, in particular blue eyes and fair skin complexion, hyperkeratosis and solar exposure (outdoor work) in increasing the relative odds ratio for lip cancer controlling simultaneously for the other factors.

REFERENCES

1. Dardanoni L, Gafà L, Paternò R, et al. A Case-Control Study on Lip Cancer Risk Factors in Ragusa (Sicily). Inter J Cancer 1984; 34: 335-337.

2. Keller AZ. Cellular Types, Survival, Race, Nativity, Occupations, Habits and Associated Diseases in the Pathogenesis of Lip Cancer. Am J Epidem 1970; 91: 486-499.

3. Lindqvist C. Risk Factors in Lip Cancer: A Questionnaire Survey. Am J Epidem 1979; 109: 521-530.

4. Lindqvist C. Risk Factors of Lip Cancer: A Critical Evaluation Based on Epidemiological Comparisons. Am J Public Health 1979; 69; 256-260.

5. Wiklund K. Swedish Agricultural Workers: A group with a Decreased Risk of Cancer. Cancer 1983; 51: 566-568.

6. Lindqvist C, Teppo L. Epidemiological Evaluation of Sunlight as a Risk Factor of Lip Cancer. Br J Cancer 1978; 37: 983-989.

7. Spitzer WO, Hill GB, Chambers LW, et al. The Occupation of Fishing as a Risk Factor in Cancer of the Lip. New Engl J Med 1975; 293: 419-424.

Occupational Epidemiology. H. Sakurai et al., editors

A CANCER MORTALITY STUDY OF PRODUCTION WORKERS IN A PAINTS AND COATINGS INDUSTRY IN ITALY

P.A. BERTAZZI*, S. GUERCILENA*, A. TIRONI*, C. ZOCCHETTI*, L. RADICE*, A.C. PESATORI*, F. MERLUZZI*, and A.M. COLOMBI**

* Institute of Occupational Health, University of Milan, Via San Barnaba 8, 20122 Milano, Italy. ** PPG Industries Inc., Pittsburgh, PA, USA

INTRODUCTION

Several investigations on paint production workers and painters carried out in different countries raised the suspicion of an increased cancer risk pertaining to working in these occupations. Exposure in painting trades is complex. Some of the compounds involved are established or suspected carcinogens (e.g., benzene, chromates, azo-dyes, PAH's, formaldehyde). A recent evaluation of the available studies concluded that there is sufficient evidence of carcinogenicity for exposure as a painter; data for exposure in paint manufacture were instead considered inadequate for evaluation (1).

MATERIAL AND METHODS

The cancer mortality experience of a cohort of employees at one of the largest coatings and paints industry in Italy was examined. All the 1,614 male workers employed for at least four months since the beginning of operations were enrolled. Their mortality experience was examined in the period 1948-1987. Individual job histories were available for all but 81 workers. Given the number of solvents used and the frequent changes in production processes, it was not possible to attribute exposure to specific solvents to individual jobs. The use of benzene per se was discontinued in the mid-fifties. A policy to refuse benzene contamination of toluene and xylene was established in 1980. Toluene, xylene, and technical hydrocarbons (kerosene) make-up 50% of solvents consumption. Different kind of resins were manufactured inside the plant, the far largest majority being represented by alkidic, epoxy-acrilic, and melamine based polymers. The pigments used were numerous. The yearly consumption of chromates was around

100 tons. Azo-dyes were used in small quantities (from 16 to 20 tons/year). Carbon black derived from combustion products was used up to the mid sixties and gradually but not completely substituted by pure carbonium preparations. More then 150 jobs were identified, and then grouped in the exposure categories reported in the table. Workers were assigned to the first job held which corresponded in 94% of the cases to the longest one. Quantitative levels of exposure were not available. All workers in production had a significant exposure to solvents. Expected deaths specific by age (5 years), period (5 years) and cause were computed from the mortality rates of the corresponding population of a nearby town (120,000 inhabitants). The ratio of observed to expected death (SMR) were calculated for each cause, taking age and calendar period into account. The departure of the SMR values from unity was tested assuming a Poisson distribution of the numerator.

RESULTS

Vital status ascertainment was successful for 96.4% of the cohort members. In table I, results for workers in the production areas are reported. When examined as a whole cohort, they exhibited nonsignificantly increased SMR values for cancer of the esophagus and the bladder, and cirrhosis. Overall mortality among subjects exposed to 'solvents only' was higher than expected. They also experienced an increased mortality owing to hematologic neoplasms (two non-Hodgkins limphomas), and cirrhosis; the number of deaths was small, however, and the SMR values statistically nonsignificant. Workers in the resins department were exposed to both solvents and resins, and exhibited a general pattern of increased mortality. The seven-fold increased risk of esophageal cancer (two deaths only) barely reached statistical significance. Noteworthy were also the increased risks of bladder and colorectal cancer, albeit based on two deaths. Workers employed in the paint manufacturing area were exposed to solvents, resins and pigments and their mortality turned out to be below expectations for virtually every cause. To three out of six bladder cancer cases no specific job could be assigned; they had however worked in the production areas of the plant, and made up a statistically significant increase in the exposure category 'unknown'.

Workers in this production unit had a remarkably low mortality from lung cancer, despite the reported use of chromate pigments and talc, which is possibly contaminated with asbestos fibers. Previous studies revealed an increased lung cancer risk for painters (2-8) but not production workers (7-11), with one single exception (12).

TABLE I

Mortality from selected causes, 1948-1987, of workers employed in the production of paints and coatings

Cause of death (ICD VIII)	Solvents Only		Solvents & Resins		Solv. Res. & Pigments		Unknown		Total	
	Obs.	SMR	Obs.	SMR	Obs.	SMR	Obs.	SMR	Obs.	SMR
All causes	44	120	43	100	92	88	19	120	198	99
All cancers	10	94	14	103	26	77	9	177	59	94
Esophagus (150)	1	391	2	703*	1	122	-	-	4	272
Stomach (151)	-	-	2	113	3	75	1	156	6	76
Colorectal (153-4)	1	127	2	200	1	41	-	-	4	88
Lung (162)	2	61	3	66	6	53	2	119	13	62
Bladder (185)	-	-	2	343	1	68	3	1418*	6	221
Hematologic (200-9)	2	297	1	113	1	44	-	-	4	96
Cirrhosis (571)	5	238	4	138	7	102	1	95	17	132

* $p < 0.05$

An increased bladder cancer risk was found in some (13-17) but not other (3-5) studies on painters and on paint manufacturers (9,10). Mortality owing to hematologic neoplasms was found to be elevated among either painters (3-5,18) or manufacturers exposed to lacquer (9). Suggestions of increased risk of esophageal cancer were found among painters (19,20). Cancer of the rectum was found to be elevated in two studies (3,9). There are also studies suggesting an increased risk of cirrhosis (6,10). No cases of prostatic cancer or multiple myeloma were found in our study.

The reported results have, thus, some support from the literature. Conclusions are difficult, however, either for sample size or exposure definition problems. Analisys by duration of exposure, years since first exposure, year of and age at first exposure failed to reveal consistent trends in mortality. Credible hypotheses to be further explored are, nonetheless, the following: working in paint production might entail an increased risk of cancer of the esophagus and the bladder; exposure to solvents in this industry might be associated with an increased mortality from hematologic neoplasms and, possibly, cyrrhosis.

REFERENCES

1. International Agency for Research on Cancer (1989) IARC Monographs on the Evaluation of Carcinogenic Risks to Humans Vol 47. IARC, Lyon
2. Engholm G, Englund A (1982) Advan Modern Envir Toxic Series vol II: 173-185
3. Whorton MD, Schulman J, Larson SR et al (1983) JOM 25: 657-660
4. Matanoski GM, Stockwell HG, et al (1986) Scand J Work Environ Hlth 12: 16-21
5. Chiazze L, Ference LD, Wolf PH (1980) JOM 22: 520-526
6. Dalager NA, Mason TJ, Fraumeni JF et al (1980) JOM 22: 25-29
7. Milne KL, Sandler DP, Everson RB, Brown SM (1983) Am J Ind Med 4: 565-575
8. Stockwell HG, Matanoski GM (1985) JOM 27: 125-126
9. Morgan RW, Claxton KW, Kaplan SD et al (1985) JOM 27: 377-378
10. Lundberg I (1986) Scand J Work Environ Health 12: 108-113
11. Kjuus H, Skjaerven R, et al (1986) Scand J Work Environ Health 12: 193-202
12. Bertazzi PA, Zocchetti C, Terzaghi GF et al (1981) Med Lav 6: 465-472
13. Cole P, Hoover R, Friedell G (1972) Cancer 29: 1250-1260
14. Schoenberg J, Stemhagen A, Mogielnicki A et al (1984) JNCL 72: 973-981
15. Miller A (1977) Cancer Research 37: 2939-2942
16. Jensen OM, Wahrendorf J, et al (1987) Scand J Work Environ Hlth 13: 129-134
17. Claude J, Frentzel-Beyme R, Kunze E (1988) Int J Cancer 41: 371-379
18. Lindquist R, Nilsson B, Eklund G et al (1987) Cancer 60: 1378-1384
19. Englund A (1980) J Toxicol Environ Health 16: 1267-1273
20. Viadana E, Bross IDJ, Houten L (1976) JOM 18: 787-792

© 1990 Elsevier Science Publishers B.V. (Biomedical Division)
Occupational Epidemiology. H. Sakurai et al., editors

OCCUPATION AND SMOKING AS RISK FACTORS IN NASAL AND NASOPHARYNGEAL CANCER

URICH BOLM-AUDORFF[1], CHRISTA VOGEL[2], HANS-JOACHIM WOITOWITZ[2]

[1] Ministry of Social Welfare, Department of Occupational Safety, Division of Occupational Medicine and Division of Epidemiology, P.O. Box 3140, D-6200 Wiesbaden 1, Fed. Rep. Germany
[2] University of Giessen, Institute and Outpatient Clinic of Occupational and Social Medicine, Aulweg 129, D-6300 Giessen 1, Fed. Rep. Germany

INTRODUCTION

Since the middle of the 1960s, a connection between work in wood processing and a raised risk of tumors of the nose and paranasal sinuses has been discussed in the literature. With the exception of two case reports and an analysis of the Hamburg and Saarland cancer registers, no studies on this topic have been carried out so far in West Germany (2-4). We therefore decided to carry out an epidemiological case control study with inclusion of all new cases in the federal state Hessia.

METHODS

In July 1984, all 65 otorhinolaryngological and all eight pathology departments in Hessia hospitals were requested by letter to communicate to us their patients with tumors of the nasopharyngeal region. The cases had to fulfill the following criteria:

- histologically verified tumors of the nose and paranasal sinuses (ICD 160) and the nasopharynx (ICD 147)
- first diagnosis in a Hessian hospital between January 1 1983 and December 31 1985
- age over 20 years

A total of 66 patients comprising 40 men and 26 women with the above tumor diagnosis was reported. The average age was 61 ± 8 years. In 62 patients, a detailed interview with regard to the previous occupational and disease history could be carried out, also with reference to smoking habits in 57 cases. This corresponds to a response rate of 94% and 86% respectively. Every interviewed tumor patient was paired with a control subject comparable in terms of age (± 5 years), sex and domicile. The control subjects were patients who had received inpatient treatment because of a bone fracture incurred in private life. Accidents at work or on the way to work were excluded. We assume that the patient group with privately

TABLE I: Occupational risk factors of nasal and nasopharyngeal cancer

Risk factor	Exposed cases (n)	Exposed controls (n)	Relative risk (n)	95% confidence interval
Wood dust				
ever exposed	7	2	3.8	0.8 - 17.2
duration of exposure ≥ 5 years	7	1	7.8*	1.3 - 48.1
latency ≥ 20 years	6	2	3.2	0.7 - 15.3
Leather dust				
ever exposed	2	--	--	--
Welding fumes				
ever exposed	4	2	2.1	0.4 - 11.5
duration of exposure ≥ 5 years	3	1	3.1	0.4 - 27.2
latency ≥ 20 years	3	1	3.1	0.4 - 27.2
Pesticides				
ever exposed	4	5	0.8	0.2 - 0.3
duration of exposure ≥ 5 years	4	5	0.8	0.2 - 0.3
latency ≥ 20 years	4	5	0.8	0.2 - 2.0
Other dusts**				
ever exposed	12	8	1.6	0.6 - 4.3
duration of exposure ≥ 5 years	12	8	1.6	0.6 - 4.3
latency ≥ 20 years	11	8	1.5	0.5 - 4.3

* $p < 0.05$
** stone dust, building site dust, cereal dust

incurred fractures is largely free from distortions with regard to the occupation practiced. After the interview was available, the relative risk from occupational and extraoccupational risk factors was determined (5). Furthermore, the 95% confidence interval of the relative risk was calculated on the basis of a chi-square test (6).

RESULTS

Of the 66 tumor patients, 54 had a tumor of the nose and paranasal sinuses and 12 had a nasopharyngeal tumor. In histological terms, these comprised 21 squamous cell carcinomas, 10 undifferentiated carcinomas, 9 lymphomas, 7 adenoid cystic carcinomas, 5 adenocarcinomas and 14 other malignant tumors.

Table 1 shows the relative risks due to occupational risk factors. After exposure to wood dust for at least five years, a relative risk of 7.8 (95% confidence interval, 1.3-48.1, $p < 0.03$) was found for malignant tumors of the nose and paranasal sinuses as well as of the nasopharynx. Of the seven tumor patients exposed to wood dust, four mainly displayed an exposure to oak and beech wood dust, including two patients with an adenocarcinoma of the nose and paranasal sinuses. On the other hand, two of the seven tumor patients were mainly exposed to a softwood exposure and one patient to a mixed exposure. In the case group, an exposure to leather dusts and welding fumes was found which was more frequent and lasted longer than in the control group, although the differences were not significant.

Chronic rhinitis was associated with a relative risk of 6.6 (95% confidence interval 1.6-26.7, $p < 0.01$) after a latency of at least one year. After a latency of at least ten years between the beginning of the chronic rhinitis and the diagnosis of the tumor, a significantly raised relative risk could no longer be demonstrated. Cigarette smoking was associated with a raised relative risk of 1.9 with regard to squamous cell carcinoma of the nasopharyngeal region, but not with regard to other nasopharyngeal tumors. A positive dose-effect relationship was found between the dose of cigarette smoke and the relative risk of squamous cell carcinomas of the nasopharyngeal region (never smoked: relative risk = 1.0, $<$ 10 pack years: relative risk 1.8, 10-19 pack years: relative risk 1.8, $\geq$ 20 pack years: relative risk 2.7).

DISCUSSION

The study confirms a raised tumor risk in the nasopharyngeal region in employees working in the wood processing industry. It was striking that the typical combination of adenocarcinoma of the nose and paranasal sinuses after prior exposure to oak and beech wood dust was only present in two patients, whereas the other tumor patients exposed to wood dust showed a different histology. In our opinion, this result is compatible with the hypothesis that a raised tumor risk is also induced by other woods, and this applies not only to adenocarcinomas of the nose and paranasal sinuses, but also to other histological types. In recent years, several study groups have been able to show that a raised risk is also present with regard to squamous cell carcinomas of the nose and paranasal sinuses in the wood processing industry (7-11).

Since 1988, adenocarcinoma of the nose and paranasal sinuses caused by oak and beech wood dust has been a recognized occupational disease in West Germany. An occupational disease was recognized in 32 patients with adenocarcinoma of the nose and paranasal sinuses in a kind of special ruling between 1984 and 1987. The figures for 1988 and 1989 have not yet been published. At present, it is being discussed whether squamous cell carcinomas of the nose and paranasal sinuses must be recognized as an occupational disease.

REFERENCES

1. IARC (1981) Wood, leather and some associated industries, IARC Monographs on the evaluation of the carcinogenic risk of chemicals to humans, Vol. 25, Lyon
2. Kraus H, Krumpe R (1979) In: Verhandlungen der Deutschen Gesellschaft für Arbeitsmedizin, Gentner, Stuttgart, pp 151-152
3. Wolf J, Hartung M, Schroeder HG, Kleinsasser O, Compes PC, Valentin H (1988) Arbeitsmed Sozialmed Präventivmed 23: Supl 10
4. Bolm-Audorff U, Vogel C, Ziegler H, Stegmaier C, Fehr R, Woitowitz HJ (1985) In: Verhandlungen der Deutschen Gesellschaft für Arbeitsmedizin, Gentner, Stuttgart, pp 553-557
5. Lilienfeld AM, Lilienfeld DE (1980) Foundation of epidemiology, Oxford University Press, New York
6. Miettinnen O (1976) Am J Epid 103:226-235
7. Hernberg S, Westerholm P, Schultz-Larsen K, Degerth R, Kuosma E, Englund A, Engzell U, Hansen HS, Mutanen P (1983) Scand J Work Environ Health 9:315-326
8. Voss R, Stenersen T, Oppedal R, Boysen M (1985) Acta Otolaryngol 99:172-178
10. Fukuda K, Shibata A (1988) Cancer Res 48:1651-1652
11. Shimizu H, Hozawa J, Seito H, Murai K, Hideto H, Takasaka T, Togawa K, Konno A, Kimura Y, Kikuchi A, Ohkouchi Y, Ohtani I, Hisamichi S (1989) Laryngoscope 99:58-61

Occupational Epidemiology. H. Sakurai et al., editors

A COHORT STUDY OF CANCER MORTALITY IN COPPER MINERS

CHEN RUOLING[1] and HU MENGXUAN[2]
1)School of Public Health, Anhui Medical University, Hefei, Anhui, P. R. of China
2)School of Public Health, Sun Yat-sen University of Medical Sciences, Guanzhow, P. R. of China

INTRODUCTION

It is well known that there was a highly increased risk of cancer mortality in metal miners (1-3), eg: iron, tin, and uranium miners. However, little study of cancer mortality in copper miners was reported. In order to evaluate the risk of cancer death in copper miners, a cohort study was carried out at the copper mines of Tongling city, Anhui province of China from Jan. 1, 1970 to June 30, 1985.

MATERIAL AND METHODS

The cohort consisted of all male workers in the copper mines, who were employed for at least one year between Jan. 1, 1970 and June 30, 1985. Women were excluded since the number was too small to make an analysis. From the worker's occupational records provided by the mines, we collected the information about name, date of birth, date of employment, date of retirement or leaving, kind of work, date and cause of death. It was checked that the records were written carefully and kept completely in the mines. Since it was important document for each workers, loss or destruction of the record had hardly occured.

All the certifications of deaths were examined at Tongling hospital. The diagnosis of cancer deaths were based on X-ray or pathological result. The causes of deaths have been classified according to the 9th revision of International Classification of Diseases.

The data were processed on Cromenco computer and analysed by the program we had written. The standardized mortality ratios (SMRs) were calculated in 1985 calendar-year and five year age-group specific mortality rate of male in Tongling city, and their statistical significance were tested according to Poission distribution.

RESULTS

There were 7031 miners in this cohort, and 77503.5 person-years were calculated (follow-up rate was 97% according to maximum person-years method). A total of 584 deaths was observed, which is significantly greater than the expected number (380.8). The different causes of deaths are shown in table 1. The cancer deaths accounted for 33.56% for the total deaths (ranked first place), and the SMR for all sites of cancer was increased. Among the cancer deaths only the risks of stomach cancer and lung cancer deaths were significantly high. It was also found that the average age of cancer deaths in the copper miners was 54.64 years old, younger than that of male in Tongling city by 3.99 years.

TABLE 1
THE OBSERVED AND EXPECTED DEATHS AND SMRS IN THE COPPER MINERS

Cause of Death (ICD 9th revision code)	Deaths		SMR
	Obs	Exp	
All causes of death	584	380.83	153**
Pulmonary tuberculosis (11)	23	14.51	159**
All sites of cancers (140-208)	196	157.46	124**
Esophagus (150)	31	26.74	116
Stomach (151)	69	48.13	143**
Liver (155)	26	29.27	89
Lung (162)	42	28.50	147*
Disease of circulatory system (390-459)	91	131.03	69**
Rheumatic heart disease (390-398)	47	56.58	83
Hypertensive disease (401-405)	16	6.53	245**
Cerebrovascular disease (430-438)	42	72.86	58**
Disease of respiratory system (460-519)	126	36.52	345**
Silicosis (502)	95	7.00	1358**
Disease of digestive system (520-579)	16	19.60	82
Cirrhosis of liver (571)	11	9.78	112
Industrial injury (800-959)	67	16.23	413**
Accident injury (E800-E989)	34	26.69	115

* $p<0.05$, ** $p<0.01$

According to the length of exposure and the time since first exposure, the observed and expected cancer death numbers were calculated (seen in table 2). The SMR tended to increase with both the

TABLE 2

CANCER DEATHS BY THE LENGTH OF EXPOSURE AND THE TIME SINCE FIRST EXPOSURE IN THE COPPER MINERS

Length of exposure (years)	Time since first exposure (years)									
	1-- Obs(Exp)	5-- Obs(Exp)	10-- Obs(Exp)	15-- Obs(Exp)	20-- Obs(Exp)	25-- Obs(Exp)	30--35 Obs(Exp)	Total Obs(Exp)	SMR	SMR+
1--	1(3.46)	0(0.12)	0(0.04)	0(0.02)	0(0.01)	0(0.00)	0(0.00)	1(3.65)	27	73 (1--, 5--, 10--)
5--		4(3.99)	0(0.21)	0(0.11)	0(0.09)	0(0.13)	0(0.09)	4(4.62)	87	
10--			4(7.61)	1(1.10)	3(0.37)	0(0.19)	0(0.06)	8(9.33)	86	
15--				24(20.92)	3(5.46)	5(3.33)	1(0.29)	33(29.99)	110	128* (15--, 20--)
20--					54(37.35)	21(14.87)	5(5.96)	80(58.19)	137*	
25--						41(32.86)	11(12.53)	52(45.39)	115	135* (25--, 30--35)
30--35							18(6.29)	18(6.29)	286	
Total	1(3.46)	4(4.10)	4(7.86)	25(22.15)	60(43.28)	67(51.39)	35(25.22)	196(157.46)		124**
SMR	29	97	51	113	139*	130	139			
SMR+	58 (1--, 5--, 10--)			130* (15--, 20--)		132* (25--, 30--35)				

* p<0.05, ** p<0.01

SMR+ was calculated in those combined groups.

length of exposure and time since first exposure. If the miners who had worked in underground were chosen to be analysed , there would be 61844 person-years and the SMR of cancer was elevated to be 134 (obs=177, exp=129.77; $p<0.01$).

DISCUSSION

The Tongling copper mine is one of the largest copper mines in China. It has been greatly developed since 1949. In the underground of the mines the levels of radioactivity was measured to be 0.55×10^{-11} curie/l, under the permission standard of China, and the dust density was approximately 10 mg/m^3.

The results of our study revealed an excess of cancer deaths in the copper miners. According to the earlier age of cancer deaths and the relation of dose-response between the length of exposure and risk of cancer (4), it could be considered that some occupational factors in the copper mines might contribute to the excess of cancer deaths. Although some surveys showed that the increased risk of cancer was generally attributed to exposure of the miners in metal mines to radon daughters (1,3,5,), it seems unlikely that the radiation exposure could explain the excess of cancer deaths in the copper miners since there was no remarkable radioactivity in the Tongling copper mines. Because the miners exposed (inhaled) a great deal of the ore dust via respiratory/digestive tract which contained Silica, Iron, Ca, S, Copper, Zn, ect and the risks of lung cancer and stomach cancer deaths were significantly highest among all cancer, dust exposure may be considered as an etiologic factor.

REFERENCES

1. Wagoner JK, Miller RW, Lundin FE, Fraumeni JF, Haij ME (1963) New Eng J Med 269:284-289
2. Boyd JT, Doll R, Faulds JS, Leiper (1970) Br J Ind Med 27: 97-105
3. Howe GR, Newcombe HB, Miller AB, Abbatt JD (1986) JNCI 77: 357-362
4. Richard Doll (1985) Int J Epidemiol 14:22-31
5. Radford EP, St. Clair Renard KG (1984) New Eng J Med 310: 1485-1494

Occupational Epidemiology. H. Sakurai et al., editors

CASE-CONTROL STUDY ON SILICOSIS AND LUNG CANCER

PIERLUIGI COCCO, PLINIO CARTA, PASQUALE BARIO, PIERINA MANCA AND DUILIO CASULA.
Istituto di Medicina del Lavoro dell'Università degli Studi di Cagliari
Via S. Giorgio, 12 - 09124 - Cagliari (Italy).

INTRODUCTION.

Some experimental studies have shown an association between lung cancer and the fibrogenic reaction following exposure to silica in rats by inhalation and by intratracheal instillation (1-3). Epidemiological studies on workers exposed to silica in different workplaces provided inconsistent results (4-5). A follow-up study of silicotic patients is being conducted by our Institute (6). So far, a small non significant excess of mortality for lung cancer has been found, neither related to the severity of the radiological aspect of silicosis nor to duration of exposure to silica. Thus, a retrospective study was planned to evaluate the strength of this association.

MATERIAL AND METHODS.

In the period 1967-83, 13.207 workers complaining of Occupational Diseases were admitted to the Institute of Occupational Medicine of the University of Cagliari (Italy), which is the only referral center for those diseases in the entire island of Sardinia. Over a half of the claims were related to exposure to dust in mines (lead and zinc, coal, other ores) and quarries, historically the main industrial activity in Sardinia.

A record-linkage with the list of lung cancer patients, discharged in the period 1974-83 from the Department of Chest Surgery of a local hospital, allowed to identify 78 male lung cancer cases.

In all cases, the diagnosis of lung cancer followed the admission to the Institute of Occupational Medicine. We randomly selected from the list of our patients of the same sex and year of birth (± 5 years) 2 controls for each case. Vital status and cause of death of controls were ascertained from population registry and death certificates in the communities of residence. For those who had died elsewhere, the cause of death was obtained where the death had occurred. Two controls found to have died of lung cancer were replaced by the nearest patient in the list of the same sex and year of birth.

A chest X-ray was routinely carried out at the Institute of Occupational Medicine. Those of the present study population were reviewed by a radiologist according to the 1980 ILO Classification of Pneumoconiosis (7). All subjects having small radiological opacities equal or over 1/0 degree of profusion were considered silicotic. Standard interviews administered upon admission to the same Institute provided information about occupational history and smoking for both cases and controls. Unfortunately, only current smoking status was available. The classification criteria for exposure to silica were derived from environmental surveys on Sardinian mines and other dusty work places conducted in the period 1973-83 (8-9). Previous levels of exposure to silica were estimated using available environmental data and historical information on technological changes.

An estimate of lifetime exposure to silica was derived from the work history for each study subject. The study population was thereby divided in three categories of exposure to silica (low, medium, high) following the tertiles of its distribution.

RESULTS.

Pathology was available for 46 of the 78 cases. The diagnosis of the remaining 32 patients was based on chest X-ray, bronchoscopy, citology of the sputum and bronchial secrete. As shown in Table 1, squamous cell carcinoma was the most common histological type. The mean latency period between the diagnosis of silicosis and that of lung cancer was 9.8 years (sd = 4.3). It was longer among non smokers (12.0 $\pm$ 7.1 years; n = 2) than smokers (9.5 $\pm$ 4.1; n = 13).

A 2.4 fold increase of the lung cancer risk with borderline statistical significance was found in silicotic patients (ILO Categories 1/0 or more) after adjusting for smoking and lifetime cumulative exposure to silica (Table 2). The risk did not show significant variations according to the level of cumulative exposure to silica. Cumulative exposure to silica by itself apparently did not influence lung cancer risk either in silicotic patients or in those negative for silicosis (ILO categories 0/-, 0/0, 0/1). In both groups the odds ratio showed a non-significant negative trend.

CONCLUSIONS.

The results of this study show a possible link between silicosis, but not silica exposure by itself, and lung cancer. However, because of the lack of statistical power, inadequate smoking histories and limited silica exposure data, further studies are required in order to confirm and explain the mechanism of this association.

The inconsistency of the results of epidemiological studies on this issue has been stressed in a recent IARC monograph (5). Difficulties have arisen from low comparability of referent populations, rare availability of data on smoking and other potential confounders.

Other factors, known as occupational carcinogens, can accompany silica in different workplaces (e.g. low levels of ionizing radiations, polycyclic aromatic hydrocarbons, arsenic). Their role, either indipendent or associated to silicosis in a multistep model of lung cancer development, deserves detailed investigation.

TABLE 1

CASES OF LUNG CANCER BY PATHOLOGY, CURRENT SMOKING STATUS AND PREVIOUS RADIOLOGICAL FINDINGS.

Lung cancer pathology	n.	Current smokers	Silicosis	
			yes (a)	no (b)
Squamous cell carcinoma	31	28	8	23
Adenocarcinoma	8	5	1	7
Oat cell carcinoma	5	5	-	5
Large cell carcinoma	2	2	-	2
Unavailable	32	27	6	26
Total cases	78	67	15	63

a: ILO categories 1/0 or more.
b: ILO categories 0/-, 0/0, 0/1.

TABLE 2

RELATIVE RISKS OF LUNG CANCER IN SILICOTIC SUBJECTS, BY CUMULATIVE EXPOSURE TO SILICA.

Cumulative exposure to silica	OR	95% C.I.	Silicosis cases	Silicosis controls
low	2.5[a]	0.5 - 13.2	3	2
medium	2.1[a]	0.7 - 6.8	7	9
high	3.1[a]	0.6 - 16.4	5	6
all	2.4[b]	1.0 - 6.2	15	17

a: Adjusted by smoking (two categories).
b: Adjusted by smoking and cumulative dose of exposure to silica (three categories).

This work has benefited from the financial aid of the Commission of European Communities under contract 7248-32-010.

REFERENCES.

1. Dagle GE, Wehner AP, Clark ML, Buschbom RL (1985) In: Goldsmith DF, Winn DM, Shy CM (eds): Silica, Silicosis and Cancer. Controversy in Occupational Medicine. Praeger, Philadelphia, pp 255-266.
2. Groth DH, Stettler LE, Platek SF, Lal JB, Burg JR (1985) In: Goldsmith DF, Winn DM, Shy CM (eds): Silica, Silicosis and Cancer. Controversy in Occupational Medicine. Praeger, Philadelphia, pp 243-253.
3. Holland LM, Wilson JS, Tillery MI, Smith DM (1985) In: Goldsmith DF, Winn DM, Shy CM (eds): Silica, Silicosis and Cancer. Controversy in Occupational Medicine, Praeger, Philadelphia, pp 267-279.
4. Goldsmith DF, Guidotti L, Johnston DR (1982) Am J Ind Med 3: 423-440.
5. IARC Monographs (1987) Silica and Some Silicates. IARC, Lyon, vol. 42.
6. Carta P, Aru G, Barbieri MT et al (1988) Med Lav 79: 431-443.
7. International Labour Organization (1980) ILO - UICC, Geneve.
8. Casula D, Cherchi P et al (1982) Valdes, Cagliari.
9. Casula D, Carta P, Sanna Randaccio F (1984) In: ILO (ed) VI International Conference of Pneumoconiosis, Bochum, vol II, pp 1107-1112.

Occupational Epidemiology. H. Sakurai et al., editors

549415

THE ROLE OF THE CENTRAL NERVOUS INVOLVEMENT IN OCCUPATIONAL CANCER RISK OF PERSONS EXPOSED TO ORGANIC SOLVENTS

RAINER FRENTZEL-BEYME
Institute of Epidemiology and Biometry, German Cancer Research Center
P.O. Box 101949, D-6900 Heidelberg (Federal Republic of Germany)

Introduction:

Results from prospective psycho-social and behavioral research indicate

1. an influence of the status of mood, such as longlasting hopelessness, on the subsequent risk of cancer;
2. mental stimulation by social activity, non-medical drug use, pharmaka or even nicotine seems to reduce the risk of cancer;
3. mental understimulation, such as endogenous depression, induced by behavioral difficulties in solving social conflicts but also as a result of chronic use of sedative medication, increases the risk of cancer (1).

A definite involvement of the brain is very likely, and especially the brain stem and its connections to the limbic system - the brain of the brain - and to the pituitary gland are entirely on the subcortical level. Solvents used in the occupational environment not only cause damage on the clinically relevant level but have been implicated with a specific action on the subcortical structures, as elegantly shown by the examples of styrene-induced dopamine modulation and the neuroendocrine effects after styrene exposure such as prolactin and thyreotropin responses (2, 3).

Toxic encephalopathy after solvent exposure is still a more controversial issue than toxic polyneuropathy (4), although the acute narcotic effect of occupational exposure to organic solvents has long been known. Different discrete brain areas may not be equally sensitive to different organic solvents (including the effects of ethanol ingestion), which could obscure the results of analyses performed on the whole brain. A relation between mental symptoms and exposure to organic solvents, however, seems to be a plausible presumption (5).

Clinical and neurological evidence of an influence of organic solvents on the central and peripheral nervous system is abundant and is also being referred to again in this volume. Newly acquired knowledge concerns the neurobehavioral effects of longterm exposure to organic solvents (6, 7, 8). Results from cohort studies for cancer risks in the occupational field seem to indicate that future concepts will have to consider the influence of a central nervous involvement of several kinds.

Occupational epidemiology and the CNS:

Epidemiological evidence only will form the basis of reference in an attempt to identify damage to the CNS (in its identifiable form of chronic mental depression) as one important confounder, if not the crucial link between exposure to narcotics and cancer incidence in otherwise differing occupational cohorts. Occupational cancer is mostly considered to be quite specifically linked with aetiologically plausible causal exposures. In several industrial exposures, though, a multiplicity of targets of increased risks, indicated by increased incidences of cancer types obviously unrelated to the exposure under study, need to be considered from the viewpoint of a promoting effect of narcotic exposure. In an editorial of the British Journal of Industrial Medicine on evidence for human carcinogenicity of vinyl chloride on different target organs (9), unexpected associations of VC with melanoma, cancers of the colon, thyroid, brain and kidneys became of interest – to my view even suggestive of a more general mode of action of the narcotic gas VC, in the presence of other carcinogens. The concurrent exposure of the cohort to dichloroethane, a material known as a solvent with an affinity to the CNS, which has been shown to have a direct and systemic carcinogenic action in the animal experiment, has to be considered. The yield of a variety of tumours after oral application (gavage) does not preclude an effect on the CNS of this solvent. If in such experiments only genotoxicity is examined, CNS damage of such narcotic compounds as dibromethane or dichloroethane may be missed. Von Metzler and Nitsch (10) have shown that psychoactive pharmaka considerably change the cancer incidence and survival after exposure to classical carcinogens, and that their action during the experiments may be monitored accordingly.

In the studies on persons exposed to the production of man made mineral fibers, several cohorts displayed a series of lethal cancers in excess, such as cancers of the bladder, buccal cavity, pancreas, brain, i.e. in organs difficult to relate to fiber exposure; and in one incidence study where buccal cancer was found in excess but possibly related to "lifestyle factors". In these studies, alcohol always could be implicated as a probable additional risk factor. In one study of MMMF workers exposed to rock wool fibres and the raw material involved (11), an internal unexposed reference cohort enabled the identification of deaths clearly in excess of expectation from causes such as malignant neoplasms, expecially specific localizations (as pancreas), neoplasms of "benign" character or of unspecified nature (80% of them located in the brain), mental disorders, and violent deaths with suicide as the foremost cause.

Internal comparisons between exposed and non-exposed workers in the same factory are probably the optimal approach for the identification of risks. In Table 1 observed deaths in both cohorts are given, cases of the ICD-No. 780-796 of whom additional specific information could be obtained being shown in parentheses (illustrating the amount of additional information after intense efforts even without a cancer registry). The relative risk (RR) and confidence intervals are given for some relevant causes of death.

Causes of death in a cohort exposed to rockwool-exposure and in a reference cohort

	Exposed cohort				Reference Cohort		
Cause (ICD)	Observed	Expected	SMR	C.I.	Obs.	RR	C.I.
All causes (000-999)	315	286	110	98-123	290	0.86*	0.68-1.10
Neoplasms							
All malignant (140-209)	80(83)**	63.1	127(132)	101-157	64(68)	1.03*	0.67-1.57
Cancer of the							
Stomach (151)	13	9.7	134	75-223	17	0.65	0.27-1.55
Pancreas (157)	6	2.5	239	97-497	0	6.76+	1.01-45.2
Larynx (161)	2	0.9	229	38-757	2	0.8	
Lung (162)	21	17.4	121	77-181	15(16)	1.41	0.17-11.73
Benign and unspecified nature (210-239)	10	3.0	336	171-600	1	2.89+	1.14-7.32
Mental disorders (290-315	7	3.1	228	100-452	7	0.62	0.02-16.21
Nervous system and sensory organs (320-389)	8	10.6	76	35-144	1	6.28	0.9-43.86
Symptoms and ill def. conditions (780-796)	23 (11)	8.6	268(128)	174-397	8	1.07	0.53-2.81
Violent deaths (E800-E999)	52(57)	39.8	131(143)	98-170	40	1.14	0.88-1.46
Suicide (E950-959)	19	13.5	141	88-216	10	1.64	

* stratified by 10-year age groups, otherwise by 25-year age groups
** "Extra" cases from death certificate information ICD-796 with additional information on c.o.d.
\+ $p < 0.05$

Higher frequencies of cancer in other studies included localizations in the larynx (12), oral cavity and pharynx (13, 14) and bladder (14). All these cancers can be related to alcohol consumption. Alcohol related excess deaths in the German MMMF cohort (mental disorders, alcoholism, suicides, road accidents) appeared to indicate a particular lifestyle of the cohort of fiber workers. The cohort study of Geneva painters (15) compared cancer mortality and incidence with a control cohort of electricians, showing once again a variety of cancer types which are in excess among painters and which could be related to alcohol intake, but also to solvent exposure, among them hormone-related types, such as testicular cancer. An analysis of official causes of disability indicated not only an excess of alcoholism but also of nervous as well as personality disorders in painters, compared with electricians. Alcohol-related causes of death were markedly in excess. The higher cancer risk, however, again impresses in that a multiplicity of lethal but equally of about 60% more incident cancers not leading to death indicate the importance of research into the relationship of brain damage and cancer risk, not only on the level of mortality but by using cancer registries. Testicular cancer may be related to painting and solvents following recent reports from the USA (16, 17) a finding reproduced in a case-control study in Germany where paints and lacquers were associated with a fivefold risk (18). The conceivable influence of solvents upon the pituitary gland is recommended for further study.

How far, with painters, either the exposure to narcotic solvents becomes a reason for "induced addiction", or addiction to alcohol correlated with a choice of occupations with solvents exposure, is not clear.

Conclusions:

Checkoway (19) suggested in case of a lack of regular, monotonically increasing risk gradients that this may be evidence of a converse healthy worker effect, possibly due to atypical lifestyle or previous employment characteristics. The physiologically most important aspect of chronic exposure to both solvents and alcohol is their narcotic or sedative effect, respectively, on central nervous functions. To consider the promoting action of this specific effect in those cancer "risks" so far implausible, it should be adjusted for in the same way as tobacco smoking. The hypothesis being that depression, especially in its masked form, is related to central nervous understimulation, the relation to diminished vital functions of the organism as a consequence is to be considered in future studies, including the assessment of resistance against acute, subacute and chronic diseases. This has been shown for cancer in general (11) not only in animal experiments, but also for different human populations (1, 20). Missing are follow-up studies for cancer incidence of workers exposed to determined quantities of solvents or of mentally injured subpopulations of such cohorts. If longlasting mental depression is related to a decreased resistance and defence, the chronically depressed subgroups from occupational cohorts, such as solvent exposed painters, oil refinery, chemical or metal workers, should be at a higher risk of diseases, especially of cancer. This should apply to persons in different cultural, racial and environmental settings and should not depend on occupational carcinogenic exposure exclusively. To test this hypothesis, the most effective and adequate approach is seen in imitating the experiment by a prospective study of solvent exposed populations of varying regional origin, varying duration of employment and different degrees of depression, e.g. by cohort studies following up specific, cross-sectionally well examined groups. One intermediate outcome of a follow-up study of pertinent cohorts being the actual incidence of mental depression, as well as prevalences of clinical and neuroimmunological parameters (such as studied before in solvent-exposed groups), the required long-term outcome could be the incidence of chronic diseases, such as cancer at non-specific sites. Always, the consideration of personality type in a prospective fashion will be an asset for the interpretation of results (20).

References:

1. Grossarth-Maticek, R, Eysenck, HJ, Vetter, H: Personality type, smoking habit and their interaction as predictors of cancer and coronary heart disease. Personal. Individ. Diff. 9, 479-495, 1988
2. Mutti, A, Vescovi, PP, Falzoi, M et al.: Neuroendocrine effects of styrene on occupational exposed workers. Scand. J. Work., Environ 10, 225-228, 1984
3. Arfini, G, Mutti, A, Vescovi, P, et al: Impaired dopaminergic modulation of pituitary secretion in workers exposed to styrene: Further evidence from PRL response to TRH stimulation. J. Occup. Med. 29, 826-830, 1987
4. Seppäläinen, AM: Neurophysiological aspects of the toxicity of organic solvents. Scand. J. Work Environ Health 11, Suppl. 1, 61-64, 1985
5. Fidler, AT, Baker, EL, Letz, RE: Neurobehavioral effects of occupational exposure to organic solvents among construction painters. Int. J. Industr. Med. 44, 292-308, 1987
6. Elofsson, SA, Gamberale F, Hindmarsh, T et al.: Exposure to organic solvents. A cross-sectional epidemiologic investigation on occupationally exposed car and industrial spray painters with special reference to the nervous system. Scand. J. Work Environ Health 6, 239-273, 1980
7. Flodin, U, Edling C, Axelson, O: Clinical studies of psychoorganic syndromes among workers with exposure to solvents. Amer. J. Industr. Med. 5, 287-295, 1984
8. Baker, EL, Letz, RE, Eisen, EA, et al.: Neurobehavioral effects of solvents in construction painters. J. Occup. Med. 30, 116-123, 1988
9. Storetvedt Heldaas, S, Langård, SL, Andersen, A: Incidence of cancer among vinylchloride and polyvinyl chloride workers. Brit. Ind. Med. 41, 25-30, 1984
10. von Metzler, A, Nitsch, C: Carcinogenesis and the central nervous system. Cancer Det. Prev. 9, 259-277, 1986
11. Claude, J, Frentzel-Beyme, R: Mortality of workers in a German rock-wool factory - A second look with extended follow-up. Scand. J. Work Environ. Health 12, Suppl. 1, 53-60, 1986
12. Bertazzi, PA, Zocchetti, C, Riboldi, L et al: Cancer mortality of an Italian cohort of workers in man-made glass-fiber production. Scand. J. Work Environ. Health, 12, Suppl. 1, 65-71, 1986
13. Moulin, JJ, Mur, JM, Wild P, et al.: Oral cavity and laryngeal cancers among man-made mineral fiber production workers. Scand. J. Work Environ. Health 12, 27-31, 1986
14. Simonato, L, Fletcher, AC, Cherrie, J et al: The man-made mineral fiber European historical cohort study. Extension of the follow-up. Scand. J. Work Environ Health 12, Suppl. 1, 34-47, 1986
15. Guberan, E, Usel, M, Raymond, L et al.: Disability, mortality, and incidence of cancer among Geneva painters and electricians: a historical prospective study. Brit. J. Indust. Med. 46, 16-23, 1989
16. Garland, FC, Gorham, ED, Garland, CT et al.: Testicular cancer in US navy personal. Amer. J. Epidemiol. 127, 411-414, 1988

17. Levin, SM, Baker, DB, Landrigan, PJ et al.: Testicular cancer in leather tanners exposed to dimethylformamide. Lancet, II, 1153, 1987
18. Frentzel-Beyme, R, Wurster, KH: Epidemiologische Befunde bei Testistumoren. Techn. Rep. 10/1989 DKFZ Heidelberg, 1989
19. Checkoway, H: Methods of treatment of exposure data in occupational epidemiology. Med. Lav. 77, 48-73, 1986
20. van der Ploeg, HM, Kleijn, WC, Mook, J, et al.: Rationality and antiemotionality as a risk factor for cancer: Concept differentiation. J. Psychosomatic Res. 33, 217-225, 1989

Occupational Epidemiology. H. Sakurai et al., editors
549 416

MORTALITY OF UK TIN MINERS 1941 TO 1986

J T HODGSON AND R D JONES

Epidemiology & Medical Statistics Unit, Health & Safety Executive, Magdalen House, Stanley Precinct, Bootle L20 3QZ, United Kingdom.

The mortality of 2,059 underground tin miners and 476 surface workers was analysed for the period 1941 to 1986. Table 1 shows cause-specific mortality in relation to cumulative time underground. Clear positive associations (p for trend <0.001) are shown for lung cancer, silicosis and silico-tuberculosis. There is no indication of any association for stomach cancer, ischaemic heart disease or respiratory disease other than silicosis. There is a statistically significant deficit of respiratory disease among those with no underground time (3 deaths, 10.8 expected). The excess of leukaemia mortality in the 10-20 years group taken alone is on the edge of statistical significance (p = 0.054), but if the expected values for longer exposures are included the SMR falls to 283 (3/1.04, p=0.13). Setting aside the mortality figures for the three causes with a clear association with time spent underground, mortality from all other causes shows no such association.

TABLE 1 MORTALITY - SMR+ AND (OBSERVED DEATHS) IN RELATION TO CUMULATIVE TIME UNDERGROUND

Cause	Time Underground (years)					
	NIL	<5	5-10	10-20	20-30	30+
All causes	93 (84)	102 (167)	154** (123)	156** (175)	150* (77)	189** (55)
Stomach Cancer	204 (5)	117 (5)	134 (3)	145 (5)	129 (2)	224 (2)
Lung Cancer	83 (8)	91 (15)	172 (14)	176* (21)	355** (17)	447** (15)
Leukaemia	117 (1)	85 (1)	382 (2)	469 (3)	- (0)	- (0)
Respiratory disease other than pneumoconiosis	28* (3)	93 (17)	186* (17)	127* (18)	94 (7)	104 (4)
Silicosis and silico-TB	-	4.3% (7)	17.5% (14)	33% (37)	36% (18)	13.8% (4)
All causes other than lung cancer, silico-TB and silicosis	94 (76)	99 (145)	133 (95)	117 (117)	90 (42)	140 (36)

* p<0.05 ** p<0.01 + % excess mortality for silico-TB and silicosis

In order to analyse the expression of risk in time, the lung cancer mortality was broken down by final cumulative exposure and time since last exposure (Table 2).

TABLE 2: LUNG CANCER SMR AND (OBSERVED DEATHS) BY FINAL CUMULATIVE EXPOSURE AND TIME SINCE LAST EXPOSURE

Final Cumulative Exposure (Years underground)	Time since last exposure (years)					
	2.5	5	10	15	25	40
Nil	109 (5)	- (0)	- (0)	135 (1)	326 (2)	- (0)
<5	73 (1)	96 (1)	154 (2)	192 (3)	77 (5)	69 (3)
5-15	101 (4)	221 (4)	305 (5)	177 (3)	157 (7)	150 (3)
15-25	210 (6)	342 (4)	555 (5)	309 (2)	- (0)	
25+	320 (14)	446 (5)	728 (5)	- (0)		

The results show a clear pattern. Within each exposure group the SMR increases with increasing time from final exposure, reaching a maximum around 10 years from final exposure, and then declines. The peak SMRs increase with increasing exposure.

The shape of this response suggests an exposure/response model in which the effect of a year of exposure increases to a maximum in the following years and then declines. The fact that exposure levels in the study population are thought to have been constant over time (a belief supported by the absence of significant cohort differences), means that modelling the expression in time of the effect of exposure is simplified. To characterise the pattern of risk in time a 3-parameter model was used in which it is assumed that following a year of exposure there is a period of zero effect followed by a period of linearly increasing effect followed by a period of exponentially decreasing effect (Figure 1). The three parameters determining this pattern are the durations of the periods of zero and of increasing effect, and the halving time of the final exponential decrease. We will refer to these parameters as the lag, rising time and effect half-life respectively. In a given year of risk the contributions of previous years' exposures to the current effect are assumed to be additive.

Maximum likelihood estimates of the three parameters were determined by searching over a grid for the values of lag, rising time and effect half-life which optimised the fit. These were: lag, 10.5 years; rising time, 0.8 years; effect half-life, 4.3 years. Figure 2 shows the deviance curves around the minimum for each of these three parameters. These curves allow approximate 95% confidence intervals for the estimates to be calculated: they are the intervals spanned by the points at which the deviance curves increase by 3.8 from the minimum value. This gives a 95% CI of (8.3, 13.5) for the lag; (0,7.8) for the rising time; and (1.3, 15.5) for the effect half-life.

Figure 1: Risk profile for unit exposure

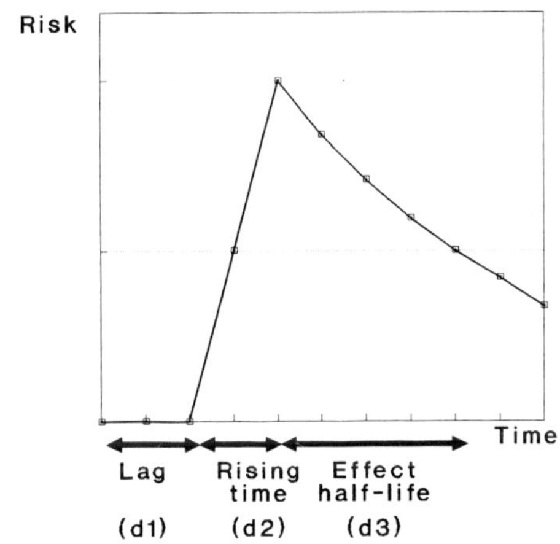

Figure 2: Deviance profiles as a function of lag, rising time and effect half-life

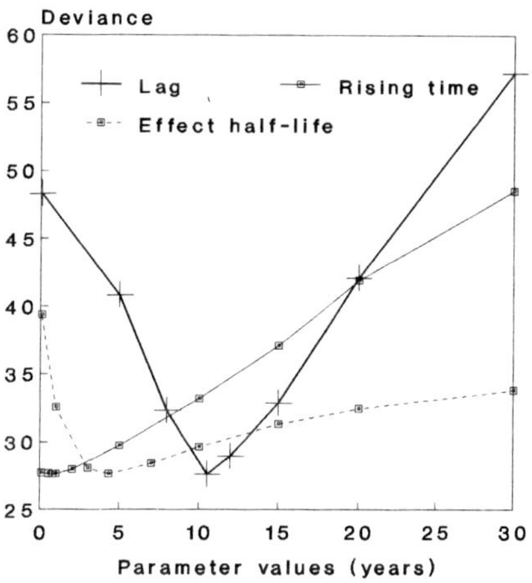

There were no measurements of radon levels in the mines from the relevant period. The earliest available measurements date from 1968. These early measurements suggest that a conservative estimate of the prevailing levels would be 10 WLM/year. On this basis the model indicated by our analysis of this data is:-

$$\text{Relative Risk} = 1 + 0.045\int_{t_o}^{t_s} r(t)w(t)dt$$

Where r(t) is the dose rate in WLM/year; t_o is the time in years since cessation of exposure; t_s is the time since first exposure; and w(t) is the risk profile function shown in Figure 1 with $d_1 = 10.5$, $d_2 = 0.8$, $d_2 = 4.3$. The implications for risk assessment of this model - which we will call the HSE model - compared with the model developed by the US Biological Effects of Ionising Radiation (BEIR) Committee (1) are shown in Figure 3.

Figure 3: Predicted lifetime relative risks based on HSE and BEIR models under different exposure conditions

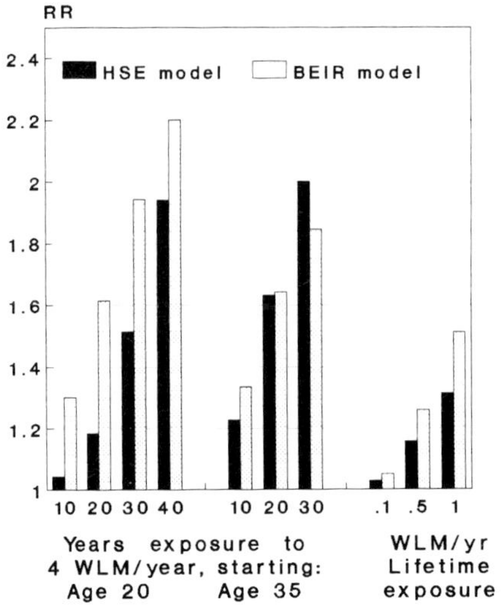

Overall the HSE model predicts rather lower risks than the BEIR model. For example the relative excesses predicted for lifetime exposures are about 70% higher on the BEIR model. For doses received at working ages the differences vary depending on the age at exposure. The differences are greatest for short exposures at young ages: the BEIR excess relative risk is 7 times the HSE model value for exposure from age 20 - 30. This difference drops as the exposure period lengthens into older ages, and for exposures from age 20 - 60 the BEIR excess relative risk is only slightly higher. For exposures starting at older ages the differences are less marked: BEIR 40% higher for exposure from age 35 to age 45; BEIR 30% lower for exposure from age 35 to age 65.

The differences between the present model and the BEIR model are of two sorts: the difference in overall risk, and the different profile of risk thorough time. As regards the difference in overall level, one might look to uncertainties in the estimation of past exposures for an explanation. But within this study the uncertainties relating to the assumed average dose of 10 WLM/ year are on the upward side and a revision of this assumption upwards would lead to a greater discrepancy with the BEIR model. Turning to the temporal expression of risk, the present data has the advantage of 45 years follow-up - 15 years longer than any of the data underlying the BEIR model. On biological grounds it seems more plausible that the pattern of risk should be linked to the time of exposure than that there would be fixed changes in risk at specific ages regardless of how far into the past the exposure responsible for the risk was situated.

Acknowledgements We gratefully acknowledge the invaluable assistance of Dr Joan Davis of the Institute of Cancer Research who established detailed job histories for these miners. We also thank the management and unions at the mines; the staff of the NHS Central Register; our support staff - particularly Anne Fletcher, Gwen Lee and Madeleine Naylor -; and Dr Michael O'Riordan, Colin Muirhead and Darren Dixon of the NRPB and our HSE colleague Peter Thomas, for helpful comments.

Reference: (1) Committee on the Biological Effects of Ionising Radiation (BEIR IV). Health risks of radon and other alpha-emitters. Washington DC National Academy Press 1988.

Occupational Epidemiology. H. Sakurai et al., editors

CASE-CONTROL STUDY ON OCCUPATIONAL RISK FACTORS IN NASAL CANCER

A.LECLERC*, D. LUCE*, M.GERIN**, A.CASAL*

* INSERM Unité 88 - 91 Bd de l'Hôpital - 75013 Paris France
** Faculté de Médecine - Université de Montréal - Canada

Cancers of the nasal cavity and sinuses are rare, but these tumors have been associated with several occupations and industrial exposures. A case control study was performed in France to assess the effect of formaldehyde and other occupational exposures (wood, leather, textile, nickel, chromium, paints and lacquers...) in these cancers. The first results, restricted to the analysis of occupational titles, are reported in the present paper.

SUBJECTS AND METHODS

Cases were patients diagnosed with primary malignancies of the nasal cavity and sinuses between January 1, 1986 and February 29, 1988 in 27 hospitals. Two hundred and seven cases were included in the study.

Two control groups were selected. Hospital controls (n=323) were patients with cancers of 15 different sites, diagnosed in the same period as the cases, in the same or in nearby hospitals. The second group of controls (n=86) was selected from lists of persons provided by the cases. The two sets of controls were grouped in the analysis.

All cases and controls were interviewed by specially trained physicians. Socio-economic factors, data on alcohol and tobacco consumption and occupational history were collected.

Age-adjusted odds-ratios and 95% confidence limits were calculated.

RESULTS AND DISCUSSION

The distribution of cases and controls by sex, age, smoking habits and alcohol consumption is shown in Table 1. Alcohol and tobacco were not found to be associated with nasal cancer.

Table 2 shows the distribution of cases by sex, site of cancer and histological type.

Table 1
Distribution of cases and controls, by sex, age, smoking habits and alcohol consumption

	Cases (n=207) %	Controls (n=409) %
Sex		
Men	80.7	78.2
Women	19.3	21.8
Age		
≤ 50	18.4	22.0
51-60	31.4	30.1
61-70	26.6	29.7
> 70	23.7	18.3
Smoking habits		
Smokers	23.7	23.5
Exsmokers	34.3	39.9
Nonsmokers	42.0	36.7
Alcohol consumption		
≤ 1 glass/day	25.6	28.6
1-3	30.4	27.1
3-7	25.6	28.1
> 7	18.3	16.1

Table 2
Distribution of cases by sex, histological type and site of cancer

Site	Squamous cell carcinoma		Adenocarcinoma		Other		Total	
	Men	Women	Men	Women	Men	Women	Men	Women
Nasal Cavity	13	1	8	1	7	7	28	9
Maxillary sinus	27	10	3	1	6	4	36	15
Ethmoidal sinus	18	5	71	3	11	6	100	14
Unidentified	1	2	0	0	1	0	2	2
Total	59	18	82	5	25	17	166	40

Cases and controls were assigned to a given occupation when they had been employed in this occupation for more than 6 months. For men, when all histological types were combined, only construction workers and woodworkers had a significant excess risk of nasal cancer. Among women, no odds-ratio was statistically significant.

Table 3 shows the odds-ratios and the 95% confidence intervals for selected occupations (blue-collar workers) in men, by histology. The elevated risk of nasal cancer in woodworkers was specifically associated with adenocarcinoma. For construction workers, the risk was higher for squamous cell carcinomas, but a borderline significant excess risk was found for adenocarcinomas. An excess of squamous cell nasal cancer was also observed for farmworkers.

Table 3
Odds ratios among men by selected occupations

	SQUAMOUS CELL CARCINOMA		ADENOCARCINOMA	
	OR	95 % CI	OR	95 % CI
Farm workers	2.23	[1.14- 4.76]	0.51	[0.28-1.90]
Metallurgy mechanic	0.49	[0.25- 1.09]	0.48	[0.26-1.04]
Construction, (woodworkers excluded)	2.50	[1.33- 4.98]	1.71	[0.99-3.30]
Construction, woodworkers	2.28	[0.68-10.75]	17.70	[7.06-41.69]
Miners	1.99	[0.66- 8.30]	0.37	[0.22-4.48]
Food industry	1.65	[0.73- 5.03]	0.58	[0.22-2.53]
Processing industry	0.96	[0.56- 3.49]	0	
Woodworkers (except construction)	0.48	[0.24- 2.29]	26.85	[13.54-51.29]
Textile, leather	1.81	[0.73-4.80]	0.38	[0.20-2.63]
Drivers	1.00	[0.49-3.21]	0.24	[0.15-1.64]
Store keepers, transport workers	0.40	[0.20-1.81]	0.96	[0.46-2.33]

Occupational risk factors were also examined by site of cancer. Among men, a significant excess risk of nasal cavity cancer was observed for coal miners (OR=12.6; 95% CI=3.9-38.5). Odds-ratios for maxillary sinus cancer were significantly above 1 for food industry workers (OR=2.8; 95% CI=1.2-8.9),non wood construction workers(OR=3.7; 95% CI=1.8-8.4) and for farmworkers (OR=2.3; 95% CI=1.1-6.0). The excess risk was more specifically associated with squamous cell carcinoma of the maxillary sinus for food industry workers (OR=3.8; 95%CI=1.6-12.9) and for farmworkers (OR=2.9; 95% CI=1.2-8.1). Most cases employed in food industry were bakers. Among woodworkers (outside the contruction industry) the risk of adenocarcinoma of the nasal cavity and of the ethmoidal sinus were very high (OR=29.5 ; 95% CI=4.7-102.1 and OR=29.5 ; 95% CI=13.6-57.6, respectively). Among contruction woodworkers, the higher risk was observed for adenocarcinoma of ethmoidal sinus (OR=18.9; 95% CI=7.5-45.8), but the risk was also found to be significantly elevated for squamous cell carcinoma of this site (OR=7.5; 95%CI=2.4-44.5).

For women, the risk of squamous cell carcinoma was significantly elevated among textile workers (OR=2.5; 95% CI=1.1-11.9), especially for ethmoidal sinus (OR=14.5; 95% CI=1.1-34.9) and among farmworkers (OR=4.9; 95% CI=1.2-33.9), especially for maxillary sinus (OR=8.4; 95% CI=1.9-60.4).

The results are consistent with previous findings. The association between risk of nasal adenocarcinoma and work in the furniture industry has been well documented. There is also some evidence of excess risk for non adenocarcinoma and for woodworkers outside the furniture industry [1]. The excess risk of nasal cancer in construction workers has been reported previously [2,3]. Several studies have shown an association of nasal cancer with work in the textile industry [3-5]. Acheson found a significant excess of cases of nasal cancer among coal miners, bakers and pastry makers [5]. An excess risk for farmers was also noted [3,6,7]. Further analysis based on occupational exposures will help to clarify the present findings.

REFERENCES

1. International Agency for Research on Cancer. IARC monograph on the evaluation of the carcinogenic risk of chemicals to humans. Wood,leather and some associated industries. Vol 25, Lyon : IARC, 1981.

2. Roush G. C., Meigs J. W., Kelly J. et al. Sinonasal cancer and occupation : a case-control study. Am J Epidemiol 1980; 111 : 183-193.

3. Ng T. P. A case-referent study of cancer of the nasal cavity and sinuses in Hong-Kong. Int J Epidemiol 1986 ; 15 : 171-175.

4. Brinton L. A., Blot N. J., Becker J.A. et al. A case-control study of cancers of the nasal cavity and paranasal sinuses. Am J Epidemiol 1984 ; 119 : 896-906.

5. Acheson E. D., Cowdell R. H., Rang E. H. Nasal cancer in England and Wales : an occupational survey. Br J Ind Med 1981 ; 38 : 218-224.

6. Takasaka T., Kawamoto K., Nakamura K. A case-control study of nasal cancers - an occupational survey. Acta Otolaryngol (Stockh) 1987 ; Suppl. 435 : 136-142.

7. Olsen J. H. Occupational risks of sinonasal cancer in Denmark. Br J Ind Med 1988 ; 45 : 329-335.

The study was conducted with contribution from 27 services :
Bordeaux : Hôpital des enfants (Pr L. Traissac) ; Centre Hospitalier Pellegrin-Tripode (Dr D. Stoll) ; Fondation Bergonié (Dr Renaud-Salis, Dr Faucher) ; Hôpital St André (Dr H. Demeaux). Caen : Centre François-Baclesse. Lille : CHR-Hôpital régional (Dr Chevalier) ; CHR-Centre Oscar Lambret (Dr Lefebvre) ; CHR-Hôpital B (Pr A. Desaulty). Lyon : Hôpital de la Croix-Rousse (Pr J. Gaillard) ; Centre Léon Bérard (Dr Gignoux). Nancy : Hôpital de Brabois (Dr A. Brunet) ; CHR (Dr R. Beurton). Strasbourg : Centre Paul Strauss (Pr Methlin) ; Clinique Ste Barbe ; Hôpital Hautepierre (Pr Klotz) ; CHR (Pr Conraux). Nantes : Hôtel Dieu (Pr Beauvillain). Paris : Institut Curie (Dr J. Brugère) ; Hôpital Boucicaut (Dr Ngo) ; Hôpital Claude Bernard (Pr Gehanno) ; CHI de Créteil (Dr Juvanon) ; Centre René-Huguenin, Saint-Cloud (Dr Mahé) ; CHI de Montfermeil (Dr Peytral) ; Institut Gustave-Roussy, Villejuif (Dr Schwaab). Toulouse : CHU Toulouse-Rangueil (Pr J.J. Pessey) ; Centre Claudius Regaud, CRAC (Pr N. Daly). Tours : CHRU, Hôpital Bretonneau (Pr Beutter).

Occupational Epidemiology. H. Sakurai et al., editors

MORTALITY OF MALE WORKERS EXPOSED TO BENZIDINE AND BETA-NAPHTHYLAMINE

KENJI MORINAGA*, ICHIROH HARA**, SATOSHI YUTANI***

* The Center for Adult Diseases, Osaka, Higashinari-ku, Osaka 537, Japan
** Public Health, Kansai Medical University, Moriguchi, Osaka 570, Japan
*** Osaka Prefectural Institute of Public Health, Osaka 537, Japan

INTRODUCTION

It is in 1940 that the first case of occupationally induced bladder tumor appeared in the Japanese literature (1). After World Wor II, the production of benzidine and beta-naphtyhlamine had been rapidly growing and peaked in 1955, mainly due to the export to the People's Republic of China (2).

Osaka had two industries which had been manufacturing these two chemicals. During the 1950s, many workers had developed acute toxic symptoms from these substances (3). After 1965, many employees were found to have sufferred from bladder tumors and among them,some patients had subsequent primary cancers (4).

This study attempts to demonstrate the cancer mortality and incidence experience of workers exposed to benzidine and beta-naphthylamine in Japan.

SUBJECTS AND METHODS

In 1978, information was assembled about employees exposed to benzidine and beta-naphthylamine who had worked in two facilities which had manufactured these two chemicals in Osaka. Records including name, sex, present address, date of birth and date of initial contact and of cessation of exposure were collected for each worker who had engaged in the manufacturing or handling benzidine and/or beta-naphthylamine. The entire cohort consisted of 887 male workers. We present the results of the retrospective cohort study of 794 male employees whose initial exposures started after 1945 and who were alive at the time of January 1, 1970. The diseased men were traced by linking with records registered at the Osaka Cancer Registry and the Hyogo Cancer Registry and all death certificates in Osaka prefecture. Persons who were living in the other prefecture than in Osaka were checked through public offices. The observed numbers of death were compared with the expected deaths, calculated by multiplying the person-years of observation within 5-year age interval for the years 1970-1974, 1975-1979, and 1980-1984 of the male Osaka population (5).

Attack rate of urinary tract tumors was calculated. The incidence of these tumors was examined between the initial exposure and the end of 1984 among the entire cohort.

RESULTS AND DISCUSSIONS

The number of person-years for the subjects was 11494. Among 794 employees, 68 deaths were ascertained, but we could not get death certificates for two cases. Mean death age was 60 years old. The number of deaths for all causes by age and year was shown in Table 1. Fifteen deaths were attributed to the genitourinary tumors on death certificates. Their mean death age was 58. Table 2 summarizes the mortality experience for the study cohort. Standardized mortality ratio for all causes of death was 0.64, which reflected "healthy worker effect". Only urinary tract tumors showed excess deaths. A nonsignificant increased

Table 1 Deaths by age and year for all causes of deaths

Age/Year	1970～74	1975～79	1980～84	Total
30～34	1	0	0	1
35～39	2(1)	1	0	3(1)
40～44	0	3(1)	0	3(1)
45～49	0	2	2(1)	4(1)
50～54	1(1)	6(1)	2	9(2)
55～59	1	4(2)	4	9(2)
60～64	2(2)	7(2)	4	13(4)
65～69	1	12(2)	3	16(2)
70～74	0	1(1)	3	4(1)
75～79	0	1(1)	3	4(1)
80～84	0	0	2	2
Total	7(4)	38(10)	23(1)	68(15)

( ) indicates the number of deaths from genitourinary tumor

Table 2 Standardized mortality ratio for main causes of deaths by two groups; exposed to benzidine and/or beta-naphthylamin and to benzidine only

		B and/ BNA		B only	
Causes of death	ICD 8	Obs.	Obs./Exp.	Obs.	Obs./Exp.
All causes	001-999	68	0.64	35	0.72
All malignant neoplasms	140-209	29	0.88	14	0.93
Cancer of stomach	151	7	0.58	3	0.55
Cancer of intestine,rectum	153-154	3	1.37	3	2.97
Cancer of lung	162	5	0.98	3	1.34
Cancer of urinary tract	188-189	9	11.84($p<0.01$)	3	8.82($p<0.05$)
All benign tumors	210-239	7	5.00($p<0.01$)	6	9.28($p<0.01$)
All circulatory diseases	390-459	25	0.46	9	0.51
Unknown		2	----	1	----

Obs.:Observed deaths, Exp.:Expected deaths, B:benzidine, BNA:beta-naphthylamine risk of intestine, rectum and lung cancer was observed for those only exposed to benzidine.

Table 3 Number of incident cases of genitourinary tumors among employees engaged in the manufacture and attack rate per 1,000 person-years

Category	B	BNA	B + BNA	Total
Number of subjects	191	111	55	157
Person-years	4546.2	2743.3	1147.8	8437.3
Number of incident cases	23	15	9	47
Attack rate / 1,000	5.06	5.47	7.84	5.57

B:benzidine, BNA:beta-naphthylamine

Among the subjects who had been mainly engaged in the manufacturing, 47 incident cases of genitourinary tumors were found till the end of 1984. Table 3 shows the attack rate by 3 exposure groups; benzidine only, beta-naphthylamine only, and both. There were not so different between the former two groups, but the last had about 1.5 times greater attack rate than the former.

Among the entire cohort, 8 cases of multiple primary cancers have been found (Table 4). All cases were histologically diagnosed. In our previous study, we reported 11 multiple primary cancer cases among the employees who worked in 14 of 15 industries that manufactured these aromatic amines in Japan (4). At that

Table 4 Multiple primary cancers among the workers exposed to benzidine and/or beta-naphthylamine

Case No.	B or BNA	Duration of exposure	1st primary cancer: Site	1st primary cancer: Age at diagnosis	1st primary cancer: Latent period	2nd primary cancer: Site	2nd primary cancer: Age at diagnosis
1.	BNA	8Y 8M	Bladder(TCC)	62	18Y	Maxillary Sinus(SCC)	66
2.	BNA	1Y 1M	Bladder(TCC)	64	26Y	Esophagus(SCC)	76
3.	B	6Y 6M	Bladder(TCC)	53	13Y	Lung(AD)	65
						Prostata(AD)	66
4.	B	1Y 4M	Bladder(TCC)	62	22Y	Rectum(AD)	65
5.	BNA	1Y 1M	Bladder(TCC)	61	20Y	Lung(SCC)	76
						Prostata(AD)	76
6.	B	24Y 7M	Bladder(TCC)	63	30Y	Lung(Sm)	76
7.	B	11Y 5M	Renal pelvids(TCC)	41	27Y	Bile duct(AD)	53
8.	B	2Y 3M	Bladder(TCC)	62	25Y	Lung(AD)	63

B:benzidine Y:year TCC:transitional cell carcinoma
BNA:beta-naphthylamine, M:month SCC:squamous cell carcinoma
AD:adenocarcinoma, Sm:small cell carcinoma

time, we presented 4 cases in this cohort. Now we have 4 additional cases. Our speculation presented before still remains that these findings may suggest a pluripotential action of these carcinogen, especially benzidine (4).

ACKNOWLEDGEMENTS

We wish to thank the Osaka Cancer Registry and the Hyogo Cancer Registry for their kind cooperation.

REFERENCES

1. Nishimura I (1940) On aniline tumors of the bladder (case report). Jpn J Urol 29:733-749, (in Japanese).
2. Hara I (1985) A history of occupational urinary tumors in Osaka. Rodo no Kagaku 40(5):52-56, (in Japanese).
3. Hara I, Hayashi M (1959) Studies in the occupational benzidine intoxication in a dyestuff factory. Rodo Kagaku Kihoh 7:39-47, (in Japanese).
4. Morinaga K, Oshima A, Hara I (1982) Multiple primary cancers following exposure to benzidine and beta-naphthylamine. Am J Ind Med 3:243-246
5. Monson RR (1974) Analysis of rerative survival and proportional mortality. Comp Biomed Res 7:325-332

Occupational Epidemiology. H. Sakurai et al., editors

549419

CANCER MORTALITY AMONG MALE FARMERS IN FINLAND DURING 1979-1985

NOTKOLA VEIJO, HUSMAN KAJ, KURPPA KARI
Kuopio Regional Institute of Occupational Health,
P.O. Box 93, 70701 Kuopio (Finland)

INTRODUCTION

The aim of this study was to analyse the cause-specific cancer mortality of male farmers by type of farm in Finland during 1979-1985. Male farmers are particularly exposed to various organic and microbial dusts, endotoxins and pesticides, which might be connected to different kinds of cancers. In earlier studies in other countries, farmers have been shown to have an elevated risk of certain types of cancer, such as cancer of the lymphatic and hematopoietic systems, stomach, prostate, brain, lip, skin and connective tissue (1). In Finland and in some other countries the total mortality of farmers has been lower than average, but the mortality of farm workers worldwide has been high (2, 3). However, the number of farm workers in Finland is small and cancer mortality can not be studied in a register - based study.

SUBJECTS AND METHODS

This study was based on the Finnish farm register. The male population included in the farm register on 31 December 1978 was defined as the population at risk. The Finnish farm register is a basic register for official farm statistics. It was built up on the information from the general farm census of 1969. The register includes all farms with a totality of cultivated land (field and garden area) surpassing hectare. Up-dating information is collected each year with a postal questionnaire.

Information about the owner, occupation of the owner, and size of the farm was taken from the farm register of 1978. Information concerning the type of farm was collected separately from the farm register of 1977.

Data on all deaths during 1979-1985 (i.e. cause of death, etc) were obtained from death certificates recorded in the Finnish register on causes of death. The International Classification of Diseases (ICD), eighth revision, was used for the classification of deaths. Only the underlying cause of death was available in the data on causes of death.

The following causes of death (ICD-8) were considered: all neoplasms (ICD 140-239) and ICD 150, 151, 153, 154, 155, 156, 157, 161, 162, 163, 170, 171, 172, 173, 174, 185, 188, 189, 191, 200, 201, 202, 203, 204, 205).

Only the men aged 35-84 years whose occupation was listed as farmer in the farm register were included. The study population thus defined numbered 117 047 persons.

The data by type of farming were classified as follows: (i) all farmers, (ii) cattle farms (dairy, pig and poultry farms), (iii) other animal husbandry, and (iv) no animals.

Because of the small numbers of deaths, the age-standardized mortality rates have been calculated with the use of indirect age standardization.

RESULTS

It was shown that, compared to the mortality of all men, the cancer mortality of farmers was generally low (Table 1, Figure 1). If the cancer mortality were close to average, the p-values would be equally distributed between zero and one, and the stars in the figure would be close to the diagonal. However, there are more values close to one than to zero, so the cancer mortality among farmers is evidently low (Figure 1).

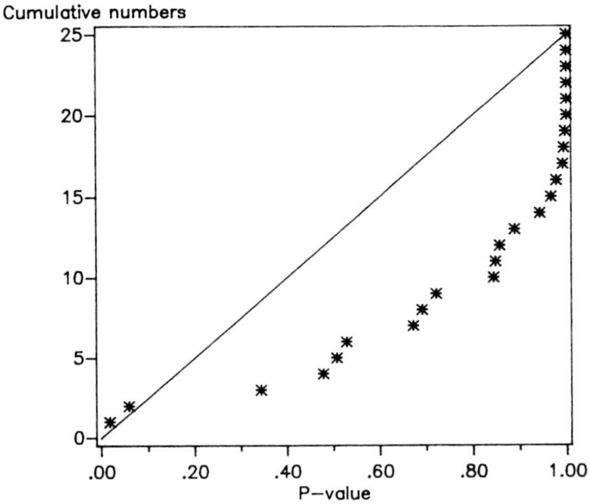

Fig. 1. Cumulative distribution of cancer p-values (1-sided) among farmers in Finland.

However, the mortality due to malignant skin neoplasm was systematically increased and the mortality due to Hodgkin's disease was also statistically significantly increased among Finnish farmers. There was no clear difference in cancer mortality by type of farm in Finland (Table 1).

TABLE 1. STANDARDIZED MORTALITY RATIOS IN 1979-1985 OF ALL NEOPLASMS (ICD-8, 140-239), MALIGNANT SKIN MELANOMA (172) AND HODGKIN'S DISEASE (201) FOR MALE FARMERS AGED 35-84 BY TYPE OF FARM IN FINLAND.

	Observed	Expected	SMR	95% CI
All neoplasms[1)]				
All farmers	2779	3634.21	0.76	0.73-0.79
Cattle farms	1571	2121.48	0.74	0.70-0.78
Other animal husbandry	353	501.42	0.70	0.63-0.77
No animals	855	1013.44	0.84	0.78-0.90
Malignant melanoma of skin (172)[2)]				
All farmers	48	37.66	1.27	0.91-1.63
Cattle farms	26	22.79	1.14	0.70-1.58
Other animal husbandry	9	5.34	1.68	0.58-2.78
No animals	13	9.55	1.36	0.62-2.10
Hodgkin's disease (201)[2)]				
All farmers	31	20.49	1.51	0.98-2.04
Cattle farms	21	12.16	1.73	0.99-2.47
Other animal husbandry	1	2.94	0.34	0.00-1.01
No animals	9	5.40	1.67	0.58-2.76

1) All males in Finland in 1982 used as reference
2) All males in 1981-83 used as reference

DISCUSSION

The reason for the generally low cancer mortality among farmers in Finland might be twofold. Firstly, male farmers in Finland do not smoke as much as the general male population in Finland. Secondly, in Finland pesticides are used in much smaller quantities and less often than in many other countries with warmer climates. The low cancer mortality among male farmers might also be explained by selection, or the healthy worker effect. It is not clear why the mortality due to Hodgkin's disease and the malignant skin neoplasm was increased. According to earlier studies, however, both of these malignancies are more common among farmers than among the general population.

REFERENCES

1. Blair A, Malker H, Cantos KP, Burmeister L, Wiklund K (1985) Cancer among farmers: A review. Scand J Work Environ Health 11:397-407

2. Notkola V, Husman K, Laukkanen V. Mortality among male farmers in Finland 1979-83 (1987) Scand J Work Environ Health 13:124-8

3. Marin R. Occupational mortality 1971-80 (1986) Central Statistical Office of Finland. Helsinki. Study No 129.

Occupational Epidemiology. H. Sakurai et al., editors

549420

DIOXINS AND CANCER MORTALITY - REANALYSIS OF THE BASF-COHORT

FRIEDEMANN ROHLEDER
Private Epidemiologist, Friedr. Hebbel Str.13, D-4712 Werne, FRG

INTRODUCTION

At the end of 1953 a group of people were exposed to dioxins after a run-away reaction in a trichloro-phenol-process at the BASF plant in Ludwigshafen. The building E 206, in which an accident occurred on the 17th of November, was situated about 3 kilometer northwest of the centers of the cities of Mannheim and Ludwigshafen with a population of about 430000 at that period. The winds in this area however come predominantly from southwest. Nowadays the BASF-accident is referred to in the lay press as a Seveso-like accident.

Three epidemiologic studies were published about the sequels of the accident (Tbl.1). The latest study of the long term consequences of the accident was reported by Lehnert and Szadkowski (L./Sz.). In their historical cohort study on behalf of the liability association or the „Berufsgenossenschaft" (BG) of the chemical industry they concluded that dioxins and especially 2,3,7,8-TCDD did not cause human malignancies. Their analysis became the foundation for a series of expert opinions in which compensation was denied to exposed workers suffering from cancer.

Table 1: Epidemiologic Studies about a Dioxin-accident at the BASF-plant 1953

Author	Year	Statement	Finding	References
Frentzel-Beyme	1981		Excess of benign and malignant neoplasia	AJE 114:425
Thiess, Frentzel-Beyme, Link	1982	The Cohort of 75 Persons ...	Excess mortality of gastric cancer	Am.J.Ind.Med. 3:179-189
Lehnert, Szadkowski	1985	153 Employees were exposed	Exc. mort. of all malignancies in "Chloracne"-group	Arb.Soz.Präv.Med. 20:225-232

REANALYSIS

Data Sources

The most obvious difference of the L./Sz.-study to the previous studies and case-reports is the enlargement of the exposed group. Therefore the suspicion was patent, that someone tried to dilute the effects of the dioxins. Following the advise of MARSH and ENTERLINE (1) verification of the completeness and correctness of the study population was indicated (Tbl. 2). The court-cases of some exposed workers facilitated a reanalysis of the data. On request of the author the court ordered the BG to hand over the same data L./Sz. had used for their study. They stated in a parliamentary hearing that they had received their data from the BG. The BG however admitted that the medical department of the BASF had assembled the study group. Since the BG should have notified the State Medical Officer (STMO) of every case, he ought to have a complete list of exposed workers. On request of the court the STMO supplied a list of all workers known to him. The study of L./Sz. has kindled controversy within the German scientific community. The BG felt therefore compelled to compile its own data on

Table 2: Sources of Data about exposed Persons of the Accident

"BASF-DAT"	"STMO-DAT"	"BG-DAT"
153 People	110 People	122 People
Source:	Source:	Source:
Medical Department of the BASF	Information from the BG to the STMO	Information from the BASF to the BG

the exposed group for independent study by a group of scientists. This data set has been added to the other files already received. The data are based on the notifications of the company to the BG. Thus they also do not represent an independent data set.

Comparison of Data-sets

STMO-DAT could be linked with BASF-DAT using date of birth and the available three first letters of name and given name (Tbl. 3). Since the cutaneous signs of systemic toxicity are regarded as a specific indicator of exposure, it is difficult to understand, why 17 cases with these signs were excluded from BASF-DAT. There are oral reports of coworkers and relatives about cancer cases in this group. As there were no means to substantiate these claims and equal information was not available for the 17 cases, they had to be excluded from the analysis as in the study of L./Sz. One wonders that the STMO had not been notified of the three cases with cutaneous signs.

BG-DAT could be linked with BASF-DAT in a step-by-step manner (Tbl. 4). Because in single cases the possibility of a mismatch can not be excluded with certainty, these data were not suitable for analysis either. From this comparison it is at least clear that the 20 supervisors cannot be regarded as exposed.

Table 3: Comparison of BASF-DAT and STMO-DAT

STMO-DAT (n=110)		BASF-DAT (n=153)
24 not in BASF-DAT:	86 in both data sets:	67 not in STMO-DAT: of these
of these according to BG-DAT 17 with cutaneous signs of intoxication, i.e. "Chlorakne" or Dermatitis	70 with and 16 without cutaneous signs	6 belonging to other BG 20 supervisors of demolition in 1968 3 with and 38 without cutaneous signs

Table 4: Comparison of BASF-DAT and BG-DAT

BG-DAT (n=122)		BASF-DAT (n=153)
32 not in BASF-DAT:	90 in both data sets:	63 not in BG-DAT: of these
of these 27 with and 5 without cutaneous signs of intoxication	71 with and 19 without cutaneous signs	9 belonging to other BG 20 supervisors of demolition in 1968 5 with and 29 without cutaneous signs

Table 5 sheds some doubt on the validity of the classification of the cutaneous signs of toxicity by comparing the information in BG-DAT with BASF-DAT . Instead of falling on the diagonal as one would expect, there are discrepancies. 18 out of 27 cases assigned as „dermatitis only" are „Chlorakne"-cases according to BG-DAT. 23 out of 55 „Chlorakne"-cases according to BG-DAT are misclassified in BASF-DAT. There is even a cancer case in BASF-DAT classified as free of cutaneous signs, who in fact is a „Chlorakne"-case according to BG-DAT. L./Sz. used the cutaneous signs of toxicity as a substitute for the unmeasured dose of dioxins. As they did not find a dose-response relationship, they rejected any relationship between dioxin and cancer. They found however a significant excess mortality of all malignancies within their

Table 5: Comparison of cutaneous signs for 90 Matched Pairs in BASF-DAT and BG-DAT

		Cutaneous signs as in BG-DAT: "Chlorakne"	Dermatitis	No cut. signs	Miss. Data	Sum
Cutaneous	"Chlorakne"	32	5	1	1	39
signs as in	Dermatitis	18	8	1	-	27
BASF-DAT:	No cut. signs	5	5	8	6	24
	Missing data	-	-	-	-	0
	Sum	55	18	10	7	90

„Chlorakne"-group[1]

In BG-DAT the ICD-number 799 (ill defined or not localized causes of death) is assigned to 18 out of 52 cases, which is an incredible 34.6 % (Data not shown). Why this cause of death is assigned so often, whereas BASF-DAT and/or the official ICD know well defined causes of death needs further explanation.

EPIDEMIOLOGIC REASONING

At this point one hesitates to analyze this data further without thorough revision. Epidemiologic data on the relationship of human malignancy and dioxin-exposure nevertheless are scarce and gave conflicting results. This is chiefly because exposure could not be quantified in epidemiologic studies so far. This data at least describe the experience of a „highly" exposed group, as can be jugded from recent analyses of body fat by RAPPE or by SCHECTER (2).

In addition, the exposure of the group was almost as in a „point source epidemic" and the observation period extends over nearly 30 years. On the other hand all the demonstrated discrepancies seem to make this data set unsuitable for analysis. Here one has to invoke epidemiological reasoning: Epidemiologic data have never been and will probably never be perfect; what epidemiology is all about, is to draw relevant conclusions in such a situation.

1. The data to be analyzed were compiled by the affected company itself.
2. Exposed cases were excluded by those who did the compiling.
3. The cutaneous signs of exposure cannot be validly substituted as an indicator of exposure level. The classification of cases is not valid in this regard.
4. The cause of death might be debatable in single cases.
5. There are still cases in BASF-DAT who certainly were not exposed and therefore will dilute any excess mortality associated with dioxin-exposure.

In conclusion, all the mentioned mistakes tend to diminish an association if one exists. If nevertheless an association emerges, then it might not be as clear as one would wish. Nobody can deny though, that there is an identifiable association. There is then only one assumption to be made to justify the analysis of BASF-DAT. The assumption is, that the medical department of the BASF has not assembled the data with the purpose to pretend an association between dioxin exposure and human malignancy although there is none.

METHODS

All the data sets described were stored in the authors personal computer. The comparison between data sets was done with a professional data bank system. The data analysis follows the person-years principle. Since an internal, not exposed reference group was not available, the standardized mortality ratio (SMR) was used as an estimator of relative risk. The male death rates of the Federal Republic of Germany in groupings of five years of age from the respective ICD-period were used as reference mortality rates[2]. The Poisson-test was calculated to give a measure of the error probability of the findings.

---

[1] In order to invalidate this finding L./Sz. invented an irreproducible confidence intervall for their SMR of 2.67 (.774 - 11.86), which is in conflict with their significant test result.

[2] I am grateful to Dr. N.Becker of the German Cancer Research Center for supplying these mortality rates to me.

FINDINGS

The analysis comprises 131 people, whom the medical department of the BASF has pointed out as exposed. It disregards any groupings according to cutaneous signs of exposure. The end of the observation period is the 31 august 1983 as in the study of L./Sz (Tbl. 6). There is no excess mortality of all causes and no „healthy worker effect" . There is no excess mortality of all natural causes of death. There is an increased mortality due to all human malignancies however, as was found by L./Sz.. If one considers the discussion about dioxins as promotors of neoplastic growth, then one would expect to see such an unspecific increase of tumors of all sites.

Table 6:
Observed and expected mortality of 131 Exposed[1] in BASF-DAT

Cause of Death ICD-No.[2]	Ob- served	Ex- pected	SMR	p-value
All Causes 000-995	43	41.42	1.04	0.4123
All natural Causes 000-799	35	37.54	0.93	0.6827
All malignancies 140-209	17	9.05	1.88	0.0117*[3]
Respiratory Cancer 161-163	8	3.01	2.66	0.0121*
Cancer of Digestive Tract 140-155	7	2.75	2.55	0.0224*
Malignancies unspecified 190-199	2	2.17	0.92	0.6371

[1] 20 Supervisors, 2 Women are excluded
[2] 7th, 8th Revision, list A, 9th Revision, list B
[3] * significant at α = 5 %

If one is willing to group the ICD-category 161: neoplasms of the larynx, 162: neoplasms of trachea, bronchi and lung and 163: other and unspecified neoplasms of the respiratory organs into one class, then one observes with eight such cancer death versus 3.01 expected cases a significant SMR of 2.66. This is an organ-specific excess of death and increases the probability that there is an association between dioxin exposure and human malignancy. If one combines in the same manner the ICD-categories 140 - 155 to a class: neoplasms of the digestive tract, one also finds a significantly increased SMR of 2.55. Given the small size of the cohort, the power of this study - that is the chance to find a difference, if one exists - is small. For example the power to find the raised SMR's was not even 50 %.

CONCLUSIONS

1. This analysis adds further evidence to an association between dioxin exposure and human malignancy;
2. Occupational cohort studies - especially of the historical type - should not be regarded as valid, unless there is company-independent confirmation of their completeness and correctness;
3. The true mortality and especially the morbidity experience of persons, who were highly exposed to dioxins following the BASF-accident, still remains to be studied with adequate methods.

Acknowledgements:
No grants were received for this study; however I am gratefull to those victims of the accident and those colleagues and friends who were helpful during the progress of the work.

References:

1. Marsh GM, Enterline PE (1981) Letter to the Editor, J. Occup. Med. 23:76-77
2. Schecter A, Ryan JJ (1987) Polychlorinated Dibenzo-para-dioxin and Dibenzofuranlevels in human adipose tissues from sick workers 32 years after occupational exposure to 2,3,7,8-TCDD in 1953 in Germany, Chemosphere, in press

Occupational Epidemiology. H. Sakurai et al., editors
549421

THE ANALYSIS OF RELATIONSHIP BETWEEN COAL WORKERS' PNEUMOCONIOSIS AND CARCINOMA

GUOAN SHEN AND HONG LI
Sichuan Institute of Labour Hygiene and Occupational Diseases, Chengdu, CHINA

INTRODUCTION

The relationship between coal workers' pneumoconiosis (CWP) and carcinoma has already aroused common concern among people. In order to research the relationship between CWP and carcinoma, this paper analysed the death frequency and proportion of all carcinoma including lung cancer, liver cancer, esophagus cancer and stomach cancer among the patients and deaths of CWP in five mines of Sichuan Province during 1963 to 1986 through retrospective study.

MATERIAL AND METHODS

The sources of materials

By using unified survey methods and registration table, 3 866 CWP cases (person-years=37 107.5) from 1963 to 1986 were collected in five mines in Sichuan Province. Among which 1 050 deaths were analysed for their death causes and 122 cases were found to have died of carcinoma including cases of 44 lung cancer, 27 liver cancer, 16 esophagus cancer, 7 stomach cancer and 28 other kind of cancer.

Reliability

All of CWP cases were diagnosed by Pneumoconiosis Diagnosis Groups of local areas accoding to the Standard of Silicosis Diagnosis of our country established in 1963. All CWP deaths were registrated by doctors of labour hygiene of each mine. 71.93 percent of the deaths were diagnosed on the basis of pathological cytology and radiographs. Among them, 40 cases' death causes were unknown, accounting for 3.81 percent. All deaths were diagnosed at least at the hospitals of counties or mines.

Statistical method and index

Standardized Mortality Ratios (SMRs) were calculated respectively according to the male controls with different age mortality of carcinoma including lung cancer, liver cancer, esophagus cancer and stomach cancer in carcinoligical epidemiology survey of the whole country and Chongqing City from 1973 to 1975.

Proportional Mortality Ratios (PMRs) were calculated respectively according to the male controls with different age death proportion of carcinoma including lung cancer, liver cancer, esophagus cancer and stomach cancer of carcinological sampling survey of Chongqing, Chengdu and Fuling in Sichuan Province from 1973 to 1975.

Aged groups are divided by the interval of 5-years old.

Both SMRs and PMRs were tested following Poisson distribution confidence table.

RESULTS

The total results of SMRs and PMRs of carcinoma including lung cancer, liver cancer, esophagus cancer and stomach cancer for CWP calculated according to different age groups are shown in table I.

TABLE I

OBSERVED AND EXPECTED DEATHS BY CARCINOMAS, SMRS AND PMRS FOR CWP (N=3 866, PERSON-YEARS=37 107.5)

	Observed	Expected		SMR		Expected	PMR
		(1)	(2)	(1)	(2)	(3)	(3)
All carcinomas	122	76.8	73.2	161**	167**	170.78	71
Lung cancer	44	6.9	11.6	643**	378**	22.57	195**
Liver cancer	27	16.8	18.6	161*	146	35.52	76
Esophagus cancer	16	17.4	17.1	92	94	50.05	32
Stomach cancer	7	20.5	9.4	32	74	29.44	24

(1)Compared with the population of whole country.
(2)Compared with the population of local area (Chongqing).
(3)Compared with the population of three local areas.
* $p<0.05$; ** $p<0.01$.

The SMRs in table I showed that, the all carcinomas mortality of CWP in five mines was significantly higher than that of the population of the whole contry and of local area. But from the PMR, no significant difference of carcinoma deaths between observed population and controled population was found.

Both SMRs and PMR of lung cancer showed that it's incidence in CWP were significantly higher than that in controled population.

The SMR of liver cancer showed that it's incidence in observed population was significantly higher than that in the population of the whole country, but no significant difference was found when compared with the population of local area. The PMR showed no increase of liver cancer.

The incidence of esophagus cancer and stomach cancer of CWP were lower than that of the general population.

DISCUSSION

Great attention has long been paid to whether the incidence of carcinoma among CWP was high and in which position did the carcinoma have a high incidence. But there are always different viewpoints.

This report has analysed the death frenquency and relative death proportion for CWP with carcinomas in five mines of Sichuan Province through retrospective study and by using SMRs and PMRs, the two statistical indexes often used in occupational epidemiological research. The result shows that the SMRs calculated based on the mortality of carcinomas, with the general male mortality of the country and Chongqing as the controls, was respectively 161 and 167($p<0.01$), namely, the carcinomas deaths among CWP were higher than that of the general population in both the whole country and the local area (Chongqing). But the PMR calculated based on three local areas was 71($p>0.05$). No increase of carcinomas deaths among CWP was found. The main cause of the difference between SMRs and PMR of carcinomas among CWP might be the different statistical methods and controls.

However, results are almost the same when two above methods were used to analyse the death frenquency and relative death proportion of lung cancer among CWP. The SMR calculated based on the controls of the country and local area were separately 643 and 378 ($p<0.01$). The PMR calculated based on the population of three local areas was 195 ($p<0.01$). This indicates CWP patients are high dangerous population of lung cancer indeed. Our former survey showed[1-3], the incidence and death of lung cancer among CWP had a tendency to happening earlier and go straight up with the extension of working years. The mortality of lung cancer of drillers were higher than that of the coal-cutting miners. The mortality of lung cancer in CWP during 12 years after 1975 was higher than that during 12 years before 1974. The mortality of lung cancer in coal miners with simple pneumoconiosis was higher than that with complicated pneumoconiosis. The cause might be the latters' early death. But among coal miners, no significant difference of lung cancer incidence was found between pneumoconiosis group and non-pneumoconiosis group. Meanwhile it had been found that the mortality of lung cancer in dust cohort was higher than the mortality in control cohort when ruling out the effects of smoking habit and smoking history (M-H test). So the high mortality of lung cancer in CWP was thought to be mainly related to occupational exposure to dust. Coal mines' dust could absorb and gather carcinogens of the air and might played a auxiliary role. High incidence may also relate to the pathological changes of pneumoconiosis and chronic bronchitis of coal miners[4], or to the increase of cholesterol in lung as well[5]. Of course, owing to different areas and sourses of materials, there might have been no consistency as to the relationship between CWP and lung cancer till now. In addtion, the CWP in this study were observed from 1963 to 1986, but the controls were observed from 1973 to 1975. It may bring about some bias to results as well.

REFERENCES

1. Shen GA(1988)Study on relationship between coal workers' pnemoconiosis and lung cancer. Occup Hyg and Dis 3(3):1-3
2. Wang JW and Shen GA(1988)A cohort study on coal miners' lung carcinoma of Weiyuan mine. Occup Hyg and Dis 3(3):4-6
3. Lin J and Shen GA(1988)Hygienic survey on underground work environment of Weiyuan mine. Occup Hyg and Dis 3(4):4-7
4. Shen GA and Xu PY(1987)Pathological observations on coal miners' bronchial lung carcinoma. Chinese J Ind Hyg and Occup Dis 5:339-343
5. Shen GA, Lin J and Li P(1987)Quantitative analysis of biochemical components and inorganic elements of coal miners' lung carcinoma tissue. Chinese J Prev Med 21:133-136

Occupational Epidemiology. H. Sakurai et al., editors

A RETROSPECTIVE COHORT MORTALITY STUDY OF WORKERS AT AN ELECTRIC CAPACITOR PLANT UTILYZING POLYCHLORINATED BIPHENYLS

T Sinks, AB Smith, G Steele, R Rinsky, K Watkins
Division of Surveillance, Hazard Evaluations, and Field Studies, National Institute for Occupational Safety and Health.
4676 Columbia Parkway R-10, Cincinnati, Ohio, 45226, USA.

Polychlorinated biphenyls (PCBs) are a class of compounds composed of biphenyl molecules with a varying number of substituted chlorine atoms. They were manufactured in the United States from 1929 until 1977 where they were widely used as a dielectric compound in electrical capacitors and transformers. Evidence for human carcinogenicity has not been well established. Previous reports of humans exposed to PCBs have reported moderate increased risks of liver and biliary cancer, cancer of the rectum, hematopoietic malignancies, and malignant melanoma.[1-3]

Presented here are the results from a retrospective cohort mortality study of workers at an electric capacitor manufacturing plant using PCBs from 1958-1977. Aroclor (Monsanto trade name) 1242 was used from 1959 to 1971 and Aroclor 1016 was used after 1971. Ten percent of the workforce was directly involved in capacitor manufacturing and had the greatest potential exposure to PCBs. However, environmental monitoring in 1977 demonstrated that the entire workforce had been exposed to PCBs.[4] Other chemical exposures at the plant included toluene, xylene, methyl ethyl ketone, trichloroethylene, and 1,1,1, trichloroethane.

Methods and Materials

Included in the analysis were 3575 white workers ever employed at this facility between January 1, 1957, when the plant opened, and March 31, 1977, the year when PCB use was discontinued. All white workers were included, regardless of their job or exposure to PCBs. Workers whose race was unknown were assumed to be white. Job histories were used to identify the date of first employment and the date of last employment. The last day of employment was March 31, 1977 or the actual last day of employment, whichever was earlier. Excluded from analysis were 14 nonwhite workers and 55 others for whom dates of birth or hire were missing.

Vital status was determined through the Social Security Administration (SSA). Copies of death certificates were acquired and the underlying cause of death determined by a qualified nosologist according to the International Classification of Diseases in effect at the time of death. Those whose vital status was unknown and those who died after June 30, 1986 were considered to be alive.

Person-years at-risk of dying were accumulated for each worker starting January 1, 1957 or on their first day of employment at the plant whichever occurred later and continued until the date of death or the study end date (June 30, 1986), whichever occurred first. The NIOSH life table computer program was used to combine sex and race-specific person-years at-risk into five-year calendar time periods and five-year age groups.[5] Expected numbers of cause-specific deaths were calculated by multiplying the age, sex, and calendar time specific United States mortality rates by the corresponding number of person-years at-risk. Person-years at-risk were additionally stratified into five-year employment and latency categories. The number of observed cause-specific deaths was divided by the number of expected cause-specific deaths to yield a Standardized Mortality Ratio (SMR). Ninety-five percent confidence intervals around the SMR were calculated using an approximation based on the Poisson distribution.[6]

Results

A total of 3575 persons were included in the final cohort; 191 were known to have died and 3384 were considered to be alive at the study end date. Overall mortality was less than expected as was the number of deaths due to all cancers combined.(Table 1) Fewer deaths were observed than expected for cancers of the digestive system with the exception of cancer of the biliary passages, liver, and gall bladder (1 observed: SMR=1.14; 95% CI 0.01 - 6.18). The number of observed deaths from cancer of the hematopoietic tissues (7) was equal to the number of deaths expected from this cause. The SMR for deaths due to cancer of the skin was significantly elevated (8 observed: SMR=4.06; 95% CI 1.75 - 8.01). All eight skin cancer deaths had an underlying cause of death from malignant melanoma. The SMR for cancer of the brain and nervous system was also elevated (5 observed: SMR=1.80, 0.58 - 4.22), but this elevation was not statistically significant. Death from diseases of the heart, the respiratory system, accidents, and violence were all well below expected.

All melanoma deaths occurred at least five years after employment began and the risk of mortality remained relatively stable after 5 years of latency.(Table 2) Two malignant melanoma deaths occurred in individuals with less than six months duration of employment and two others had worked between six months and five years. The SMR for skin cancer mortality was greatest for person-years accumulated with 10-14 years of duration of employment (3 observed, 0.23 expected).

All five brain cancer deaths occurred five or more years after initial employment.(Table 2) One brain cancer death occurred in an individual with

Table 1
Summary of Observed and Expected Deaths
All Whites Combined

Underlying Cause of Death	Observed Deaths	Expected Deaths	Ratio	95% C.I. Lower - Upper
All Causes	191	283.5	0.67**	0.58 - 0.78
All Cancers	54	63.4	0.85	0.64 - 1.11
Site Specific Cancers				
Buccal Cavity & Pharynx	0	1.6	----	
Digestive Organs & Peritoneum	8	13.8	0.57	0.25 - 1.14
Biliary Passages, Liver and Gall BLadder	1	0.9	1.14	0.01 - 6.18
Pancreas	2	2.8	0.70	0.08 - 2.55
Rectum	1	1.2	0.81	0.04 - 7.29
Respiratory System	15	20.2	0.74	0.42 - 1.23
Urinary System	2	2.5	0.81	0.49 - 1.35
Lymphatic & Hematopoietic	7	7.2	0.97	0.39 - 2.01
Skin@	8	2.0	4.06**	1.75 - 8.01
Brain and Nervous System**	5	2.8	1.80	0.58 - 4.22
All other sites combined	5	8.4	0.60	0.19 - 1.39
Diseases of the Heart	59	85.4	0.69**	0.52 - 0.89
Diseases of the Respiratory System	10	12.3	0.81	0.39 - 1.50
Accidents	27	41.3	0.65*	0.43 - 0.95
Violence	14	21.5	0.65	0.36 - 1.09

* - p less than 0.05; ** - p less than 0.01.
@ - Expected number of deaths were calculated using mortality rates for basal cell carcinoma, squamous cell carcinoma, and malignant melanoma combined. All observed skin cancer deaths were malignant melanomas.
**- Cancer of the brain and central nervous system included the following ICD codes: ICD 193 (6th & 7th revision); ICD 191, 192 (8th & 9th revision).

Table 2: Distribution of Observed and Expected Deaths by Latency and Duration of Employment:. All Whites Combined

LATENCY	1 day- 4 years	5 years- 9 years	10 years- 14 years	15 years- 19 years	20+ years	Total
Cancer of the Skin						
Observed	0	2	3	2	1	8
SMR		5.96	6.38*	3.86	2.32	4.06**
Cancer of the Brain						
Observed	0	2	1	2	0	5
SMR		4.03	1.57	2.97		1.80

DURATION OF EMPLOYMENT	1 day- 5 months	6 months- 4 years	5 years- 9 years	10 years- 14 years	15 years +	Total
Cancer of the Skin						
Observed	2	2	1	3	0	8
SMR	3.76	2.74	3.45	12.82**	0.00	4.06**
Cancer of the Brain						
Observed	1	0	1	2	1	5
SMR	1.39		2.37	5.82	3.65	1.80

Expected number of skin cancer deaths calculated for basal cell carcinoma, squamous cell carcinoma, and malignant melanoma combined. All observed skin cancer deaths were malignant melanoma.

Cancer of the brain and central nervous system included the following ICD codes: ICD 193 (6th & 7th revision); ICD 191, 192 (8th & 9th revision).
* - p less than 0.05; ** - p less than 0.01

less than six months duration of employment. The remaining four deaths occurred in workers with five or more years employment. The SMR for brain cancer was greatest for person-years accumulated with 10-14 years duration of exposure (2 observed, 0.34 expected).

The excess mortality from skin cancer and brain cancer was observed for both men and women. White men were at excess risk of mortality from skin cancer (6 observed: SMR=3.63; 95% CI 1.32 - 7.90) and cancer of the brain and central nervous system (4 observed: SMR=1.76; 95% CI 0.48 - 4.50). White women were also at excess risk of death from skin cancer (2 observed: SMR=6.63; 95% CI 0.70 - 22.57) and cancer of the brain and central nervous system (1 observed: SMR=2.01; 95% CI 0.05 - 11.21).

Discussion

The major finding of this study was the dramatic excess mortality from malignant melanoma. It is interesting to note that the death certificate of a ninth cohort member had malignant melanoma listed as a contributory cause. This excess mortality from malignant melanoma should be interpreted with caution. First, the results presented here reflect the risk of death for the entire cohort and do not take into account specific exposures to PCBs. Second, none of the previously reported cohort studies of capacitor plant workers found deaths caused by malignant melanoma.[2,3,7] Although the association between exposure to PCBs and malignant melanoma has been described previously, details regarding study methods, workplace exposures, latency, and duration of exposure were not reported and it is not possible to adequately assess this report.[4] Third, the increased malignant melanoma death risk seen in this cohort may have been the result of non-occupational risk factors specific to the geographic location of the plant. This seems unlikely, however, since melanoma mortality rates for the county where the plant is located have not been increased relative to state or national rates.[8]

The excess risk of mortality from cancer of the brain and nervous system has not been previously reported for capacitor manufacturing workers exposed to PCBs. The excess reported here was not statistically significant and may represent a chance finding. It should be noted that three additional workers in this cohort are known to have died having had brain cancer. Brain cancer was a contributory cause of death for one worker, the underlying cause of death in a second worker who died after the study end date, and the underlying cause of death in a a third worker excluded because of race.

This analysis had several limitations. Two assumptions were made that may have resulted in a conservative estimate of the malignant melanoma mortality risk for this cohort. We considered those whose vital status was unknown (13%) to have been alive until the study-end date, possibly missing additional deaths and over-estimating the person-years at-risk. We also assummed as white, those whose race was unknown. This would over-estimate the expected number of melanoma deaths if a substantial proportion of the cohort was not white.

In summary, this study found an excess of mortality from malignant melanoma and brain cancer in a cohort of 3575 capacitor manufacturing workers exposed to PCBs. This finding was consistent for both men and women. Future plans include the utilization of a job-exposure matrix based on environmental and biological PCB measurements collected at the plant in 1977.

References

1. Bertazzi PA, Riboldi L, Pesatori A, Radice L, Zochetti C. Cancer Mortality of electrochemical workers exposed to PCBs. Am.J.Ind.Med. 1987;11:165-176.

2. Brown DP. Mortality of workers exposed to polychlorinated biphenyls - an update. Arch Env Hlth. 1987;42:333-339.

3. Bahn AK, Rosenwaike I, Herrmann N, Grover P, Stellman J, O'Leary K. Melanoma after exposure to PCBs. NEJM, August 19, 1976:430.

4. Smith AB, Schloemer J, Lowry LK, Smallwood AW, Ligo RN, Tanaka S, Stringer W, Jones M, Hervin R, Glueck CJ. Metabolic and health consequences of occupational exposure to polychlorinated biphenyls. British Journal of Industrial Medicine. 1982;39:361-369.

5. Waxweiler RJ, Beaumont JJ, Henry JA, Brown DP, Robinson CF, Ness GO, Wagoner JK, Lemen RA. A modified life-table analysis system for cohort studies. JOM. 1983;25:115-123.

6. Rothman KJ, Boice JD. Epidemiologic Analysis with a Programmable Calculator. US Dept HEW. Pub. No 79-1649. 1979

7. Gustavsson P, Hogstedt C, Rappe C. Short-term mortality and cancer incidence in capacitor manufacturing workers exposed to polychlorinated biphenyls (PCBs). Am.J.Ind.Med. 1986;10:341-344.

8. Riggan WB, Van Bruggen J, Acquavella JF, Beaubier J, Mason TJ. U.S. Cancer Mortality Rates and Trends, 1950-1979. NCI/EPA Interagency Agreement on Environmental Carcinogenesis. Sept, 1983.

Occupational Epidemiology. H. Sakurai et al., editors

EPIDEMIOLOGIC CONSIDERATIONS ON LUNG CANCER RISK OF PNEUMOCONIOSIS PATIENTS AT 11 'ROSAI' HOSPITALS IN JAPAN

KEN TAKAHASHI[1], TOSHITERU OKUBO[1], KEIZOU CHIYOTANI[2] and KEN-ICHI SAITOH[2]

[1]Department of Environmental Epidemiology, University of Occupational and Environmental Health, Kitakyushu City, Japan
[2]Rosai Hospital for Silicosis, Tochigi Prefecture, Japan

MATERIALS AND METHODS

A joint survey project by 11 'Rosai' hospitals was organized in 1979 to examine the lung cancer mortality of pneumoconiosis patients[1]. 'Rosai' hospitals are specialized in the treatment of pneumoconiosis and other occupational diseases and injuries. Although there is no obligation for pneumoconiosis patients to be sent to these hospitals, they have played an important part in the treatment of the disease.

Pneumoconiosis patients in these hospitals who were qualified for the workmen's compensation as of the beginning of 1979 and who qualified thereafter were followed-up for five years, until the end of 1983. Female patients were excluded from the study and a total of 3,335 hospitalized male pneumoconiosis patients formed the cohort. As type of pneumoconiosis, silicosis and anthracosilicosis accounted for 96.5% of all pneumoconioses.

Age adjusted expected numbers were calculated by the person-years method using mortality of the general male population as the reference. The first year of follow-up for each patient was excluded from the calculation of person-years, and deaths occurring within that period were not counted.

RESULTS

Mortality from major causes of death is shown in Table 1. All cause mortality is elevated to an O/E ratio of 2.83 at the significant level. This is mainly attributed to the 345 deaths due to respiratory insufficiency due to pneumoconiosis. The relevant numbers for this cause are not shown because referent mortality rates were not available although reasonably assumed to be small. Among cancer deaths, the O/E ratio for lung cancer is highest at 4.80 and statistically significant.

Table 1 Mortality from major causes of death

Cause of death	O	E	O/E	95%CI
All causes	581	205.4	2.83	2.69-2.97
Neoplasms (140-208)	129	63.0	2.05	1.80-2.30
Esophagus(150)	7	3.1	2.26	1.12-3.39
Stomach(151)	26	19.3	1.35	0.89-1.80
Liver(155)	6	7.0	0.86	0.10-1.61
Pancreas(157)	7	3.4	2.06	0.97-3.14
Lung(162)	60	12.5	4.80	4.23-5.37
Leukemia(204-208)	2	1.1	1.82	0.00-3.73
Ischemic heart diseases (410-414)	8	16.1	0.50	0.00-1.00
Cerebrovascular diseases (430-438)	28	42.2	0.66	0.36-0.97

Table 2 Mortality for lung cancer (ICD 162) by smoking category

Smoking category	Person-years	O	E	O/E	95%CI
Never smoked	1229.3	4	1.8	2.22	0.73-3.71
Ex-smoker	3883.0	23	4.6	5.00	4.07-5.93
Current smoker	5894.5	33	6.1	5.41	4.60-6.22

Table 3 Summary of matched case-control comparisons by exposure, work history and industry

Exposure, work history, and industry	Total pairs (n=72)		Epidermoid cancer subgroup pairs(n=38)	
	Odds ratio	Chi square	Odds ratio	Chi square
Silicosis	5.67	9.80	12.00	9.31
Duration (years) of dusty work on the surface:				
≥ 10	0.67	0.40	1.00	0.00
≥ 20	1.00	0.00	2.00	0.33
≥ 30	0.75	0.14	0.50	0.33
Age (years) at first engagement in dusty work:				
< 20	1.73	2.13	1.83	1.47
< 30	1.90	2.79	1.50	0.60
< 40	2.00	0.33	1.00	0.00
Grade of pneumoconiosis by radiographic category:				
> 2	1.25	0.22	1.67	0.50
> 3	1.00	0.00	1.20	0.09
4	0.90	0.05	1.20	0.11
Work history:				
Quarrymen	1.33	0.57	1.83	1.47
Quarrymen or coal miners	0.57	1.64	0.50	1.33
Quarrymen, coal miners or other mine workers	2.00	1.00	3.00	1.00
Kilnmen or casters	∞	6.00	∞	3.00
Industry:				
Mining	1.83	1.47	1.67	0.50
Mining or tunnelling	1.75	0.82	1.50	0.20
Ceramics	∞	6.00	∞	3.20

In the cohort, the proportion of current smokers and ex-smokers combined was 10% higher than in the general population. Lung cancer mortality was classified according to smoking status as shown in Table 2. The highest O/E ratio was observed in the current smokers at 5.41, statistically significant. Ex-smokers showed a 5.00 O/E ratio, also statistically significant. Those who had never smoked had a 2.22 O/E ratio, though statistically not significant. The general male population consists of approximately 60% current smokers and 10 to 20% ex-smokers, the composition of which is reflected in the lung cancer mortality rate used as the reference. Thus it can be assumed that for the O/E ratio of non-smokers, the expected number is overestimated and the O/E ratio underestimated. The presence of some risk factor other than smoking was suggested from this table.

There was no dose-response relationship between lung cancer mortality and duration of dusty work or radiographic categories.[2]

A nested case-control study was performed to evaluate in detail the various risk factors for lung cancer such as exposure conditions and work histories. There were 73 lung cancer cases whose deaths were due to lung cancer and satisfied the diagnostic criteria for this analysis. The controls were selected from the cohort according to the following matching criteria: 1) pneumoconiosis patient in the same hospital, 2) alive at the time of death of the subject in the case-control study, 3) within ± three years of the subject's age at the time, 4) in the same dichotomous smoking category (never or ever smoker). A control case could not be found for one lung cancer case.

The results of the nested case-control analysis are shown in Table 3. Comparisons were repeated separately for the epidermoid cancer subgroup, which accounted for 57.5% of all the histological types of the lung cancer cases. As the type of pneumoconiosis, silicosis showed a significantly elevated odds ratio. When restricted to the epidermoid subgroup, the odds ratio was twice that of the total group. There was no clear tendency for difference in duration, age, or radiographic categories. Among the various work histories, a significantly elevated odds ratio was observed for kilnmen or casters. Among the type of industry, the ceramics industry showed a significantly elevated odds ratio.

DISCUSSION

These results were presented by Chiyotani, our co-worker, at the seventh International Pneumoconioses Conference in 1988. There are several sources of bias that were identified in this study which requires evaluation from an epidemiologic point of view.

To cope with the problem of selection bias, we excluded from the calculation the first follow-up year of person-years and the deaths occurring within that period. This procedure was meant to avoid the inclusion of cases with already diagnosed serious diseases, such as cancer, into the cohort. The results showed that lung cancer was the only cause of death for which the mortality was clearly elevated when compared to the reference. It is therefore inferred that the factor of high-risk patients being accumulated in specialized hospitals had been controlled by this method.

Comparison with the general population could have been misleading for two reasons. One is the influence by the likelihood of hospitalized pneumoconiosis patients to receive frequent X-ray check-ups in the course of their diseases and thus lead to early detection of lung cancer cases. This possibility will deviate the O/E ratio downward as long as effective treatment is initiated. The other is the influence by the complication of two serious and deteriorating diseases, i.e. lung cancer and pneumoconiosis. Surgery indications or therapeutic measures for lung cancer could be affected so as to shift in disfavor the expected survival curve of the "general" lung cancer patient. This possibility, had it occurred, will, in turn deviate the O/E ratio upward.

In summary, an excess of lung cancer was found in a cohort study of hospitalized pneumoconiosis patients. Several sources of bias were identified and evaluated but no single source of such bias could explain the observed elevated risk.

REFERENCES

1. Chiyotani K, et al (1983) In: VIth International Pneumoconiosis Conference, Volume 1: pp 228-236. Excess risk of lung cancer deaths in hospitalized pneumoconiotic patients.

2. Chiyotani K, et al (1987) Jap J Trauma Occup Med 35:554-561

Occupational Epidemiology. H. Sakurai et al., editors

NATURAL KILLER CELL ACTIVITY IN WORKERS EXPOSED TO OCCUPATIONAL CARCINOGENS

TAKESHI TANIGAWA*, SHUNICHI ARAKI*, SUMIKO ISHIZU**, TAKAHARU ARAKI***
KAZUHITO YOKOYAMA*
*) Department of Public Health, School of Medicine, University of Tokyo, 7-3-1, Hongo, Bunkyo-ku, Tokyo 113 (Japan)
**) Occupational Health Service Center, Shiba, Minato-ku, Tokyo 108 (Japan)
***) Center of Occupational Medicine, Tokyo Labor Accidence Hospital, Omoriminami, Ota-ku, Tokyo 143 (Japan)

Natural killer (NK) cells are a subpopulation of lymphocytes with the capability to lyse a variety of aberrant cells independent of the major histocompatibility complex. In recent years, evidences are accumulating that NK cells have an important role in inhibition of tumourigenesis (1). At present, however, there are few systemic reports on NK cells in workers at a high risk for occupational cancer. In this study, we measured the number as well as the activity of NK cells in the peripheral blood of workers with history of occupational exposure to aromatic amines and chromate.

SUBJECTS

<u>Workers exposed to aromatic amines</u>

Subjects were 63 males exposed to benzidine or beta-naphthylamine (aromatic amines, AA) until 1972. Thirty-one of these subjects, aged 54 to 70 (mean 62), had been previously treated for bladder cancer and then cured (ex-cancer AA workers). The remaining subjects, aged 43 to 69 (mean 58), had not been diagnosed as bladder cancer (non-cancer AA workers). Control subjects were 33 healthy male volunteers aged 42 to 64 (mean 54).

<u>Workers exposed to chromate</u>

Subjects were 23 male retired workers with a past history of occupational exposure to chromate (Cr workers); ages ranged from 53 to 74 (mean 64). Control subjects were 12 healthy males aged 41 to 64 (mean 53).

None of the subjects and controls had signs and symptoms indicative of infection at the time of the study or had used medications which might affect immunological parameters. Smoking habits in ex- and non-cancer AA workers, and Cr workers were not significantly different from those in their control groups.

METHODS

Peripheral blood mononuclear cells (PBMC) were isolated from heparinized peripheral blood by Ficoll-Conray density centrifugation. NK cell activity was determined by the ^{51}Cr release assay using K562 as target cells (2). Target cells were labelled with ^{51}Cr, washed and suspended in 10 % FCS-RPMI1640 medium. 10^4 of target cells was mixed with varying numbers of PBMC in a microculture plate at the effector to target (E:T) ratios of 5:1, 10:1, 20:1, and 40:1. The plate was incubated for 4 hours. Radioactivity released into the supernatant (X) was then counted by a gamma counter. The spontaneous (S) and maximal (M) ^{51}Cr releases were determined by incubating labelled target cells with medium alone and with 1% Triton X-100, respectively.

The percent specific cytolysis was calculated as (X - S) x 100 / (M - S) (%). Using the regression equation of these values to the logarithm of the E:T ratios, "one" lytic unit (LU) was defined as the number of effector cells required for 33.3% specific cytolysis of 10^4 target cells (N). The gross NK activity in peripheral blood was expressed as $10^7/N$ (LUs/10^7 cells).

To determine the relative frequency of NK cells, PBMC were incubated with FITC-conjugated monoclonal anti-Leu-11a antibody (Becton Dickinson), and analyzed by a Coulter EPICS V flowcytometer. Leu-11a positive cells are shown to represent lymphocytes with NK activity (3). "Unit NK cell activity" was approximated by dividing the gross NK activity (LUs/10^7 cells) by a percentage of Leu-11a positive cells.

RESULTS

Workers exposed to aromatic amines

There was no significant difference in the gross NK activity among three groups (TABLE I) . The mean percentage of Leu-11a positive cells in lymphocytes in AA workers, however, was significantly higher than that in the control group (Fig. 1) . Between ex-cancer and non-cancer AA workers, no difference was observed. As a result, both ex-cancer and non-cancer AA workers showed significantly reduced "unit NK cell activity" as compared with the control group (Fig. 2) .

TABLE I
THE GROSS NK ACTIVITY IN EX- AND NON-CANCER AA WORKERS AND CONTROLS

Subjects	Median	Range
Ex-cancer AA workers	43.7	0.03 - 177
Non-cancer AA workers	20.1	0.5 - 269
Controls	47.1	3.7 - 104

AA= aromatic amines

Workers exposed to chromate

The mean gross NK activity was significantly higher in Cr workers than in the control group (Fig. 3). Peripheral blood cells of Cr workers were lymphocytopenic as compared with controls. Cr workers had significantly elevated proportion of Leu-11a positive cells than controls, although there was no significant difference in absolute number of Leu-11a positive cells (TABLE II). There was no significant difference in "unit NK cell activity" between Cr workers and controls.

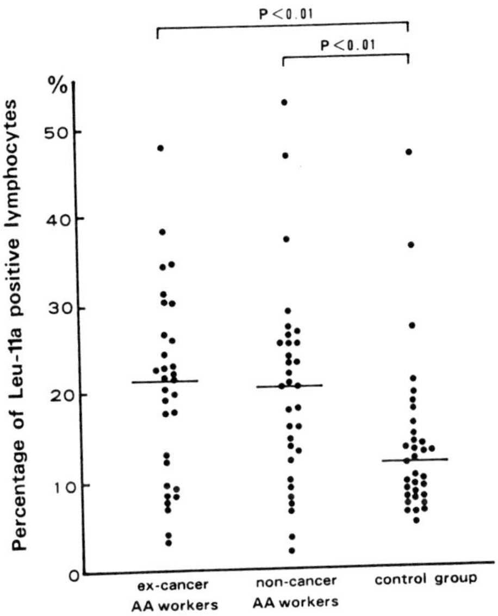

Fig. 1. Percentage of Leu-11a positive cells in in lymphocytes in AA workers and controls. Transverse lines are median values.

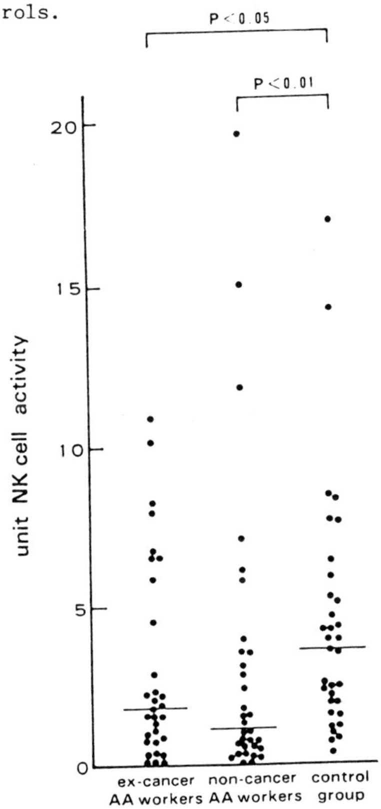

Fig. 2. Unit NK cell activity in AA workers and controls. Transverse lines as Fig. 1.

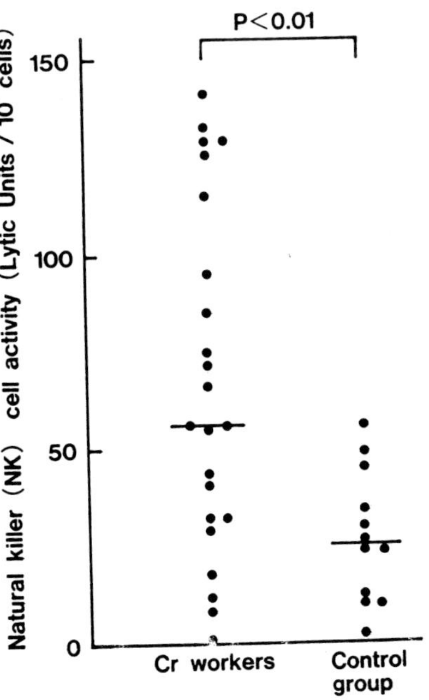

Fig. 3. The gross NK activity in Cr workers and controls. Transverse lines as Fig. 1.

TABLE II

DIFFERENCES IN NUMBERS OF LYMPHOCYTES AND LEU-11A POSITIVE CELLS BETWEEN CR WORKERS AND CONTROLS (MEDIAN VALUES WITH RANGES IN PARENTHESES)

	Cr workers	Controls
lymphocytes:		
Proportion to leukocytes (%)	33 (18-44)*	41 (28-54)*
Number per 1mm^3 of whole blood	2100 (1200-3400)**	3300 (2000-4500)**
Leu-11a positive cells:		
Proportion to lymphocytes (%)	10.3 (3.9-42.6)*	5.1 (1.7-20.9)*
Number per 1mm^3 of whole blood	270 (60-1000)	140 (50-550)

** $p<0.001$, * $p<0.01$ (Wilcoxon rank sum test).

DISCUSSION

We found the abnormalities on NK cells in both high risk groups. There, however, were some differences in the details (TABLE III).

The common finding in two groups was the increased relative Leu-11a positive cells. It is already reported that Leu-11a positive cells are also increased in overt bladder cancer and lung cancer patients. It thus seems that this finding is extended into the high risk populations before overt cancer patients.

"Unit NK cell activity", on the other hand, was decreased in AA workers but not in Cr workers. This difference between AA and Cr workers might reflect the degrees of risk for cancers, in which the former has by far greater risk than the latter.

TABLE III

ABNORMALITIES ON NATURAL KILLER (NK) CELLS IN AA AND CR WORKERS

	AA workers	Cr workers
Proportion of Leu-11a positive cells	increased	increased
Gross NK activity	normal range	increased
Unit NK cell activity	decreased	normal range

AA = aromatic amines

In conclusion, the combination of the measurements of the proportion of Leu-11a positive cells and "unit NK cell activity" may provide one of the predictive indicators of the risk for occupational cancers. The follow-up study of the high risk groups should clarify this point.

REFERENCE

1 Bloom BR (1982) Nature 18:214-5

2 Minato N, Takeda A, Kano S, Takaku F (1982) J Clin Invest 69:581-8

3 Lanier LL, Le AM, Phillips JH et al. (1983) JImmunol 131:1789-96

4 Tanigawa T, Araki S, Ishizu S et al. Br J Ind Med (in press)

Occupational Epidemiology. H. Sakurai et al., editors

549423

WOOD DUST EXPOSURE AND SQUAMOUS CELL CANCERS OF THE UPPER RESPIRATORY TRACT

THOMAS L. VAUGHAN, MD, MPH.

Program in Epidemiology (MP-474), Fred Hutchinson Cancer Research Center, 1124 Columbia St., Seattle, WA 98104, USA.

INTRODUCTION

Exposure to wood dust, particularly from hardwoods during furniture manufacturing, has been convincingly demonstrated to increase the risk of adenocarcinoma of the sinonasal cavity (1,2). However, a number of questions remain concerning the relationship between wood dust and cancer, including:

- Is wood dust exposure also related to squamous cell carcinoma?
- Does exposure *via* other occupations increase sinonasal cancer risk?
- Are cancers of other respiratory sites associated with wood dust?

These questions were addressed using data from two population-based case-control studies which investigated squamous cell carcinomas of the sinonasal cavity (SNC), nasopharynx (NPC), oro- and hypopharynx (OPC), and larynx (LC).

METHODS

Both studies were carried out using cases identified by the Cancer Surveillance System of the Fred Hutchinson Cancer Research Center. This population-based registry attempts to identify all cancers occurring in 13 counties of western Washington State, an area with a population of approximately three million. The first study included cases of pharyngeal cancer diagnosed between 1980 and 1983 and sinonasal cancer diagnosed between 1979 and 1983. Interviews were successfully completed for 71% of those eligible. Approximately half of the interviews were with the cancer patients themselves and half with surrogates, usually the spouse. The second study focused on the three largest counties and included cases of laryngeal cancer diagnosed between September, 1983 and February, 1987. Of eligible cases identified, interviews were completed for 81%, all but 7% with the patients themselves. After excluding non-squamous cell tumors, the following numbers of cases were analyzed: OPC - 183, SNC - 27, NPC - 21, LC - 234.

In each study, controls were selected by random digit dialing to be similar in age and sex distribution to the cases, with at least twice as many in each 5-year age-sex stratum. For the first study, 96% of households contacted were successfully screened. Of those screened households with eligible subjects, 83% completed the interview, yielding 552 available for analysis. For the second study, 95% of households were screened, and 80% of eligible subjects were interviewed, leaving 547 for analysis.

Interviews for the first study were completed by phone, and for the second, in person. Lifetime occupational histories were obtained, including a description of the duties involved in each job, as well as the associated industry. Information on additional risk factors, including smoking and alcohol history was also recorded. Jobs considered to entail significant exposure to wood dust included: carpenters, forestry and logging workers, precision woodworkers (including patternmakers, cabinet makers and other furniture makers and finishers), and woodworking machine operators.

The odds ratio was calculated as an estimate of the relative risk (RR) of disease associated with employment in wood-related occupations. Stratified analysis and logistic regression were used to control as necessary for the potential confounding effects of age, sex, race, cigarette smoking and alcohol consumption. The effects of duration of employment and a hypothesized 15 year induction period on RR estimates were also investigated.

RESULTS

In both studies, the proportion of controls with a history of ever working in a wood-related occupation was approximately 11% (Table 1). This contrasts strongly with the 26% of SNC cases who had ever held such an occupation, but only slightly with the job history of NPC cases (14%). A similar proportion of persons with OPC and LC had ever worked in such jobs (9% and 11% respectively). The same pattern held when only jobs 15 or more years before diagnosis were counted.

After adjusting for the risk factors above, the relative risk estimates and 95%

TABLE 1
HISTORY OF EMPLOYMENT IN WOOD-RELATED OCCUPATIONS

	Subject Type	Ever Employed	(%)	Employed 15+ Years Before Dx	(%)
Study #1					
	Sinonasal Cavity	7	(25.9)	7	(25.9)
	Nasopharynx	3	(14.3)	3	(14.3)
	Oro- and Hypopharynx	14	(7.7)	12	(6.6)
	Control	60	(10.9)	43	(7.8)
Study #2					
	Larynx	27	(11.5)	21	(9.0)
	Control	61	(11.2)	52	(9.5)

confidence intervals (CI) associated with ever having worked in one of the four wood-related occupations were 2.1 (0.8-5.9) for SNC, 1.1 (0.3-4.5) for NPC, 0.6 (0.3-1.2) for OPC, and 0.9 (0.5-1.5) for LC. When an induction period was taken into account, the RR for SNC increased to 2.7 (CI = 1.0-7.6) with a significant trend test for duration of work (p=0.02). For NPC the RR increased to 1.4 (0.4-5.4), whereas the overall RR's for the other two sites remained below one. When exposure was defined as long-term employment (10 or more years) taking place at least 15 years before the reference date, the RR's for SNC and NPC increased markedly, to 6.0 and 5.6 respectively, while the RR's for OPC and LC increased slightly, to 1.8 and 1.6. These data are summarized in Figure 1.

Focusing on individual occupations, the largest risk of SNC was found to be associated with a history of employment as a wood working machine operator in the lumber and wood products industry. The overall RR of 7.9 (CI=1.6-39.2) increased to 28.9 for subjects with long-term employment 15 years or more before diagnosis. None of the seven exposed SNC cases had worked as precision woodworkers (including furniture makers), in contrast to four of the controls. All exposed NPC cases had worked as carpenters, for whom an overall RR of 3.3 (CI=0.8-13.2) was calculated, with a significant trend test (p=0.02). For OPC and LC, no individual wood-related occupation was associated with increased risk.

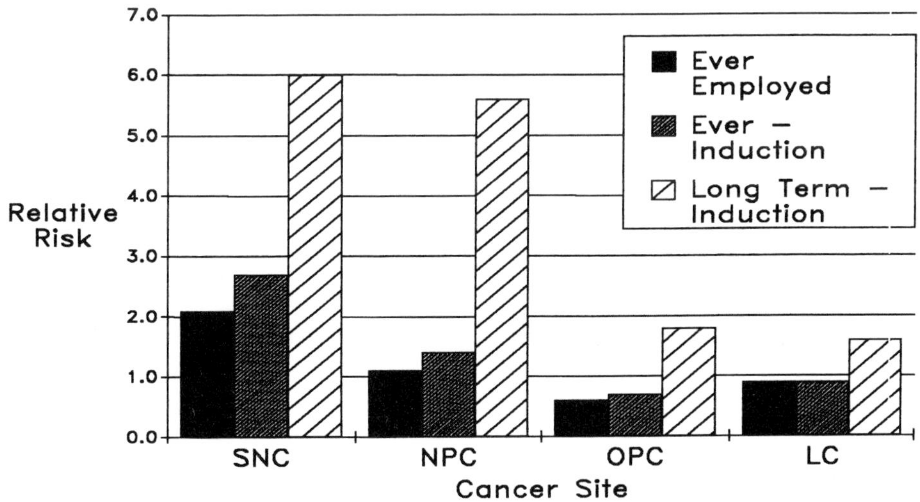

Figure 1. Relative risk of squamous cell cancer of the upper respiratory tract in wood-related occupations. RR's are adjusted for age, sex, cigarette smoking history, alcohol consumption and race as necessary. Exposure is calculated in three ways: i) including all years of employment (ever), ii) excluding the most recent 15 years (ever - induction), and iii) counting only persons with 10 or more years of employment after excluding the most recent 15 years (long term - induction).

DISCUSSION

These results support the hypothesis that wood dust exposure increases the risk of squamous cell cancer of the sinonasal cavity. In addition, they indicate that exposure in occupations other than furniture manufacturing may be etiologically relevant. The most likely type of exposure in these jobs in Washington State is to relatively large-sized softwood particles.

A number of previous studies are consistent with these findings, although not all are in agreement (reviewed in (3)). It should be noted that although the RR for adenocarcinoma associated with furniture work is probably very large (4), squamous cell carcinomas are much more common, typically representing over half of SNC tumors. From the present study, it is estimated that 11% of all SNC squamous cell cancers occurring in western Washington can be attributed to wood dust exposure occurring primarily in the wood product manufacturing industry.

There is some evidence that squamous cell carcinomas of the nasopharynx are also related to wood dust exposure. The few studies that have looked at this site support this hypothesis (3,5,6). There is very little support in this study for an association with other cancers of the upper respiratory tract. The 60 - 80% increases in risk for LC and OPC with long term exposure in the distant past are suggestive of a small effect, but can also be explained by chance.

An important conservative bias in this study is the reliance on job titles as a surrogate for wood dust exposure. The very small numbers of SNC and NPC cases available are also limiting factors. A larger multi-centered study of NPC in the U.S. is currently underway in which over 200 cases will eventually be assembled; it is hoped that this study will yield more definitive information on the risks associated with this common exposure.

REFERENCES

1. Macbeth RG (1965) Malignant disease of the paranasal sinuses. J Laryngol Otol 79:592-612.
2. Acheson ED, Cowdell RH, Rang EH (1981) Nasal cancer in England and Wales: an occupational survey. Br J Ind Med 38:218-24.
3. Vaughan, TL (In Press) re: Case-control study of nasal cancer in workers employed in wood-related industries. J Occ Med.
4. Acheson ED, Cowdell RH, Rang E (1972) Adenocarcinoma of the nasal cavity and sinuses in England and Wales. Br J Ind Med 29:21-30.
5. Hardell L, Johansson B, Axelson O (1982) Epidemiological study of nasal and nasopharyngeal cancer and their relation to phenoxy acid or chlorophenol exposure. Am J Ind Med 3:247-257.
6. Ng TP (1986) A case-referent study of cancer of the nasal cavity and sinuses in Hong Kong. Int J Epidemiol 15:171-175.

RESPIRATORY DISEASES
Pneumoconiosis

Occupational Epidemiology. H. Sakurai et al., editors

CLINICAL ASPECTS OF PNEUMOCONIOSIS IN VARIOUS DUST WORKERS

YOSHIHARU AIZAWA, TSUTOMU TAKATA, KIICHIRO HASHIMOTO, MAMORU TOMINAGA and HIROSHI TATSUMI

Department of Preventive Medicine and Public Health, School of Medicine, Kitasato University, 1-15-1, Kitasato, Sagamihara, Kanagawa 228 (Japan)

INTRODUCTION

Pneumoconiosis statistics in Japan are annually issued from the Ministry of Labor (1). The document does not describe the pictures of pneumoconiosis in detail. The clinical aspects of specific dust workers have been already described (2-4). However, the comparison of clinical pictures of all kinds of dust work has not been studied. In this study, the aspects observed in 10 types of dust work were studied on the basis of nationwide data obtained at pneumoconiosis examinations.

MATERIAL AND METHODS

Pneumoconiosis examination in Japan

Pneumoconiosis examination consists of obtaining occupational history related to dust work, a chest radiograph, clinical chest examination, examination for complications and pulmonary function tests.

Chest radiographs are classified according to the Japanese Classification of Radiographs of Pneumoconiosis. Radiographic appearances are classified into one of six categories(PR1 to PR4C).

Pulmonary function tests consist in conducting spirometry, obtaining flow volume curve and making blood gas analysis if necessary. The absence of pulmonary dysfunction is indicated by F(-), requirement for blood gas analysis as F(+) and a considerable degree of pulmonary dysfunction as F(++).

The radiograph and statements certifying the results of pneumoconiosis examination are submitted to the Chief of the Prefectural Labor Standards Office if an examinee is diagnosed as having signs of pneumoconiosis on the chest radiograph. The mode of pneumoconiosis supervision is determined by the Chief of the Prefectural Labour Standards Office on the basis of radiograph and degree of pulmonary dysfunction. No.1 supervision is for persons considered unaffected by pneumoconiosis. No.2 supervision is for those whose radiographic appearances correspond to category 1(PR1), No.3A is for category 2(PR2) and No.3B is for category 3(PR3), 4A(PR4A) or 4B(PR4B). No.4 is for those whose radiographic appearances correspond to category 4C(PR4C) or who have considerable pulmonary dysfunction due to pneumoconiosis.

Subjects

There were 260,629 examinee among 589,758 workers exposed to dust in Japan in 1985. Among them 44,531 persons were diagnosed as having signs of pneumoconiosis on the chest radiographs by physicians. Copies of 44,531 statements of the results of pneumoconiosis examination were sent to us from 47 Prefectural Labour Standards Offices from April 1, 1985 to March 31, 1986. A total of 39,670 statements was analyzed in this study following exclusion of statements not adequately documented, those with negative pneumoconiotic signs on chest radiograph diagnosed by Prefectural Labour Standards Offices or those of minor dust workers such as glass or others.

The types of dust work consisted of welding(21.6%), excavation(17.9%), pottery manufacture(17.1%), foundry(14.7%), grinding(9.4%), carbon

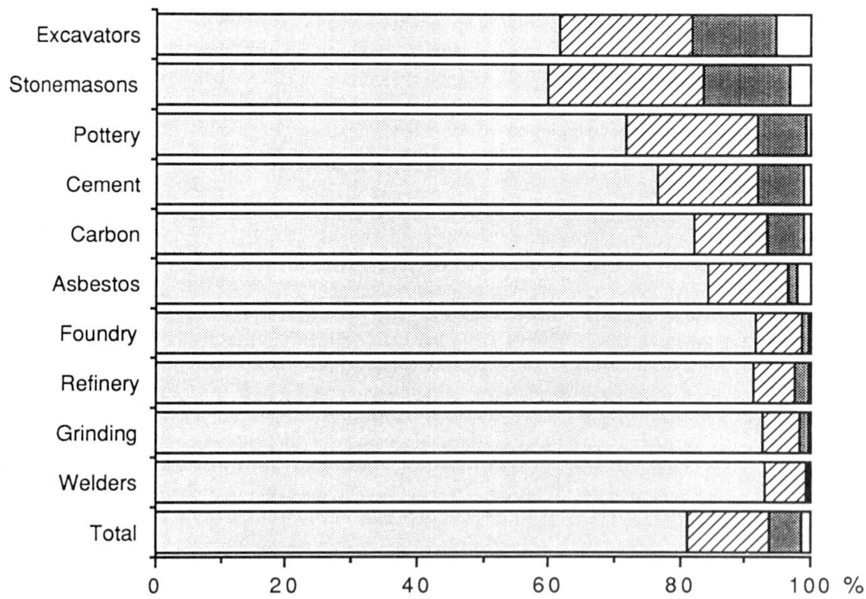

Fig. 1. Modes of supervision given to the workers or ex-workers engaged in ten types of dust work. ☐ = No.2. ▨ = No.3A. ■ = No.3B. ☐ = No.4.

manufacture(7.0%), refinery(5.6%), stone(3.4%), asbestos(1.8%) and cement manufacture(1.5%).

RESULTS AND DISCUSSION

Mode of Supervision

The No.2 mode was most frequent(93.0%) while No.3B(0.5%) and No.4(0.2%) were rarely applicable among welders. Essentially the same modes were found applicable to foundry, grinding and refinery workers. The No.2 mode was most frequent(61.6%), with No.3B(12.7%) and No.4(5.3%) being somewhat less among excavators. Stonemasons required essentially the same modes of supervision. Pottery makers and workers exposed to carbon, asbestos and cement indicated intermediate between welders and excavators.

Chest radiographs

The proportion of category 3-or-higher on chest radiograph was noticeable among excavators and stonemasons(14%), whereas it was negligible among welders, grinding, refinery, foundry and asbestos workers(<2%).

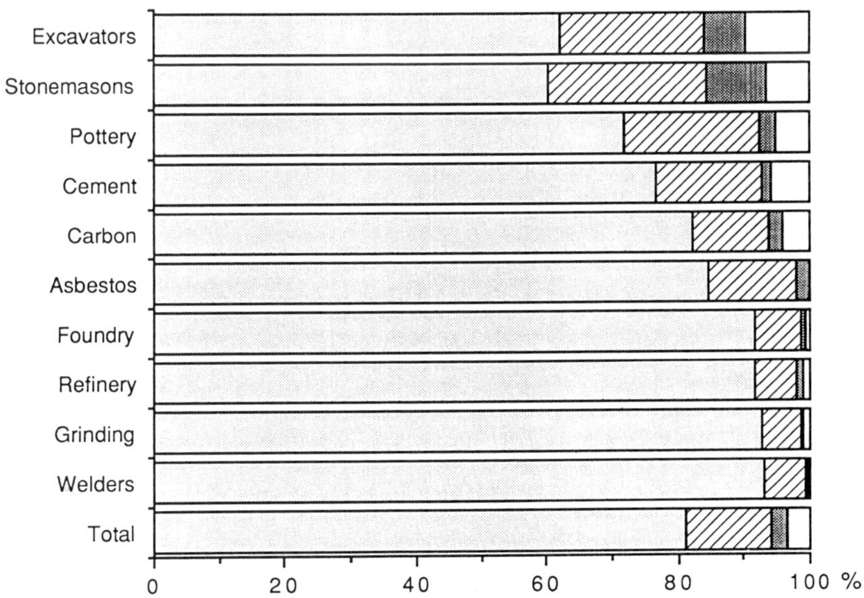

Fig. 2. Categories of chest radiographs diagnosed for the workers or ex-workers engaged in ten types of dust work. ▢ = PR1. ▨ = PR2. ▩ = PR3. ☐ = PR4.

Pulmonary dysfunction

A considerable degree of pulmonary dysfunction was applicable to 2.0-4.5% of dust workers such as excavators, stonemasons and asbestos workers, while it was negligible among welders, foundry, grinding, refinery workers (<0.5%).

Abnormal spirometry was observed in more than 25% of excavators, stonemasons and asbestos workers, while it was observed in less than 15% of foundry, refinery workers and welders. The restrictive ventilatory impairment was conspicuous in asbestos workers.

Relationship between chest radiographs and pulmonary dysfunction

The degrees of pulmonary dysfunction increased in proportion as advanced categories of profusion of small opacities on chest radiographs in all kinds of dust work.

ACKNOWLEDGMENTS

This study was supported by a grant from the Ministry of Labor in Japan. Assistance of Ms. Yumiko Sugiura and Ms. Kimiyo Yajima was greatly acknowledged.

REFERENCES

1. Ministry of Labour (1986) Annual guide of industrial hygiene in Japan. Japan Industrial Safety and Health Association, Tokyo, pp 226-228

2. Crosbie WA (1986) Arch Environ Health 41:346-353

3. Moore E, Martin JR, Edwards AC, Muir DCF (1987) Arch Environ Health 42:351-355

4. Collins HPR, Dick JA, Bennett JG, Pern PO, Rickards MA, Thomas DJ, Washington JS, Jacobsen M (1988) Br J Ind Med 45:43-55

Occupational Epidemiology. H. Sakurai et al., editors

EVALUATION OF VENTILATORY FUNCTION IN COAL WORKERS' PNEUMOCONIOSIS

CHEE KYUNG CHUNG, KYU SANG CHO, SEI KON KIM
Industrial Medical Center, Catholic University Medical College,
Seoul 137-701 (Korea)

INTRODUCTION

In Korea, anthracite has been traditionally in wide use both at home and in industries and, therefore, anthracite mining has always been the major source of pneumoconiosis. The prevalence rate of suspects or more simple pneumoconiosis in anthracite mines reaches at present 14.5 % among coalface workers and even 24.3 % among rock drillers (1, 2). Accordingly, the control of pneumoconiosis has always been a serious problem in coping with occupational diseases.

Necessary for establishing a diagnosis of pneumoconiosis are a history of exposure to coal dust and certain relatively characteristics abnormalities on the chest radiograph. The respiratory impairments due to pneumoconiosis are evaluated by lung function tests. Since the respiratory impairments do not always coincide with radiographic findings of pneumoconiosis, lung function tests are most useful in assessing the extent of disability to determine the compensation for pneumoconiosis patients. The ventilatory function tests which reflect the obstructive changes in the airways are now widely used in the evaluation of respiratory impairments of pneumoconiosis patients because the obstructive type of ventilatory impairments is at present by far the commonest change in lung functions (3).

This study was carried out to evaluated the ventilatory impairments and to find out a more sensitive test for evaluating the degree of respiratory impairments in different radiographic categories of coal workers' pneumoconiosis.

MATERIAL AND METHODS

The subjects of this study comprised 2818 anthracite coal miners who were diagnosed as pneumoconiosis on the basis of occupational history and chest radiograph. Pneumoconiosis was classified according to ILO U/C international classification of radiographs of pneumoconioses (4), i.e. 542 patients were suspects, 2128 patients small opacities and 148 patients large opacities. The subjects were aged 44.7 ± 6.8 (mean ± SD) years in suspect group, 45.2 ± 6.3 years in small opacity group and 45.4 ± 6.5 years in large opacity group. Their heights were 165.4 ± 5.5 cm in suspect group, 165.6 ± 5.3 cm in small opacity group and 165.5 ± 5.4 cm in large opacity group.

The various ventilatory parameters, such as FVC, $FEV_{1.0}$, MMF, $FVC_{t(0.25-0.75)}$, PFR, $\dot{V}_{max}$ 50 and $\dot{V}_{max}$ 75, were obtained by analyzing forced expiratory spirogram and maximal expiratory flow-volume curve which were measured by Flow-Volume Curve

Recorder in a standing position. The exercise index was obtained from MVV, exercise ventilation and minute volume at rest which were measured by spirometer and two step-test.

The concentration of the respirable dust fraction was measured by weight and its free silica content was determined by the X-ray diffraction method. The mean respirable dust concentration in the air was 3.07 ± 1.78 mg/m^3 with the mean free silica content of 1.63 ± 1.30 %.

RESULTS

The mean values of all ventilatory parameters expressed in percentage of the predicted significantly decreased from category 2 compared with those of suspects (Tab. 1). Among those paratmeters, MMF, $FVC_{t(0.25-0.75)}$, $\dot{V}_{max}$ 50 and $\dot{V}_{max}$ 75 markedly changed with the progress of pneumoconiosis. However, $FVC_{t(0.25-0.75)}$ may not be practical to perform lung function test as a reliable measurement for evaluating the ventilatory impairments because it may be more complex and difficult to calculate. In general, the ventilatory function tended to decrease gradually with the progress of pneumoconiosis.

TABLE 1

MEAN VALUES OF VENTILATORY PARAMETERS BY THE CATEGORY OF SIMPLE PNEUMOCONIOSIS

Category / Parameter	0/1 (Susp)	1/0-1/2	2/1-2/3	3/2-3/4	1/0-3/4 (SRO)
FVC, % pred	100.3 (13.7)	100.4 (13.2)	96.9 (14.2)	94.3 (13.8)	98.7 (13.7)
$FEV_{1.0}$, % pred	91.6 (16.4)	90.9 (15.7)	86.3 (17.0)	83.8 (17.9)	88.6 (16.6)
$FEV_{1.0}$/FVC, %	77.7 (9.5)	76.8 (8.7)	75.3 (9.7)	74.9 (10.0)	76.1 (9.2)
MMF, % pred	74.5 (30.1)	71.6 (28.3)	65.5 (27.8)	64.1 (28.9)	68.9 (28.4)
$FVC_{t(0.25-0.75)}$, % pred	147.3 (74.2)	150.5 (68.4)	162.3 (78.4)	165.9 (87.5)	155.8 (74.3)
PFR, % pred	90.6 (18.2)	91.2 (17.4)	87.5 (19.2)	86.1 (20.2)	89.5 (18.4)
$\dot{V}_{max}$ 50, % pred	82.6 (32.6)	79.8 (31.0)	73.5 (30.8)	72.4 (32.9)	77.0 (31.4)
$\dot{V}_{max}$ 75, % pred	77.7 (38.3)	74.9 (33.9)	71.7 (33.2)	70.5 (36.7)	73.4 (34.1)
MVV, % pred	105.6 (18.8)	106.7 (18.6)	102.5 (20.7)	98.4 (20.9)	104.5 (19.7)
EI, %	26.7 (7.7)	26.3 (7.5)	28.8 (9.2)	30.6 (9.8)	27.6 (8.5)

( ) ; Standard deviation

In pneumoconiosis patients with large opacities, the mean values of ventilatory parameters significantly decreased compared with those of suspects and small opacities. This finding was noticeable in category B and C (Tab. 2).

TABLE II

MEAN VALUES OF VENTILATORY PARAMETERS BY THE CATEGORY OF PNEUMOCONIOSIS WITH LARGE OPACITIES

Category / Parameter	A	B	C	Total
FVC, % pred	85.6±14.0	73.6±19.2	76.7±14.1	76.1±17.8
$FEV_{1.0}$, % pred	66.7±18.6	52.9±20.8	47.0±14.7	56.1±20.3
$FEV_{1.0}$/FVC, %	65.5±13.4	59.2±12.2	57.9±11.9	61.0±12.8
MMF, % pred	41.5±24.1	29.5±19.2	24.3±12.8	32.3±20.8
$FVC_{t(0.25-0.75)}$, % pred	277.7±111.1	285.9±118.5	303.9±128.9	274.2±120.8
PFR, % pred	68.4±22.5	53.3±21.3	45.5±18.0	56.4±22.7
$\dot{V}_{max}$ 50, % pred	48.1±24.1	37.0±19.4	31.9±15.5	39.5±21.5
$\dot{V}_{max}$ 75, % pred	47.6±26.8	37.9±25.9	32.4±20.2	39.8±25.5
MVV, % pred	82.5±20.4	64.7±22.0	55.7±15.5	68.5±22.6
EI, %	38.9±10.4	45.1±13.8	52.0±16.4	44.7±14.3

FVC: Forced vital capacity, $FEV_{1.0}$: Forced expiratory volume in one second, MMF: Maximal mid-expiratory flow, $FVC_{t(0.25-0.75)}$: Time to expire the middle half of FVC, PFR: Peak flow rate, $\dot{V}_{max}$ 50: Maximal expiratory flow at 50 % of expired FVC, $\dot{V}_{max}$ 75: Maximal expiratory flow at 75 % of expired FVC, MVV: Maximal voluntary ventilation, EI: Exercise index = (exercise ventilation/ MBC) x 100

The respiratory impairments of pneumoconiosis at rest do not always coincide with work capacity because of the mechanism and the reserving capacity of the lungs. Therefore, an excercise test is necessary for assessing the degree of disability to determine the compensation for pneumoconiosis patients. The exercise index(EI) and MMF were more sensitive indices than the other ventilatory parameters for evaluating the vetilatory impairments of pneumoconiosis. The proportions of patients with substandard EI and MMF were 45.8 % and 40.2 % in suspect group and 56.1 % and 47.5 % in small opacity group, whereas the proportions of patients with substandard FVC, $FEV_{1.0}$/FVC and MVV were lower than the other parameters (Tab. 3).

Table 4 illustrated the number of cases with abnormal findings of other ventilatory parameters among patients with normal FVC, $FEV_{1.0}$/FVC and MVV which are now used in the evaluation of respiratory impairments of pneumoconiosis. MMF had the highest rate in ventilatory parameters.

TABLE III

PERCENT OF PATIENTS WITH SUBSTANDARD VENTILATORY PARAMETERS IN EACH CATEGORY OF PNEUMOCONIOSIS

Category / Parameter	0/1 (Susp)	1/0-1.2	2/1-2/3	3/2-3/4	1/0-3/4 (SRO)	A-C(LO)
No of subject	542	1,252	607	269	2,128	148
FVC	6.5	6.5	11.9	14.1	9.0	56.1
$FEV_{1.0}$	28.4	29.8	40.7	40.6	35.2	91.9
$FEV_{1.0}$/FVC	17.0	18.5	25.0	26.4	21.4	75.0
MMF	40.2	43.3	52.9	54.6	47.5	91.9
$FVC_{t(0.25-0.75)}$	34.9	38.7	44.8	45.0	41.2	81.1
PFR	23.6	23.4	29.2	30.1	25.9	82.4
$\dot{V}_{max}$ 50	28.4	31.2	39.5	39.8	34.6	87.8
$\dot{V}_{max}$ 75	34.1	36.5	41.7	43.1	38.8	89.9
MVV	12.0	11.1	16.8	20.8	14.0	74.3
EI	45.8	51.2	61.1	67.7	56.1	95.3

TABLE IV

NUMBER OF CASES WITH ABNORMAL FINDINGS OF OTHER VENTILATORY PARAMETERS AMONG PATIENTS WITH NORMAL FVC, $FEV_{1.0}$/FVC AND MVV

Parameter	Case (%)		
	FVC	$FEV_{1.0}$/FVC	MVV
$FEV_{1.0}$	678(27.7)		581(25.2)
MMF	1034(42.3)	684(32.2)	900(39.0)
$FVC_{t(0.25-0.75)}$	918(37.6)	522(24.6)	766(33.2)
PFR	528(21.6)	278(13.1)	384(16.6)
$\dot{V}_{max}$ 50	710(29.5)	360(17.0)	581(25.2)
$\dot{V}_{max}$ 75	821(33.6)	473(22.3)	683(29.6)

REFERENCES

1. Moon WK, CHO KS (1985) An epidemiological study on the coal workers' pneumoconiosis in Korea. J Cathol Med College 38:951-961

2. Kim HJ, Yun IG (1985) Epidemiological study on dust conditions of rock places and prevalence of pneumoconiosis among tunnel drillers in a Korean Coalmine area. J Cathol Med College 38:975-985

3. Lee MC (1980) Relationship between pulmonary function impairments by one-second forced expiratory volume and radiographic progression in pneumoconiosis. J Cathol Med College 33:505-514

© 1990 Elsevier Science Publishers B.V. (Biomedical Division)
Occupational Epidemiology. H. Sakurai et al., editors

549424

STUDY ON THE PREDICTION OF PREVALENCE OF SILICOSIS IN SEVEN MINES AND PLANTS

JIEZHI LOU, QIAN ZHOU, GUIFAN SUN
Division of Pneumoconiosis, Department of Public Health,
China Medical University, Shenyang, Liaoning, China

INTRODUCTION

Study on the predication of prevalence of silicosis is important for future preventive work of silicosis (1-2). In this study the life table method was used to predict the trend of prevalence of silicosis in seven mines and plants, where the incidence of silicosis was high. From the middle of 1950s to the early of 1960s, these mines and plants have initiated comprehensive dust control programes focusing on wet operation. Before that, the average dust concentration was as high as 200.5-340.0mg/m³. After that, it decreased to 3.9-29.3mg/m³.

MATERIAL AND METHODS

In this paper the subjects were investigated include all of the workers exposed to dust who had physical examination card and detailed records of their occupational history as well as X-ray chest films kept by the enterprises. The time of first exposure to dust was recorded. The time of diagnosis was recorded for each silicosis patient (based on the criteria of radiographic classification of silicosis published by the Ministry of Public Health of China). During the investigation, the time of their non-silicosis related death or the time when the workers transferred from the enterprise were also recorded. For the purpose of analysis and comparison, the seven enterprises were divided into three groups, metallic mine group (a lead mine and a molybdenum mine), coal mine group (two coal mines) and plant group (a fireproof raw material workshop in a steel plant, a foundry in a factory producing heavy machines, and a raw material workshop in a glass factory). The life table method was used to calculate the accumulated prevalence rate of silicosis and average annual prevalence of silicosis in dust-exposed workers who were employed in different periods (before 1950, 1950-, 1950-, 1960-1964) up to 1981 in three groups (1). Because of non-silicosis have been found in the workers who were first exposed to dust after 1965, so it be supposed in this paper that the average annual incidence for these workers will be equal to that of 1960-1964.

Table 1 Expected number of silicosis among workers exposed to dust in different periods and in different mines and plants

Types of Plants and Mines	Dust Exposure Time	No. of Workers Exposed to Dust	Expected Number of Silicosis in Different Age Groups											Total
			25-	30-	35-	40-	45-	50-	55-	60-	65-	70-	75-	
Metallic Mine Group	pre 1950	620	—	—	—	—	2.48	40.70	46.70	37.41	8.01	3.28	1.82	140.44
	1950-	2792	—	—	—	—	16.72	108.72	53.08	23.51	7.41	6.31	1.52	217.27
	1955-	1820	—	—	—	11.00	26.64	22.25	10.76	3.14	0.64	0.18	—	74.61
	1960-	942	—	—	3.93	3.07	1.09	0.45	0.26	0.15	—	—	—	8.95
	1965-1978	2002	0.67	12.31	6.56	1.85	0.61	0.46	0.27	0.04	—	—	—	22.77
	subtotal	8146	0.67	12.31	10.49	15.92	47.54	172.58	111.11	64.25	16.06	9.77	3.34	464.04
Coal Mine Group	pre 1950	1122	—	—	—	—	3.99	62.16	68.73	52.64	14.44	3.52	1.68	207.16
	1950-	1762	—	—	—	—	11.19	150.50	85.55	64.41	21.75	3.65	1.30	338.35
	1955-	3938	—	—	—	13.24	145.58	224.77	108.32	41.28	7.37	1.65	—	542.12
	1960-	1581	—	—	54.40	53.46	15.82	7.73	4.98	2.28	—	—	—	138.67
	1965-1978	1981	1.83	107.52	46.48	18.67	5.89	4.55	2.25	0.61	—	—	—	197.80
	subtotal	10284	1.83	107.52	110.88	85.37	182.47	449.71	269.74	161.22	43.56	8.82	2.98	1412.10
Plant Group	pre 1950	147	—	—	—	—	0.43	12.59	13.63	9.69	2.13	1.03	0.74	40.24
	1950-	563	—	—	—	—	2.29	64.64	34.29	19.92	5.61	1.46	0.72	128.93
	1955-	618	—	—	—	2.04	4.26	2.81	1.14	0.40	0.10	0.01	—	10.76
	1960-	165	—	—	1.61	1.25	0.41	0.18	0.09	0.10	—	—	—	3.64
	1965-1978	1027	0.42	17.08	7.13	1.97	0.72	0.34	0.15	0.02	—	—	—	27.83
	subtotal	2520	0.42	17.08	8.74	5.26	8.11	80.56	49.30	30.13	7.84	2.50	1.46	211.40
Total	pre 1950	1889	—	—	—	—	6.90	115.45	129.10	99.74	24.58	7.83	4.24	387.84
	1950-	5087	—	—	—	—	30.20	323.86	172.92	107.84	34.77	11.42	3.54	684.55
	1955-	6376	—	—	—	26.28	176.48	249.83	120.13	44.82	8.11	1.84	—	627.49
	1960-	2688	—	—	59.94	57.78	17.32	8.36	5.33	2.53	—	—	—	151.26
	1965-1978	4910	2.92	136.91	70.17	22.49	7.22	5.35	2.67	0.67	—	—	—	248.40
	subtotal	20950	3.98	136.91	130.11	106.55	238.12	702.85	430.15	255.60	67.46	21.00	7.78	2099.54

Table 2 Expected number of silicosis in future years among workers exposed to dust in different periods and in different plants and mines

Types of Mines and Plants	Dest Exposure Periods	No. of Workers Exposed to Duse	Expected Number of Silicosis in Future Years										Total
			<5	5-	10-	15-	20-	25-	30-	35-	40-	45-	
Metallic Mine Group	pre 1950	620	39.68	38.63	35.02	20.80	6.07	0.24	—	—	—	—	140.44
	1950-	2762	55.24	54.19	49.33	38.83	18.06	1.62	—	—	—	—	217.27
	1955-	1820	15.47	15.45	15.25	13.76	9.59	4.28	0.80	—	—	—	74.61
	1960-	942	1.41	1.41	1.41	1.36	1.26	1.11	0.76	0.23	—	—	8.95
	1965-1978	2002	3.00	3.00	3.00	2.98	2.88	2.77	2.56	1.92	0.64	0.02	22.77
	subtotal	8146	114.80	112.68	104.01	77.73	37.86	10.03	4.12	2.15	0.64	0.02	464.04
Coal Mine Group	pre 1950	1122	57.78	56.68	51.95	31.04	9.32	0.39	—	—	—	—	207.16
	1950-	1762	88.98	88.17	81.80	55.47	22.84	1.09	—	—	—	—	338.35
	1955-	3938	122.08	121.99	119.75	101.74	59.42	16.17	0.97	—	—	—	542.17
	1960-	1581	22.13	22.13	22.13	21.27	19.51	17.12	11.22	3.18	—	—	138.67
	1965-1978	1881	26.33	26.33	26.33	26.06	25.20	24.08	21.99	16.29	5.12	0.07	197.80
	subtotal	10284	317.30	315.30	301.96	236.58	136.29	58.85	34.18	19.45	5.12	0.07	1424.10
Plant Group	pre 1950	147	11.38	10.98	9.88	6.11	1.85	0.04	—	—	—	—	40.24
	1950-	563	33.22	32.80	30.81	22.53	9.35	0.22	—	—	—	—	128.93
	1955-	618	2.16	2.16	2.14	1.95	1.47	0.73	0.15	—	—	—	10.76
	1960-	165	0.58	0.58	0.58	0.55	0.51	0.45	0.30	0.09	—	—	3.64
	1965-1978	1027	3.60	3.60	3.60	3.52	3.58	3.41	3.18	2.50	0.83	0.01	27.83
	subtotal	2520	50.94	50.12	47.01	34.72	16.70	4.85	3.63	2.59	0.83	0.01	211.40
Total	pre 1950	1889	108.84	106.29	96.85	57.95	17.24	0.67	—	—	—	—	387.84
	1950-	5087	177.44	175.16	161.94	116.83	50.25	2.93	—	—	—	—	684.55
	1955-	6376	139.71	139.60	137.14	117.45	70.48	21.19	1.92	—	—	—	627.49
	1960-	2688	24.12	24.12	24.12	23.18	21.28	18.68	12.28	3.48	—	—	151.26
	1965-1978	4910	32.93	32.93	32.93	32.62	31.60	30.26	27.73	20.71	6.59	0.10	248.40
	total	20950	483.04	478.10	452.98	348.03	190.85	73.73	41.93	24.19	6.59	0.10	2099.54

In addition, we investigated the age distribution of workers exposed to dust but who, as yet, have not suffered from silicosis. Using the data of life expectancy of male citizens in Shenyang, China in 1976 (3), we estimated the predicted number of silicosis patient in workers at different age groups and the trend of silicosis in future.

RESULTS

The total 26,603 workers who had exposed to dust for more than three years were investigated in this paper. Up to the end of 1981, 3,804 patients in different stages of silicosis were detected for an overall prevalence of 14.30%. The accumulated prevalence rate and the average annual prevalence rate of silicosis in dust-exposed workers who were employed in different periods (before 1950, 1950-, 1955-, 1960-1964) in metallic mine group were 42.40%, 11.23%, 3.82%, 0.62% and 1.28%, 0.40%, 0.17%, 0.03%, in coal mine group were 33.93%, 28.39%, 14.30%, 5.02% and 1.03%, 1.01%, 0.62%, 0.28%; in plant group were 51.25%, 32.91%, 1.60%, 1.05% and 1.55%, 1.18%, 0.07%, 0.07% up to 1981. The general accumulated prevalence rate and the average annual prevalence rate of silicosis were 38.20%, 21.00%, 10.76%, 3.28% and 1.16%, 0.75%, 0.47%, 0.18% respectively. On the basis of the age distribution of non-silicosis workers, life expectancy in various age groups and average annual silicosis incidence of dust exposed workers in different periods, the trend of silicosis in future was shown in table 1 and 2. Table 1 shows that the old workers over 45 years old and first exposed to dust before 1960s will be the main patients with silicosis diagnosis in future, they will account for 82.07% and 80.96% of the total predicted silicosis patients respectively. Table 2 shows that the expected new cases of silicosis in these mines and plants will be 483 in the following 5 years. Although the new cases of silicosis will fewer and fewer with the time passed, the occurence of new cases of silicosis will not decrease much within the following 15 years, it will decrease significantly in another following 20 years and decrease dramatically in another following 30 years.

REFERENCES

1. Jiezhi Lou, Tieshan Qi (1984) J of China Public Health Statistics 1 : 12
2. Jiezhi Lou, Zhengpei Yao (1984) Science and Technology of Labour Protection 4 : 9 (China)
3. Yanling Liu (1979) J of China Medical University 1 : 43

© 1990 Elsevier Science Publishers B.V. (Biomedical Division)
Occupational Epidemiology. H. Sakurai et al., editors

THE DEVELOPMENT OF COALWORKERS' PNEUMOCONIOSIS IN RELATION TO TIME UNDERGROUND, CALENDAR TIME, AND AGE IN A GERMAN COALMINE

P. MORFELD*, B. KAMPMANN*, H.-J. VAUTRIN**, C. PIEKARSKI*

* Institut für Arbeitswissenschaften der Ruhrkohle AG, Dortmund
**Bergwerk Walsum, Ruhrkohle AG, Duisburg, F.R. Germany

INTRODUCTION

In Germany the threshold limit value of silica-coal-dust in the coal mine atmosphere is under discussion again by the Senate Commission for the examination of industrial agents (14). The commission's proposals are based on results of an epidemiological study on the risk of developing coalworkers' pneumoconiosis (CWP) by Reisner et al. (9). This study can be criticized for different reasons (1, 4, 7, 12, 14).

- Validity and precision of the personal dust values being used as the main measure of exposure are debatable.
- Chest radiographs of the miners were recorded using the Johannesburg classification system of 1930 which is no longer in use. Moreover second reading was not applied.
- The study was based on tabulated data of prevalent cases. No incidence statistics were calculated.
- Data sampling stopped more than 15 years ago. The applicability of the results on today's conditions has not been proved.
- The proposed revision of the limit value is based only on data of a subgroup of Reisner's study. For statistical reasons conclusions on CWP risk are restricted to a time underground of 15 years.

To overcome these difficulties new research has been started. In this study analysis is focused on non-causal time variables. Measures of personal dust exposure are ignored on purpose.

MATERIAL AND METHODS

The study group implies all miners (n = 472) having retired from Walsum coal mine as workers in 1973-77, 1980, 1985 after at least 20 years underground. Observation time comprises 13877 person-years. 5701 chest radiographs were evaluated independently by at least two physician readers according to the 1980 ILO classification. Development of profusion was monotone in each person. The miners enter the study with the beginning of time underground. Exit is the last medical survey at the mine during time underground.

In a first step prevalences and cumulative incidences (2, 5) for all profusion categories of coalworkers' simple pneumoconiosis (CWSP) were determined for each two-year interval of time underground. The median was calculated for the prevalent cases.

In a second step for certain times in the period underground prevalences of the profusion categories were stratified for the beginning of work underground in calendar time.

In a third step the data are modelled taking age at the beginning of work underground additionally into account. A sequence of Cox models was fitted by means of backward elimination (3, 5). Time-to-response was defined as time underground. The starting model allowed for linear terms, quadratic terms and interaction of calendar time and age. Moreover risk functions were determined using unconditional logistic regression (3, 5).

RESULTS AND DISCUSSION

For time underground between 28 and 30 years a prevalence of CWSP ≥ 1/1 of 16.8 % (n = 280, .95-confidence limits: 12.6 % and 21.7 %) and a cumulative incidence of 19.3 % are found. Although risk is increasing with time underground, the upper limit of the

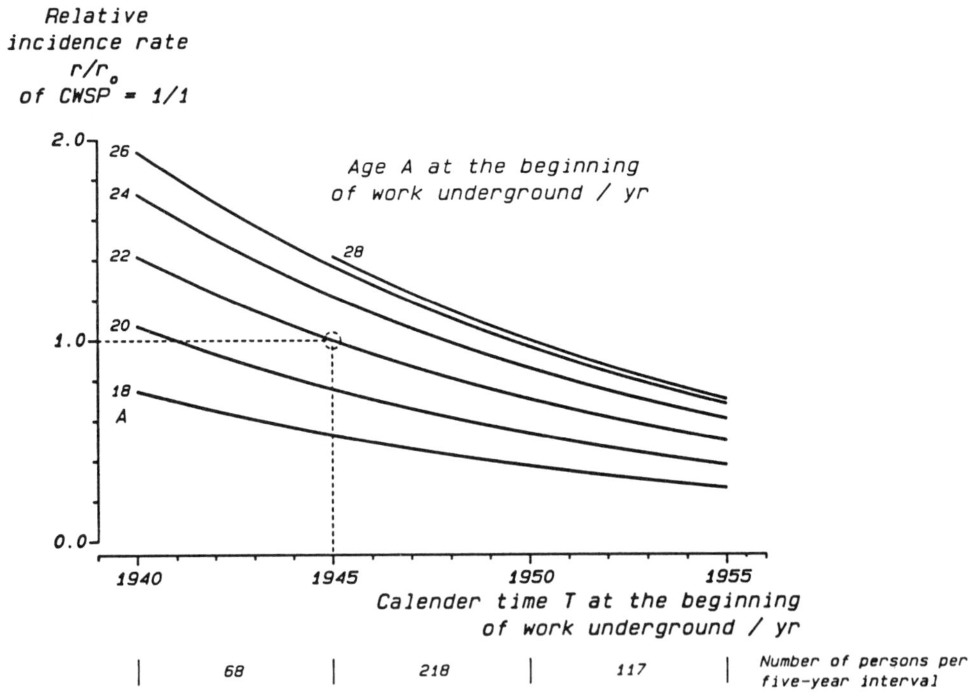

Fig. 1: Relative incidence rate of CWSP = 1/1 in the whole study group (n = 472) estimated by the final Cox PH model $\ln(r/r_0) = c_1*(T/yr - 1945) + c_2*(A/yr - 22) + c_3*(A/yr - 22)^2$.

.95-confidence interval of the median of profusion is less or equal 0/1 for a time underground less than 35 years.

Tabulating prevalences indicates that the risk is going down with calendar time: for a fixed time of 20 years underground the prevalence of CWSP ≥ 1/1 decreases from 3.8 % (beginning of work 1940-49, n = 286) to 0 % (beginning of work 1950-59, n = 155).

Relative rates of CWSP = 1/1 adjusted for calendar time and age by a Cox model are presented in Fig. 1. All effects of this reduced model are significant. The PH assumption is retained: tests of time-underground-dependent interaction yield p > 0.6.

Estimation of prevalence by means of logistic regression is shown in Fig. 2. The model confirms results yielded by stratification.

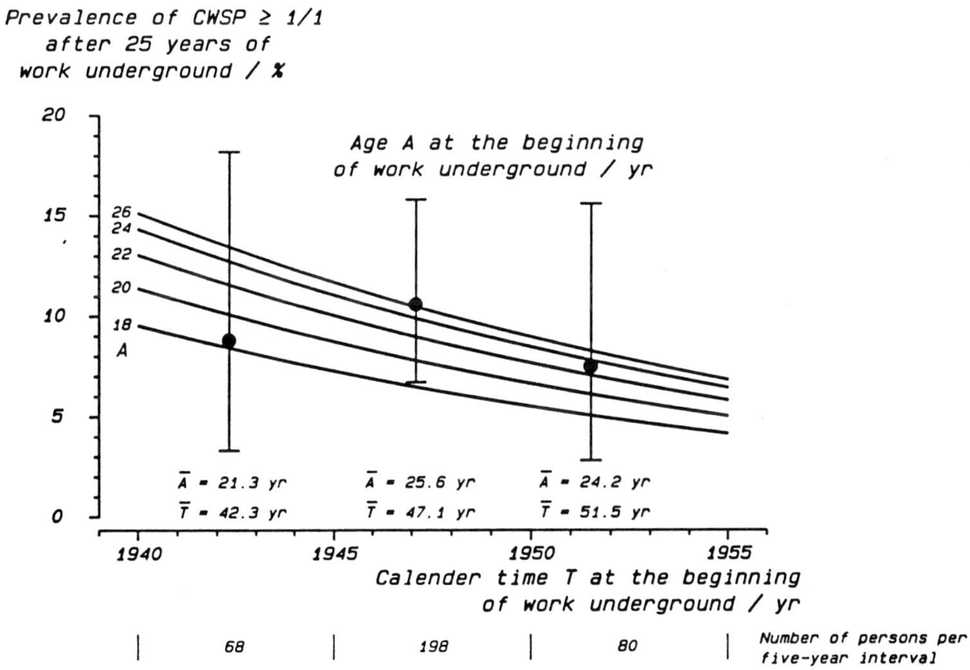

Fig. 2: Point prevalence P of CWSP ≥ 1/1 after 25 years of work underground (n = 395) estimated by the logistic model $\ln(P/(1-P)) = b_0 + b_1*(T/yr - 1900) + b_2*(A/yr) + b_3*(A/yr)^2$. Prevalences determined by stratification on T are shown as full circles for 5-yr intervals with .95 confidence-limits (binomial distribution). Mean values of T and A are given for each interval.

The original finding of Reisner et al. (9) that risk is rising with age at the beginning of work up to an age of about 30 years can be confirmed.

The risk of CWP is decreasing significantly with calendar time; this agrees with findings of other authors (8, 10, 13). Therefore current epidemiological data are necessary to estimate an adequate threshold limit value of silica-coal-dust under today's mining conditions.

REFERENCES

1. Bauer HD, Robock K (1988) Comparative measurements with different measuring instruments; problems in the evaluation of dust conditions in the hard coal mining industry. VIIth International Pneumoconioses Conference Pittsburgh (in print)
2. Coleman M, Douglas A, Hermon C, Peto J (1986) Cohort study analysis with a FORTRAN computer program. Int J Epidemiol 15:134-137
3. Dixon WJ, Brown MB, Engelman L, Frane JW, Hill MA, Jennrich RI, Toporek JD (1985) BMDP statistical software manual. University of California Press, Berkeley, Los Angeles, London
4. Kampmann B, Morfeld P, Vautrin HJ, Piekarski C (1989) Rückgang der Prävalenz der Silikose über der Kalenderzeit für sieben Abkehrjahrgänge eines Bergwerks im deutschen Steinkohlenbergbau. Verh. d. Dtsch. Ges. f. Arb.-Med. (in print)
5. Kleinbaum DG, Kupper LL, Morgenstern H (1982) Epidemiologic Research. Principals and Quantitative Methods. Von Nostrand Reinhold Company, New York
6. Morfeld P, Vautrin HJ, Kampmann B (1988) Expositionszeitspezifische Prävalenzen der Silikose für zwei Abkehrjahrgänge eines Bergwerks im deutschen Steinkohlenbergbau. Verh. d. Dtsch. Ges. f. Arb.-Med. 28:661-663
7. Prinz B, Stolz R (1988) Effect of the measuring strategy on the determination of the respirable dust concentration in the breathable air at underground workplaces. VIIth International Pneumoconioses Conference Pittsburgh (in print)
8. Reischig HL (1989) Die Entwicklung der Mischstaubpneumokoniose im Saarbergbau. Kompaß 99:58-61
9. Reisner MTR, Kotitschke G, Niesert E (1985) Pneumokoniose und Staubexposition - Epidemiologische Untersuchungen im Steinkohlenbergbau an der Ruhr über einen Zeitraum von 20 Jahren. Silikosebericht Nordrhein-Westfalen 15:445-492
10. Soutar CA (1987) Update on lung disease in coalminers. Br J Ind Med 44:145-148
11. Vautrin HJ, Morfeld P, Kampmann B (1988) Prevalences, incidence densities and cumulative incidences of pneumoconiotic changes for two groups of miners of a mine in Western German coal mining. VIIth International Pneumoconioses Conference Pittsburgh (in print)
12. Vautrin HJ, Morfeld P, Kampmann B (1989) Vergleichende Untersuchungen zur Pneumokonioseentwicklung auf einem Bergwerk der Ruhrkohle AG im Hinblick auf eine Festsetzung des Grenzwertes für quarzhaltigen Kohlengrubenstaub. Silikosebericht Nordrhein-Westfalen Band 17 (in print)
13. Vékény H (1987) Zum Problem der Bewertung der Veränderung der Silikosegefahr am Beispiel der Mecseker Kohlengruben. Zbl Arbeitsmed 37:113-116
14. Woitowitz HJ, Armbruster L, Bauer HD, Breuer H, Bruch J, Lange HJ, Rödelsperger K, Sieben J, Stalder K. (1989) Überprüfung des Grenzwertes für quarzhaltigen Kohlengrubenstaub. Zbl Arbeitmed 39:132-146

Occupational Epidemiology. H. Sakurai et al., editors

THE DOSE – RESPONSE RELATIONSHIP IN FLUORITE PNEUMOCONIOSIS

ZHANG QIFENG, XU YIN AND SHEN HANMING
Department of Preventive Medicine, Zhejiang Medical University, Hangzhou, China

INTRODUCTION

With the development of fluorite industry , more and more workers are occupationally exposed to fluorite dust , however , the harmful effects of fluorite dust on worker health have not been widely studied . In order to understand the dose – response relationship between the fluorite dust and the fluorite pneumoconiosis , a 16 – year's follow – up study was performed in a fluorite mine in China . The information about fluorite pneumoconiosis was investigated and analysed [1] .

MATERIAL AND METHODS

Dust Concentration

Established in 1942, this fluorite mine has gone through 3 mining periods relative to its different dustproof methods . In the first period (before 1962), no dustproof measure was taken ; in the second one , only a simple wet mining method was adopted (from 1962 to 1966) ; and in the third period (after 1966), comprehensive dustproof measures were carried out . The dust concentration was measured regularly and expressed in an average concentration in a 8 – hour working day . Corresponding to above 3 periods , 3 different exposure levels of dust concentration were defined . They were high , moderate and low exospure levels .

Study Population

The total population of this study was composed of 843 miners who had exact employment and examination records and had no harmful – dust exposure history before employment. They were divided into three groups according to their employment time . The number of miners in each group was 455, 249 and 139 respectively . All miners worked with a same mining procedure , which included punching , demolishing , loading and transfering . They were exposed to a mixed type of dust .

The visit was made once a year . It included physical and chest roentgenogram examinations . On roentgenogram , the pneumoconiosis was diagnosed according to the standard issued by the Government .

Statistical Methods

For each group, the following statistical indices were computed. Incidence rate stands for the probability that healthy miners will develop pneumoconiosis during a special period of time. In this paper, two kinds of incidence rate were stated in terms of two different periods, one was the yearly incidence rate as shown in Fig. 1, the other was the accumulated incidence rate(AIR) as given in table I. The latter was calculated as follows:

$$AIR = \frac{\text{Number of new pneumoconiosis over the follow-up period}}{\text{Population in each group}} \text{ per 100}$$

Other indices such as accumulated prevalence rate(APR), accumulated mortality rate(AMR) and average standing of incidence(ASI) were computed as follows:

$$APR = \frac{\text{Number of existing cases of pneumoconiosis at the end of follow-up period}}{\text{Population in each group}} \text{ per 100}$$

$$AMR = \frac{\text{Number of deaths from pneumoconiosis in the follow-up period}}{\text{Population in each group}} \text{ per 100}$$

$$ASI = \frac{\text{Sum of the cases' exposure years before incidence}}{\text{Number of pneumoconiosis cases}}$$

The χ^2 test was used to examine the difference in AIR, APR and AMR among these 3 groups[2], and the relative risk (RR) was calculated in order to determine the effect of fluorite dust upon pneumoconiosis[2]. The RR was defined as the ratio of AIR, APR and AMR for miners in low and moderate exposure groups to the corresponding rates for those in high exposure group, respectively. The 95% confidence limit (95% C. L.) was based on the difference in χ^2 statistics.

RESULTS AND DISCUSSION

The dynamic processes of the dust concentration and annual pneumoconiosis incidence rate over 18 years (1964 – 1982) were shown in Fig . 1 . It was found that the curves of the dust concentration and the incidence rate were very similar in tendency and fluctuation . Both of them had peaks in the beginning , sharply declined in the early period of the 18 years , and then they fluctuated and dropped in a small range during the late years .

In addition, there was a "time – delay" between above two curves. The delayed time represented the response time of the lungs to fluorite dust. It just corresponded to standing of incidence. In Fig. 1, if the incidence rate curve was shifted ahead a interval equal to the delayed time, it might cover the curve of dust concentration. This result indirectly revealed that the dose – response relationship between fluorite dust and fluorite pneumoconiosis really existed.

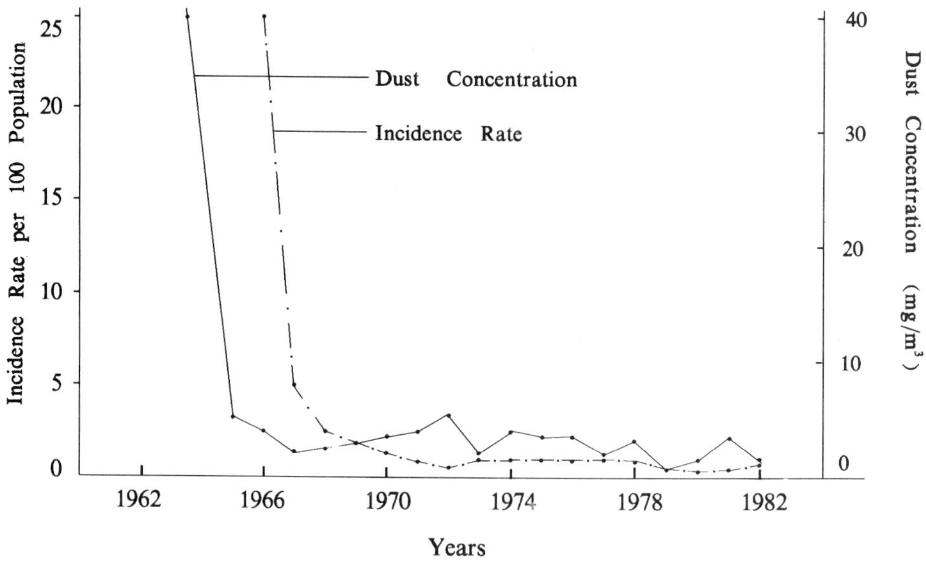

Fig. 1. Dust concentration and pneumoconiosis incidence rate, Dongfeng Fluorite Mine, 1964 – 1982.

Table I listed the data of AIR, APR , AMR and ASI in these 3 groups. It aslo gave the analysed results. The AIR in high, moderate and low exposure group was 24. 8%, 0. 8% and 0% respectively. The result of the χ^2 test indicated that the difference of AIRs among 3 groups was highly significant ($\chi^2 = 105.19$, $p < .0001$).

TABLE I

DATA OF AIR, APR, AMR AND ASI IN THREE GROUPS AND SOME ANALYTICAL RESULTS

Group	Sample	AIR (%)	APR (%)	AMR (%)	ASI (year)	RR** (1)	RR** (2)	RR** (3)
High exposure group (164. 1mg/m^3)	455	24. 8	85. 4	5. 9	4. 3	1	1	1
Moderate exposure group (8. 96mg/m^3)	249	0. 8	0. 8	0. 0	11. 9	0. 021	0. 006	0. 000
Low exposure group (1. 31mg/m^3)	139	0. 0	0. 0	0. 0	--			
χ^2 value		105. 19*	608. 13*	23. 80*		105. 01*	607. 38*	25. 58*
95%C. L.						.010 − .044	.0003−.0009	***

* The difference is statistical significant($p<0.0001$)

** RR(1), RR(2) and RR(3) indicates the RR from AIR, APR and AMR individually

*** The 95% C. L. can not be calculated for RR = 0

In high exposure group, the APR was 85. 4%, and in moderate and low exposure groups, the APR was 0. 8% and 0. 0% respectively. It was found that the APRs in these 3 groups were significantly different (χ^2=608. 13, p<. 0001).

According to the results in Table I, the AMR in high exposure group was 5. 9% and there was no death in the moderate and low exposure groups. Obviously, the difference of AMRs among 3 groups was also significant(χ^2=23. 80, p<. 0001). These results indicated that there was an association between fluorite dust and pneumoconiosis, which meant the fluorite dust was a risk factor of pneumoconiosis.

In the comparisons of AIR , APR and AMR between any two groups , the results expressed that all differences were statistical significant except for that between moderate and low exposure groups . The data of low and moderate exposure groups therefore were merged for the calculation of RR . As illustrated in Table I , comparing to high exposure group (RR = 1), the RR of merged group from AIR , APR and AMR was 0 . 021 (χ^2= 105 . 01, p< . 0001, 95% C . L . = . 010− . 044), 0.006 (χ^2= 607 . 38, p< .0001, 95% C . L . = . 003−. 009) and 0 (χ^2=25 . 58, p< . 0001), respectively . In addition , the result in Table I showed that the ASI was prolonged obviously with the decreasing of dust−exposure−level . These meant the risks of pneumoconiosis in incidence , prevalence and mortality increased with the rise of dust −exposure−level . which implied the existence of dose−response relationship between fluorite dust and pneumoconiosis .

As mentioned above , there was no significant difference in AIR , APR and AMR between moderate and low exposure groups . But it did not mean that the dose−response relationship could be ignored .

Actually , the miners in the moderate exposure group were also exposed to low dust level in their later exposure years . It was the main reason for the absence of significant difference between the two groups . In some sense , the result further confirmed the existence of the dose – response relationship between fluorite dust and fluorite pneumoconiosis .

SUMMARY

The results of this study showed that the change of each index among 3 exposure groups was highly significant. The AIR, APR, AMR but ASI decreased with the decline of dust concentration, which was related to the improvement of dustproof measures. The dose – response relationship between the fluorite dust and the fluorite pneumoconiosis was identified and it may be conducive to improving the dustproof measures and protecting the miners' health further.

REFERENCES

1. Zhang QF (1984): Social and Economic Benefits of Prevention Measure to Dongfeng Fluorite Mine. Chinese Journal of Industrial Hygiene and Occupational Diseases. 1: 18 – 24

2. Guo ZC (1988): Methods of Mathematical Statistics in Medical Research. Publishing House of People's Health. Beijing. 171 – 177, 691 – 703.

Other respiratory diseases

Occupational Epidemiology. H. Sakurai et al., editors

549425

RESPIRATORY ALLERGY IN CHEMICAL WORKERS EXPOSED TO PLATINUM SALTS

ULRICH BOLM-AUDORFF[1], HEINZ-GÜNTER BIENFAIT[1], JOACHIM BURKHARD[1], ADOLF-HERMANN BURY[2], ROLF MERGET[3], GERHARD PRESSEL[1], GERHARD SCHULTZE-WERNINGHAUS[3]

[1] Ministry of Social Welfare, Department of Occupational Safety, Division of Occupational Medicine and Division of Epidemiology, P.O. Box 3140, D-6200 Wiesbaden, FRG
[2] Heraeus GmbH, Department of Occupational Medicine, D-6450 Hanau, FRG
[3] University of Frankfurt, Department of Internal Medicine, Division of Pneumology, D-6000 Frankfurt am Main, FRG

INTRODUCTION

The sensitizing action of complex platinum salts especially potassium and ammoniumhexachloroplatinate in the respiratory tract has been known for a long time. Reviews have been reported by Parkes (1985) and Schultze-Werninghaus (1986) (1, 2). In this paper, we should like to present the results of a cross-sectional study in a platinum-processing plant.

METHODS

Altogether, 65 employees in the platinum processing sections of the plant (comprising 63 men and two women) were investigated. These employees were aged 37.2 ± 10.8 years. The mean duration of platinum exposure was 8.9 years, with variation between one and 40 years. The employees were subdivided into three groups on the basis of the level of platinum exposure with the assistance of a chemist from the plant investigated:

1. relatively high exposure (platinum refinery, n = 21)
2. moderate exposure (gold, silver, palladium, iridium and osmium refinery with bystander exposure to platinum, since they are accommodated in the same building as the platinum refinery, manufacture of catalysts, filling of noble metal preparation, n = 23)
3. relatively low exposure (alkaline dissolution of metallic platinum, plant tradesmen, n = 21).

The staff's occupational and symptom history was determined by means of a standardized questionnaire. Furthermore, an analysis of lung function including

TABLE I
Results of the allergologic investigations in 65 chemical workers with exposure to platinum salts

	Symptom status			
Type of investigation	work-related symptoms (n = 15)	symptoms not related to work (n = 10)	no symptoms (n = 40)	Total (n = 65)
1	2	3	4	5
Prick test pos. H_2PtCl_6 (n, %)	9/14[1] 64.3%	2/10 20%	1/40 2.5%	12/64 18.7%
Environmental allergens (n, %)	2/13 15.4%	4/10 40%	13/40 32.5%	19/63 30.2%
Total IgE (U/ml)	230.4 ± 296.9[2]	48.6 ± 35.4	108.2 ± 138.5	127.2 ± 189.7
Total IgE > 100 U/ml (%)	53.3[2]	10.0	40.0	38.5
Platinum-specific IgE (% binding)	10.8 ± 11.3[3]	2.4 ± 1.3	4.6 ± 3.6	5.7 ± 6.9
Histamine release (% of maximum release)	17.3 ± 20.9	15.6 ± 12.5	19.0 ± 14.8	18.1 ± 16.2

[1] $p < 0.01$ compared to column 3 and 4.
[2] $p < 0.05$ compared to column 3, not significant compared to column 4.
[3] $p < 0.05$ compared to column 3 and 4.

spirometry, flow volume curve and resistance according to the interrupter method was performed before and after the Monday shift as well as after the Friday shift. The lung function instrument "Pneumoskop" from Jäger, Würzburg, West Germany was used. In the evaluation of the lung function, predicted values of the European Community of Coal and Steel were used (3).

In the allergological investigation, a skin prick test was carried out with a 10^{-3} molar H_2PtCl_6 solution as well as with extracts of six frequent environmental allergens (tree, grass and herb pollen, dust mites, fungal spores as well as cat epithelia). A blood sample was also taken to determine total IgE and the platinum-specific IgE. In addition, the histamine release was determined after incubation of basophils the whole blood with H_2PtCl_6.

The chi-square test used for the comparison of prevalences and the t test for the comparison of mean values. The Wilcoxon test for matched pairs was used to compare the lung function at different times.

RESULTS

15 workers (23.1%) reported work-related conjunctivitis, rhinitis, coughing, expectoration or dyspnoe. The same symptoms without a strict relation to the workplace was reported by 10 workers (15.4%), in example the symptoms also occurred at home. Workplace-related symptoms were found significantly more frequently in the group of staff with high platinum exposure than in persons with moderate or low exposure ($p < 0,01$).

The results of the allergological investigations are shown in Table 1. A total of 12 out of 64 employees tested (18.7%) showed a positive prick test with H_2PtCl_6. A positive result was shown significantly more frequently in the group with work-related symptoms than in the two other groups (64.3%, 20.0%, 2.5%). On the other hand, employees with work-related symptoms more rarely showed a sensitization to allergens tested from the general environment. A higher total IgE and platinum-specific IgE, but not a raised histamine release in consequence of H_2PtCl_6 was found in employees with work-related symptoms.

The group of employees with work-related symptoms showed a normal lung function before the beginning of the working shift on Monday morning. In the course of the Monday shift and the working week, there was a fall in FEV_1 from 100.7% to 95.9% of the predicted values ($p < 0.05$) and the flow values also fell (most markedly FEF 25, from 95.1% to 73.4% of the normal values, $p < 0.05$). On the other hand, airway resistance remained unchanged. This finding can be interpreted as an indication of a discrete peripheral obstructive lung disease developing in the course of the week. In the two other groups, no alterations of lung function were shown in the course of the working week. Employees with respiratory tract symptoms not related to the workplace already have a markedly disturbed lung function on Monday morning before the working shift. In clinical terms, this group mainly comprises the staff with chronic bronchitis and non-specific bronchial hyperreactivity.

DISCUSSION

In the present study, the prevalence of typical work-related symptoms in terms of allergic conjunctivitis, rhinitis or obstructive airway disease caused by sensitization to platinum salts of 23.1% is very much less than the results of earlier years which described a prevalence of sensitization between 50.7% and 73% (4 -7). Recently, Murdoch et al. (1986) and Merget et al. (1988) reported on sensitization rates of 12.4% and 38.5% (8, 9) in the skin prick test. The latter investigation is also a study in a plant in West Germany. However, the less exposed plant tradesmen were not included in the study.

A prevalence of about 20% with a sensitization to platinum salts such as we found cannot be accepted in terms of occupational safety, since there was a large number of clinically manifest diseases amongst these employees. In the work with platinum salts, procedures with formation of dust or aerosols, e.g. blow out of filter presses with compressed air must be avoided under all circumstances. Processing of platinum salts should be carried out very largely in closed systems because of the high allergenic potency of these compounds. Furthermore it is to be noted that the German threshold limit value for platinum compounds (2 $\mu g/m^3$) was definitely maintained in the plant over a long term. This TLV is thus evidently not able to keep the prevalence of allergic airway diseases within reasonable limits and should therefore be re-examined.

REFERENCES

1. Parkes WR (1985) Occupational lung disorders. Butterworths, London, pp 432-433
2. Schultze-Werninghaus G (1986) Allergologie 9:479-486
3. Quanjer D (ed.) (1983), Bull Europ Physiopath Resp 19: Suppl 5
4. Hebert R (1966) Arch Mal Prof 27:877-886
5. Hunter D, Milton R, Perry KMA (1945) Brit J Ind Med 2:92-98
6. Massmann W, Oppitz H (1954) Zbl Arbeitsmed 4:1-4
7. Roberts AE (1951) Arch Industr Hyg 4:559
8. Murdoch RD, Pepys J, Hughes EG (1986) Brit J Industr Med 43:37-43
9. Merget R, Schultze-Werninghaus G, Muthorst T, Friedrich G, Meier-Sydow J (1988) Clin Allergy 18:569-580

Occupational Epidemiology. H. Sakurai et al., editors

THE RELATIONHIP BETWEEN LUNG FUNCTION, DUST EXPOSURE AND ENDOTOXIN EXPOSURE IN ANIMAL FEED WORKERS

DICK HEEDERIK, TJABE SMID
Departments of Environmental Health and Air Pollution, Wageningen University, P.O. Box 238, 6700 AE, WAGENINGEN, The Netherlands.

INTRODUCTION

In The Netherlands approximately 6000 people are employed in animal feed production. Several raw materials are used such as grain, pulses, waste products of the vegetable oil and starch industry.

Since 1985 a large scale study is in progress. The primary aim of this project is to study the influence of occupational dust exposure in animal feed mills on respiratory symptoms and lung function.

STUDY POPULATION

The total population consisted of 315 workers from 14 animal feed production mills. Part of this population had no occupational exposure; administrative departments of the different mills. Those exposed were divided into 8 occupational title categories. Some characteristics of the population are given in table I.

METHODS

The study consisted of:

- environmental monitoring of several dust fractions including respirable dust, thoracic dust and inspirable dust, endotoxin concentration in these dust fractions, viable fungal colony forming units.
- personal monitoring of inspirable dust exposure and endotoxin concentration in these personal samples.
- registration of respiratory symptoms with a shortened questionnaire.
- lung function measurements by normal expiratory spirometry.

Initially, results were studied in a simple tabular analysis. Differences in occupational dust exposure between various occupational titles and animal feed mills were tested in an analysis of variance. The relationship between respiratory symptoms, dust exposure and endotoxin exposure was studied in a logistic regression analysis after correcting for age and smoking habits. The relationship between lung function, dust exposure and endotoxin exposure was studied in a multiple regression analysis after a correction age, standing height and pack years smoked.

TABLE I

CHARACTERISTICS OF THE STUDY GROUP

	N	n (%)	mean (s.d.)
age (years)	315		39,4 (11,0)
height (cm)	315		178,0 (6,5)
pack years	315		274,1 (271,8)
current smokers	315	172 (55)	
ex-smokers	315	77 (24)	
non-smokers	315	66 (21)	
dust years (year)	315		11,2 (9,7)
cumulatieve dust exposure (g.day/m^3)	312		26,7 (30,9)
cumulatieve endotoxin exposure (ng.day/m^3)	312		74,7 (78,0)
current dust exposure (mg/m^3)	312		8,6 (9,9)
current endotoxin exposure (ng/m^3)	312		24,8 (19,6)
FVC	315		5,33 (0,88)
FEV_1	315		4,10 (0,87)
MMEF	315		3,72 (1,53)
PEF	315		9,73 (2,66)
MEF_{75}	315		7,69 (2,41)
MEF_{50}	315		4,75 (1,78)
MEF_{25}	315		1,62 (0,88)

RESULTS

Exposure

In total more than 550 personal samples were available for gravimetric analysis and endotoxin analysis. First an analysis of variance was performed with dust and endotoxin concentration as dependent variables and occupational title and feed mill as explanatory variables. Results showed that occupational title explained most of the variance in dust as well as endotoxin concentration. Therefore, a cumulative exposure was calculated based on the different occupational titles ever performed, the average dust exposure in that particular occupational title and the time spent in that occupational title. Trimmers had the highest mean dust and endotoxin exposure of respectively 40 mg/m^3 and 80 ng/m^3. Those who were involved in sacking and the truck drivers had the lowest mean dust exposure (3 mg/m^3) and an endotoxin concentration of 6 ng/m^3 and 30 ng/m^3.

Respiratory symptoms

No clear cut relationship were found between respiratory symptoms and cumulative and current dust or endotoxin exposure. However, statistically significant relationships were found between the number of years a worker had a worked on a dusty department and respiratory symptoms. Those who has 0-2 years of exposure had a low prevalence of cough, those with 2.5-9 and 10-16 years of exposure the highest (Odds Ratios 2.4 and 2.2 respectively), while those with the longest number of years the lowest prevalence(Odds Ratio 0.95). For wheezing and sputum a similar pattern was found. However, the prevalence of shortness of breath and dyspnea clearly decreased with increasing years of exposure. For those who were exposed longest, 17-40 years an Odds Ratio 0.20 was found compared to those with an exposure of 0-2 years.

Lung function

Lung function data gathered at the beginning of the monday work shift were analysed in a multiple regression analysis. Statistically significant relationships were found between most of the lung function variables and dust as well as endotoxin exposure after correction for the confounding variables. Such relationships were found for the cumulative exposure and the current exposure to dust and endotoxin. The relationship between endotoxin exposure and lung function appeared to be a statistically stronger one. The relationship between the cumulative endotoxin exposure (ng.day/m^3) and lung function is given in table II.

TABLE II

RELATIONSHIP BETWEEN LUNG FUNCTION AND CUMULATIVE ENDOTOXIN EXPOSURE CORRECTED FOR AGE, STANDING HEIGHT AND SMOKING

variable	R^2-model	$ß_{cumendo}$	$SE_ß$
FVC (l)	46	-0,0008	0,0005
FEV_1 (l)	56	-0,0014**	0,0005
MMEF (l/s)	41	-0,0025**	0,0010
PEF (l/s)	29	-0,0101**	0,0019
MEF_{75} (l/s)	31	-0,0085**	0,0017
MEF_{50} (l/s)	31	-0,0040**	0,0012
MEF_{25} (l/s)	43	-0,0006	0,0005

The population mean endotoxin exposure was 75 ng.day/m^3 which is equivalent to a daily endotoxin exposure of 1-5 ng/m^3. For such an occupational exposure the regression model predicted an FEV_1 decrease of 5% and a decrease for most of the flow-volume variables between 5 and 10%.

CONCLUSIONS

The personal dust exposure in animal feed mills is relatively high. Many workers are exposure above the Dutch Maximal Allowed Concentration of 10 mg/m^3. For some of the respiratory symptoms, a positive relationship with years of dust exposure was found. How-ever, for shortness of breath and dyspnea a significant reduction of the symptom prevalence was found with increasing numbers of years of exposure. This might point to a healthy workers effect. Those who develop respiratory symptoms tend to leave the industry resulting in a low prevalence for some respiratory symptoms in groups with larger exposure times. Relationships between the dust exposure and lung function were found, after allowing for confounder variables. However, the relationship between an occupational endotoxin exposure and lung function appeared to be stronger than the relationship between dust exposure and lung function. This might indicate that endotoxins play an important role in the development of lung function changes among animal feed production workers. However, we also found a statistically significant relationship between the number of colony forming units and the endotoxin concentration in samples taken at fixed points (pearson correlation 0.32; $p<0.05$; n=79). This could indicate that the endotoxin measured is a marker for other microbiological factors in the dust. The relationship between endotoxin and lung function does therefore not necessarily reflect an effect of endotoxin itself on lung function.

ACKNOWLEDGEMENTS

This study was granted by the Dutch Directorate General of Labor of the Ministery of Social Affairs and Employment.

Occupational Epidemiology. H. Sakurai et al., editors

MAXIMAL EXPIRATORY FLOW-VOLUME PATTERNS BY OYSTER-SHUCKER ASTHMA PATIENTS AND NASAL ALLERGY PATIENTS

TADAMICHI MEGURO(1), MASANA OGATA(1), BENJAMIN G. FERRIS(2)

(1)Department of Public Health, Okayama University Medical School, Okayama, Japan
(2)Department of Environmental Science and Physiology, Harvard School of Public Health, Boston, MA, U.S.A.

INTRODUCTION

Measurement of forced vital capacity(FVC) and forced expiratory volume in one second($FEV_{1.0}$) is essential laboratory means for confirming the diagnosis of obstructive airway diseases including occupational asthma (o-A). But measurement of maximal expiratory flow-volume(MEFV) is not generally used compared with that of FVC and $FEV_{1.0}$. We thought that MEFV measurement would be useful in the supervision of o-A patients and of occupational nasal allergy (o-NA) patients, because MEFV charts represent characteristic patterns[1-2] corresponding to symptoms in non-occupational asthma (no-A) patients[3-4] and in non-occupational nasal allergy (no-NA) patients[5-6]. We studied MEFV charts of oyster-shucker asthma (os-A) patients and no-A patients. Further we tried MEFV studies of no-NA patients.

MATERIAL AND METHODS

While oyster-shucking (o-s) workers inhaled sea-squirt (s-s) fluids during the work before the improvement of working environment of o-s workshop, some of them revealed asthmatic symptoms, nasal allergy symptoms, and conjunctivitic symptoms after the work at night. On the one hand, they took the hyposensitization therapy for the specific antigen, s-s extracts for five years, because high levels of specific I_gE titer of s-s extracts were confirmed. On the other hand, the average concentration of s-s fluids in the environment was remarkably lowered because of the improvement of handling procedures. Their asthmatic symptoms were remarkably improved compared with those before the improvement of working environment. During the o-s work season, MEFV measurement was performed for ten patients. Maximal expiratory flow-volume measurement was also performed for two no-A patients, and for thirty-seven no-NA patients and thirty-seven non-occupational healthy control (no-H) subjects. More than 50% of no-NA patients had house-dust as allergen.

RESULTS

NON-OCCUPATIONAL ASTHMA PATIENTS

Maximal expiratory flow-volume charts of no-A patients in provocation test are shown in Fig.1. In MEFV charts of A and B, flow rates after provocation were

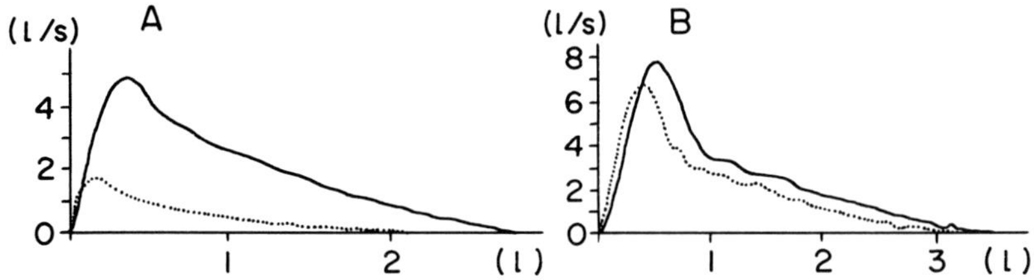

Fig.1. Maximal expiratory flow-volume charts in provocation test in non-occupational asthma patients.
A:21yr female. Antigen is house-dust. Solid line shows the MEFV chart before provocation and dotted line shows it after provocation(a fall in FEV1.0;54.7%).
B:29yr male. Antigen is ragweed. Solid line shows it before provocation and dotted line shows it after provocation(a fall in FEV1.0;13.7%).

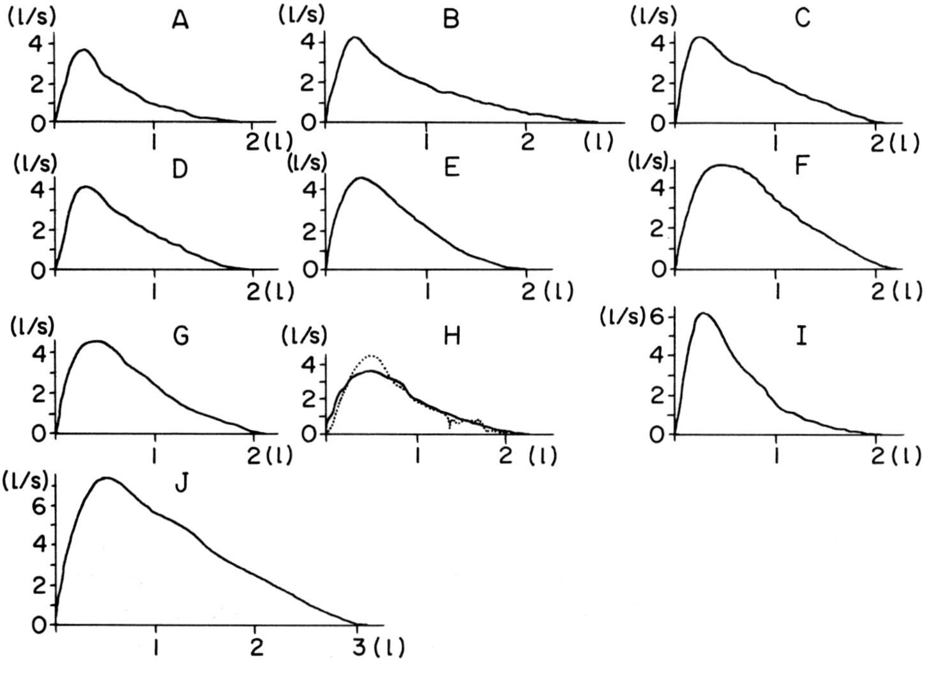

Fig.2. Maximal expiratory flow-volume charts in oyster-shucker asthma patients.

A: K.O., 70yr, female. B: A.S., 53yr, female. C: M.I., 59yr, female.
D: K.Y., 64yr, female. E: K.T., 52yr, male. F: H.M., 52yr, female.
G: N.M., 43yr, female. H: Y.N., 61yr, female. I: T.N., 64yr, male.
J: T.N., 31yr, male.

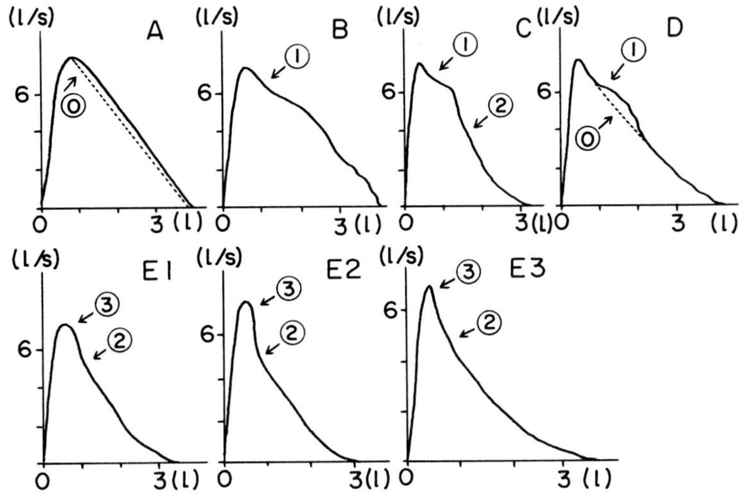

Fig.3. Five types of schemata of maximal expiratory flow-volume charts.

⓪:The broken straight line is considered to be flow changes in healthy subjects. ①:This shows short concave flow changes.②:This shows long concave flow changes. ③:This shows the slope of flow rates from peak flow rate(PEFR) (E1; a gentle slope, E2; a moderate slope, E3; a very sharp slope).

Table 1. Distribution of maximal expiratory flow-volume types in non-occupational nasal allergy patients and non-occupational healthy control subjects.

	Maximal expiratory flow-volume type								
	A	B	C	D	E	(E1	E2	E3)	Total
Nasal allergy patients	4	13	2	1	17	9	6	2	37
	10.8	35.1	5.4	2.7	45.9	24.3	16.2	5.4	100.0 %
Healthy control subjects	15	9	3	2	8	5	2	1	37
	40.5	24.3	8.1	5.4	21.6	13.5	5.4	2.7	100.0 %

lower than those before provocation all over the entire course. Thus, provocation effects are clearly observed in MEFV charts.

OYSTER-SHUCKER ASTHMA PATIENTS

Maximal expiratory flow-volume charts in o-A patients are shown in Fig.2. Five MEFV charts (A, B, C, D and H) were similar to those shown in Fig.1, but remainder five MEFV charts (E, F, G, I and J) were a little different (atypical patterns) from those shown in Fig.1. The former five MEFV charts showed sudden flow falls just after PEFR (moderate slopes), but the latter five MEFV charts did not show clear sudden flow falls. From the MEFV charts of o-s A patients, we emphasized that MEFV charts changed due to the improving their symptoms corresponding to the improvement of o-s working environment.

NON-OCCUPATIONAL NASAL ALLERGY PATIENTS

Distribution of MEFV types in no-NA patients and no-H subjects are shown in Table 1. Distribution of type B and type E in no-NA patients (35.1% and 45.9%) was higher percentage than that of no-H subjects (24.3% and 21.6%). Distribution of type A in no-NA patients (10.8%) was lower than that of no-H subjects (40.5%). Significant differences were shown in MEFV types between no-NA patients and no-H subjects. Judging from the results in o-A and no-A patients, MEFV charts in o-NA patients will show similar patterns compared with those of no-NA patients. Thus, we think that MEFV measurement will be useful for the supervision of o-NA patients and for health-care of workers in occupational nasal allergy.

Therefore, we conclude that MEFV charts are very useful for assessing the airway obstruction of occupational respiratory and nasal allergy diseases and for occupational respiratory and nasal health-effect monitoring.

ACKNOWLEDGEMENT

The authors wish to thank Prof. I.Kimura, and colleagues of the Department of Internal Medicine, and M.D. K. Nishioka of the Department of Otorhinolaryngology, of Okayama University Medical School, for help in physical examination.

REFERENCES

1. Landau LI, Phelan PD (1973) Amer Rev Resp Dis 108:593-602.
2. Tien Y, Elliott EA, Mead J (1979) J Appl Physiol 46:565-570
3. Meguro T, Tsubota N, Jitsunari H, Tanizaki K, Hosokawa M, Ogata M (1978) Okayama Igakkai Zasshi (in Japanese) 90:1479-1483
4. Meguro T, Tsubota N, Jitsunari H, Tanizaki K, Hosokawa M, Ogata M (1978) Okayama Igakkai Zasshi (in Japanese) 90:1485-1489
5. Meguro T, Ogata M, Nishioka K, Yamanaka M, Ogura Y (1983) Acta Med Okayama 37:163-166
6. Nishioka K, Meguro T, Masuda Y, Date R, Ogura Y (1987) Annals of Allergy 59:379-382

Occupational Epidemiology. H. Sakurai et al., editors

AIRFLOW OBSTRUCTION IN A CROSS-SECTIONAL STUDY OF PULMONARY FUNCTION IN WORKERS IN THE PAINT AND PRINT INDUSTRY

NG TZE PIN, ONG SAY GARK

Department of Community, Occupational and Family Medicine, National University of Singapore; Department of Community Medicine, University of Hong Kong.

INTRODUCTION

There are few studies of the pulmonary health of workers in the paint and print industries who are typically exposed to substantial quantities of solvent vapours and other chemical aerosols such as pigments (titanium dioxide, chromates), and akyl, epoxy and urethane resins. A few chemical constituents of paint products, such as isocyanates and dimethyl ethanolamine are known to cause acute (1,2) or chronic (3) airways obstruction. A recent study of spray painters in the construction industry has also suggested an increased risk of airflow obstruction that was related to the duration of exposure (4).

MATERIAL AND METHODS

We studied two exposed groups of workers within the paint and print industry: namely, 75 enamel/lacquer/print workers (age range 21-76 years) exposed to volatile solvents and other non-particulate products, and a smaller group of 16 emulsion workers exposed to titanium dioxide dust (age range 25-64 years). The unexposed referents were 124 non-production factory workers and postal workers (age range 21-67 years). These represented 86% and 92% of those eligible aged 20 years and above in the exposed and unexposed groups respectively. Pulmonary function parameters were evaluated using the best of three acceptable maximal forced expiratory manuevres performed on a closely calibrated dry-wedged bellow spirometer (Vitalograph TM with integral PFT printer), with results corrected to body temperature and pressure saturation. Heights were measured without shoes.

RESULTS

Table 1 shows the basic characteristics and measured lung function parameters of the subjects.

Table 1. Basic characteristics and lung functions of subjects

Parameters	Enamel/print	Emulsion	Unexposed
Number of subjects	75	16	124
Age,years	34.5 (12.7)	40.9 (13.8)	31.3 (8.8)
Height,cm	168 (6.3)	166 (5.4)	168 (5.5)
Never smokers	27 (36%)	6 (37%)	90 (73%)
Ever smokers	48 (64%)	10 (63%)	34 (27%)
Cigarettes per day	12.5 (7.3)	18.4 (11.8)	10.5 (6.8)
FVC,litres	3.94 (0.54)	3.85 (0.77)	3.98 (0.60)
FEV1,litres	3.31 (0.59)	3.12 (0.74)	3.48 (0.58)
FEV1/FVC,%	84 (8.9)	81 (7.0)	87 (6.6)
PEF,L/m	449 (117)	431 (101)	492 (91)
FMEF,L/s	3.87 (1.51)	3.28 (1.25)	4.83 (2.12)
FEF75-85,L/s	1.47 (0.81)	1.20 (0.63)	1.73 (0.91)

Pulmonary function parameters by exposure groups were adjusted for age, height and smoking, and compared using analysis of co-variance. Compared to unexposed referents, both enamel/print and emulsion workers had lower percent forced expiratory volume in one second / forced vital capacity (%FEV1/FVC), peak expiratory flow (PEF) and forced mid-expiratory flow (FMEF). Similar results were also seen in a separate analysis in never smokers (Table 2).

Table 2. Adjusted mean (standard error) values of pulmonary function parameters by exposure groups (all subjects and never smokers)

Parameters	Enamel/print	Emulsion	Unexposed
	All subjects		
FVC,litre	3.95 (0.05)	4.10 (0.11)	3.94 (0.04)
FEV1,litres	3.33 (0.05)	3.43 (0.10)	3.42 (0.04)
FEV1/FVC,%	84.3 (0.7)*	83.6 (1.6)	86.7 (0.6)
PEF,L/m	450 (11)**	461 (23)	490 (8)
FMEF,L/s	3.93 (0.20)**	3.80 (0.44)	4.69 (0.16)
FEF75-85,L/s	1.53 (0.09)	1.58 (0.18)	1.65 (0.07)
	Never smokers:		
FVC,litre	3.95 (0.09)	3.96 (0.19)	4.01 (0.05)
FEV1,litres	3.41 (0.07)	3.32 (0.16)	3.53 (0.04)
FEV1/FVC,%	86.4 (1.2)	84.1 (2.6)	88.0 (0.6)
PEF,L/m	454 (17)*	450 (36)	498 (9)
FMEF,L/s	4.08 (0.27)*	3.84 (0.56)	4.71 (0.15)
FEF75-85,L/s	1.66 (0.15)	1.55 (0.32)	1.81 (0.08)

* $p<0.05$ ** $p<0.01$ Compared to unexposed
@ Adjusted for age, height and daily cigarette consumption

Table 3. Smoking-adjusted relative risks of airflow obtruction for enamel/print and emulsion workers compared to unexposed workers.

	Enamel/print	Emulsion	Unexposed
Never smokers, N	27	6	90
FEV1/FVC <75%, N (%)	2 (7.4%)	1 (16.7%)	2 (2.2%)
Ever smokers, N	48	10	34
FEV1/FVC <75%, N (%)	11 (22.9%)	3 (30%)	2 (5.9%)
M-H relative risk	1.66	3.81	1.00
(95% CI)	(1.10 - 2.51)	(1.45 - 10.00)	

The smoking-adjusted Mantel-Haensel relative risks of airflow obstruction (indicated by %FEV1/FVC less than 75) was 1.66 (95% CI 1.10-2.51) in enamel/print workers and 3.81 (95% CI 1.45-10.00) in emulsion workers (Table 3). Enamel/print workers who had worked for 10 or more years had a relative risk of airways obstruction, after controlling for smoking, of 2.51 (95% CI 1.32-4.76) (Table 4).

Table 4. Smoking-adjusted relative risks of airflow obtruction for exposure duration in enamel/print workers

	>= 10 years	< 10 years
Never smokers, N	7	20
FEV1/FVC <75%, N (%)	2 (28.6%)	0 (0.0%)
Ever smokers, N	18	30
FEV1/FVC <75%, N (%)	7 (38.9%)	4 (13.3%)
M-H relative risk	2.51	1.00
(95% CI)	(1.32 - 4.76)	

CONCLUSION

The results suggest a risk of airflow obstruction for exposed workers in the paint and print industry, but further studies are needed to characterize the pulmonary effects of specific exposures within the industry.

REFERENCES

1. Cockcroft DW, Mink JT. Isocyante-induced asthma in an automobile spray painter. J Can Med Assoc 1979;121:602-604.

2. Valliers M, Cockcroft DW, Taylor DM, Dolovich J, Hargreave FE. Dimethyl ethanolamine-induced asthma. Am Rev Resp Dis 1977;115: 867-871.

3. Wegman DH, Peters JM, Pagnotto L, Fine LJ. Chronic pulmonary function loss from exposure to toluene diisocyante. Br J Ind Med 1977;34:196-200.

4. Schwartz DA, Baker EL. Respiratory illness in the construction industry:airflow obstruction among painters.Chest 1988;92,1: 134-137.

Occupational Epidemiology. H. Sakurai et al., editors
5 4 9 4 2 6

EFFECTS OF LONG-TERM EXPOSURE TO LOW CONCENTRATION OF CHLORINE ON WORKERS' HEALTH

Zhicheng Shi

(Research Center of Occupational Medicine, Third Hospital, Beijing Medical University, Beijing, China)

INTRODUCTION

Chlorine is widely used in chemical and light industries. It is a toxic and irritant chemical. Exposure to high concentrations of its vapour may result in acute poisoning, even in death. There have been a few catastrophic accidental exposures of both industrial and general populations. The risk of acute exposure was significantly reduced on account of using modern engineering procedures and proper safety protections.

Recently, more attention is paid to long-term exposure to low concentration of chlorine on workers' health. the current study is reported on this issue.

SUBJECTS AND METHODS

353 workers on a diaphragm cell chlorine production chemical plant were examined. They were divided by duration of exposure into two groups; Group A, 220 workers employed between 10-25 years; Group B, 133 workers employed for less than 10 years. Their average age was 42.4 (range 23-52). Environmental levels of chlorine in the workplaces where the electrolytic processes were conducted ranged from 2.60 — 11.0mg/m^3(mean 4.82±0.36mg/m^3). The current threshold limit value in China is 1mg/m^3.

The control group, consisting of 192 workers from the same plant, who were not exposed to chlorine. The average age was 39.7 (range 26-55).

For chlorine workers and controls included in the study, the following examination and tests were performed; questionnaire on complaints, espicially respiratory symptoms and smoking habits, clinical examination including ENT examination, chest X-ray film, pulmonary function tests comprising; FVC, VC, FEV_1, FEF_{25-75}, PEFR/H $\dot{V}_{75}$/H, $\dot{V}_{50}$/H, $\dot{V}_{25}$/H.

RESULTS

The data showed that the prevalence of upper airway complaints, such as sore throat, hoarseness, dryness in the throat and respiratory symptoms, such as shortness of breath, chest tightness and pain, wheezing, cough and phlegm. In addition, headache, weakness, sleeplessness in workers of Groups A and B were 3-8 times higher than those in controls (TAB. I).

TABLE I
Prevalence(%) of Main Symptoms

	Group A (n=220)		Group B (n=133)		Controls n=192	
Symptoms	№.	%	№.	%	№.	%
Sore throat	32	14.4	14	10.5	8	4.2
Hoarseness	18	8.1	10	7.5	6	3.1
Dryness in the throat	47	21.2	24	18.0	11	5.7
Shortness of breath	41	18.5	20	15.0	12	6.2
Chest tightness	39	17.6	24	18.0	10	5.2
Chest pain	28	12.6	12	9.0	3	1.6
Wheezing	5	2.3	2	1.5	0	0
Cough	34	15.3	16	12.0	12	6.2
Phlegm	18	8.1	10	7.5	21	10.9
Headache	42	18.9	26	19.5	24	12.5
Weakness	44	19.8	22	16.5	12	6.2
Sleeplessness	22	9.9	10	7.5	11	5.7
Dizziness	16	7.2	8	6.0	10	5.2
Poor memory	39	17.6	21	15.8	34	17.7
Poor appetite	12	5.4	6	4.5	10	5.2

The prevalence of pulmonary symptoms was highest in current smokers. The rhin-pharyngeal signs (rhinities, angina and olfactory deficiency) in workers of Group A also were higher than those in controls ($P<0.01$) (TAB. II).

TABLE II
E.N.T. Examination Findings

	Group A (n=220)		Group B (n=133)		Controls (n=192)	
	№.	%	№.	%	№.	%
Chronic rhinitis	48	21.82*	16	12.03	18	9.38
Chronic tonsillitis	40	18.18*	14	10.52	20	10.42
Olfactory deficiency	36	16.36*	8	6.02	7	3.65

* $P<0.01$ Compare with that of controls

8. 6% of workers in Group A and 2.8% workers in Group B had some abnormal changes in chest X-ray films, compared to 2. 3% of controls(TAB. III).

TABLE III
Chest X-ray Findings

Findings	Group A (n=220)		Group B (n=133)		Controls (n=192)	
	№	%	№	%	№	%
Fine irregular linear opacities	8	3.6	3	2.1	3	1.6
Small miliary opacities or small patches	5	2.3	0	0	0	0
Emphysema findings	2	0.9	0	0	0	0
Tuberculosis	4	1.8	1	0.7	1	0.5
Total	19	8.6	4	2.8	4	2.1

The results of pulmonary function tests showed that $\dot{V}_{50}/H$. FEF_{25-75} in workers of both Group A and B were lower than those in controls ($P< 0.01$); FEV_1 in workers of Group A was lower than in controls ($P<0.05$) (TAB. IV. V).

TABLE IV
Results of Spirogram Measurements (Mean±SD)

Parameter	Group A (n=220)	Group B (n=133)	Controle (n=192)
VC (L)	4.10± 0.58	4.25± 0.65	4.16± 0.46
VC(%of pred)	104.12±14.62	106.40±16.12	105.38±14.38
FVC (L)	4.12± 0.58	4.28± 0.78	4.18± 0.46
FVC (%of prea)	103.34±18.10	106.34±16.72	105.26±16.45
FEF_1	3.21± 0.54▲	3.66±0.66	3.68±0.52
FEV_{25-75}(L/S)	2.84± 0.86※	2.87±0.94※	3.31±0.83
FEV_1/FVC(%)	86.1 ±10.12	87.1±10.72	86.8±8.74
FEV_1/VCPR(%)	83.11±10.68	86.45±10.72	85.24±12.20

▲$P<0.05$ ※$P<0.01$ Compare with those of controls

TABLE V
Results of MEFV measurement (Mean ± SD)

Parameter	Group A (n= 220)	Group B (n= 133)	Controle (n= 192)
PEFR/H(L/S/M)	4.01 ± 1.31	4.24 ± 1.04	4.12 ± 1.22
$\dot{V}_{75}$/H(L/S/M)	3.54 ± 0.79	3.78 ± 0.66	3.56 ± 0.68
$\dot{V}_{50}$/H(L/S/M)	1.84 ± 0.63*	1.96 + 0.56*	2.33 ± 0.58
$\dot{V}_{25}$/H(L/S/M)	0.84 ± 0.30	0.88 ± 0.34	0.89 ± 0.32
$\dot{V}_{50}$/V_{25}(%)	2.43 ± 0.67	2.48 ± 0.53	2.46 ± 0.62

※P<0.01 compare with that of controls

Furthermore, the abnormality of pulmonary function in smokers both of Groups A and B was higher than that in nonsmokers. $\dot{V}_{50}$/H, $\dot{V}_{25}$/H, FEV_1, FEF25−75 all were significantly different between smokers and nonsmokers (P<0.1 or P<0.05)(TAB.6).

TABLE VI
Comparison of Lung Function Between Smokers and Nonsmokers

Parameter	Group A (n=220) Nonsmokers (n=102)	Group A (n=220) Smokers (n=118)	P	Group B (n=133) Nonsmokers (n=67)	Group B (n=133) Smokers (n=65)	P
FEV_1	81.5 ± 12.3	77.4 ± 10.6	<0.05	83.4 ± 11.7	80.6 ± 10.4	<0.05
FEF_{25-75}	78.4 ± 9.7	74.2 ± 8.5	<0.05	80.3 ± 10.6	76.5 ± 8.7	<0.05
$\dot{V}_{50}$/H	73.3 ± 12.4	65.7 ± 18.6	<0.01	74.6 ± 12.4	66.8 ± 10.8	<0.01
$\dot{V}_{25}$/H	75.8 ± 18.3	70.3 ± 15.7	<0.01	76.4 ± 11.3	70.2 ± 14.3	<0.01

DISSCUSION

There are few reports in literature concerning with the long-term effects of exposure to low levels of chlorine. Patil, et al (1969)[1] reported an epidemiological survey on 600 diaphragm cell workers and 382 control workers from 25 plants manufacturing chlorine in North America, which showed there was no higher incidence of abnormal chest X-rays or abnormal pulmonary function tests among diaphragm cell workers compared to controls, but exposure date showed that almost all workers were exposed to concentrations of chlorine less than 1ppm. Chester et al (1969)[2] demonstrated that a significant difference in the mean forced expiratory flow was found between subjects not exposed to chlorine and chlorine gas workers, but the effects of smoking made it impossible to attribute this reduction to exposure to chlorine alone.

Our study indicated that long-term exposure to ralative low concentration of chlorine is capable of producing lasting abnormalities of resparatory system, including symptom, pulmonary function and chest X-ray.

In general, the abnormalities rate in chlorine workers with long duration of exposure (>10 years) was higher than that in chlorine workers with short duration of exposure (<10 years). It demonstrated that there was a dose-effect relationship.

Our study also showed that exposure to chlorine and cigartte smoking may have an additive effect which played an important role in the impairment of resparatory system among the chlorine workers. The combined effect of smoking and chlorine seemed to be worse than those of either agent alone.

Comparing the pulmonary function tests with the pulmonary symptoms, as well as chest X-ray changes we found that there was good carrelation between repiratory symptoms and pulmonary function tests, but poor correlation between chest X-ray changes and pulmonary function tests. We considered the reason was that the pulmonary function of chlorine workers was essentially influenced by airway obstructive impairment, which is hardly to be seen in the chest X-ray film.

In conclusion, our study indicated that long-term exposure to relative low concentration of chlorine definitely effects workers health, espicially causes impairment of respiratory system. Therefore, occupational hygiene at workplaces should be enforced, education for workers about stopping smoking should be conducted and the respiratory state of the chlorine workers should be monitored.

REFERENCES

1. Patil, L.R.S. et al (1970) The health of diaphragm cell workers wxposed to chlorine. Am Ind Hyg Assoc J 31:678-686
2. Chester, E.H. et al (1969) The prevalence of chronic obstructive pulmonary disease in chlorine gas workers. Am Rev Resp Dis 99:365-373

Occupational Epidemiology. H. Sakurai et al., editors

549427

HIGH INCIDENCE OF PULMONARY TUBERCULOSIS AMONG PATHOLOGISTS AND PATHOLOGY TECHNICIANS IN JAPAN

MINORU SUGITA[1), YUTAKA TSUTSUMI[2)], TOSHITAKA ISHIKO[3)], MASASHI SUCHI[1)], HITOSHI KASUGA[1)]

1): Department of Public Health, Tokai University School of Medicine Boseidai, Isehara-shi, Kanagawa-ken 259-11 Japan
2): Department of Pathology, Tokai University School of Medicine
3): Department of Pathology, Kanto Teishin Hospital

INTRODUCTION

In Japan, tuberculosis was the leading cause of death between 1935 and 1950 (1), and its incidence and prevalence were very high during this period, but since then the mortality rate, incidence, and prevalence of tuberculosis have decreased remarkably (1) due to socioeconomical improvements and the appearance of specific chemotherapy. The incidence and prevalence of pulmonary tuberculosis in hospital workers, particularly among staff of pathology divisions, is assumed to be high. However, there have been no report on this subjects in Japan. In the present study, we investigated the incidence of pulmonary tuberculosis among pathologists and pathology technicians in Japan and its association with occupation.

MATERIALS AND METHODS

Subjects

Tokai University. Pathologists in the Pathology Division at Tokai University Hospital were questioned about past history of treatment for tuberculosis after 1975. As controls, employees in the Medical School and the other Schools of Tokai University were similarly questioned. The questionnaires were collected between May and June 1987.

Whole Japan. Questionnaires about past history of treatment for tuberculosis and activity in pathology services were distributed to employees in 171 pathology divisions and departments in 80 medical schools and their hospitals and in 217 non-university hospitals certified by the Japanese Society of Pathology and/or where members of the Japanese Association of Hospital Pathologists were employed. As a control, workers in departments of preventive medicine and public health (PMPH) in 80 medical schools in Japan were similarly questioned. The questionnaires were collected from July through September in 1988.

Statistical analysis

The annual incidence of tuberculosis (per 100,000 subjects), the Woolf's odds ratio (2), and Mantel-Haenszel's odds ratio (3-5) and chi-square test value with Yates' continuity correction (6) were calculated.

RESULTS

Tokai University

The number of respondents to the questionnaire, the proportion of the respondents, the number of subjects with histories of treatment for tuberculosis, the annual incidence of tuberculosis, the Woolf's odds ratio, and the chi-square test value with Yates' continuity correction for each section are shown in TABLE-I (7). The incidence was calculated as

incidence = number of patients / number of respondents / 12.5y,

where 12.5y indicates the duration in years from 1975 to July 1987. The odds ratio in TABLE-I is expressed by a reciprocal. Therefore, when the denominator is larger than 1.0, it indicates that the incidence of tuberculosis in pathologists is higher than that in the control section. TABLE-I shows a significantly higher incidence of tuberculosis among pathologists than in any of the other sections. Results of Mantel-Haenszel's analysis with the age group (≤39 and ≥40 years old) as the confounding factor were similar to the values shown in TABLE-I.

TABLE I

RESULTS OF STATISTICAL ANALYSIS IN TOKAI UNIVERSITY

Occupation	Number of respondents	% of respondents	No. of patients	Annual incidence	Woolf's odds ratio	X^2-value
Pathologists	11	91%	2	1455.	1	-----
Researchers in non-Clin. Dept.	48	94%	0	0.	1/ 25.5	4.33*
MD. in Clin. Dept.	184	48%	0	0.	1/ 97.1	18.26**
Nurses	566	74%	3	42.4	1/ 42.4	21.29**
Technicians	200	63%	0	0.	1/105.5	19.90**
Clerks in Med. Sch	271	94%	2	58.6	1/ 28.4	12.22**
Employees in other schools	726	62%	3	33.1	1/ 54.4	27.83**

Clin. Dept.: clinical departments, MD: Medical doctors,
Med. Sch: medical school, No.: Number, incidence: /100,000,
**: p<1%, *: p<5%

Whole Japan

One hundred sixty-two (94.5%) pathology divisions and departments in medical schools and their hospitals and 144 (66.4%) pathology divisions in non-university hospitals responded to the questionnaire. Based upon the number of medical schools, 91.3% of PMPH departments responded to the questionnaire. The respondent in pathology divisions and departments consisted of 1201 pathologists (medical doctor = MD), 1187 technicians, 77 non-MD researchers, 93 clerks, and 37 others, while those in PMPH departments were 336 MDs, 78 technicians, 234 non-MD researchers, 54 clerks, and 30 others.

TABLE-II shows the number of patients, the person-years, the annual incidence, and the odds ratio and the X^2 value between pathology and PMPH by occupation (8). As indicated in Table-II, the annual incidence of pulmonary tuberculosis in pathologists or pathology technicians was evidently higher than that in analogous workers in PMPH departments (odds ratio = 6.08-8.58, p<1%).

TABLE II

RESULTS OF STATISTICAL ANALYSIS IN WHOLE JAPAN

	Pathology			PMPH				
Occupation	No. of patients	person years	Annual incidence	No. of patients	person years	Annual incidence	Odds ratio	X^2-value
MD.	71	10381	$683.9/10^5$	4	3532	$113.3/10^5$	6.08M	14.98**
Technicians	58	9790	$592.4/10^5$	0	713	0.	8.58W	3.24
MD. & Tech.	129	20171	$639.5/10^5$	4	4245	$94.2/10^5$	6.77M 7.12J	17.96** 19.02**
Others	1	1303	$76.7/10^5$	0	2990	0.	6.89W	0.18
Total	130	21474	$605.4/10^5$	4	7235	$55.3/10^5$	10.98M	33.90**

MD.: Medical doctors, Tech.: Technicians, No.: Number, **: p<1%,
Others: Others than Medical doctors and Technicians,
PMPH: preventive medicine and public health, W: Woolf's odds ratio,
M: improved Mantel-Haenszel's method with age correction,
J: improved Mantel-Haenszel's method with age and occupation correction

Between pathology and PMPH groups, there were no statistical differences in incidences of pulmonary tuberculosis which had been treated before the subjects started to work in the present speciality by occupation (odds ratio = 0.82-1.04, no significance).

The annual incidence in pathologists ($683.9/10^5$) or pathology technicians who had assisted in autopsies ($823.8/10^5$) was remarkably higher (odds ratio = 5.52-6.65, p<1%) than that in technicians who had not assisted in autopsies ($125.1/10^5$).

DISCUSSION

The incidences of pulmonary tuberculosis in pathologists were significantly higher than those of the controls in both of the studies, and the incidence in pathology technicians who had assisted in autopsies was remarkably higher than that in technicians who had not assisted in autopsies. The consistency of these findings is important in order to judge etiological association between disease and occupation epidemiologically.

Difference between the incidences of pulmonary tuberculosis before start to work in the pathology and the PMPH speciality was small. The small difference before start to work contrasts with the significant difference after start to work between both of the groups.

Pathologists have many opportunities to examine cadavers with active tuberculosis at autopsy and to perform frozen section diagnosis on tissues with tuberculomas in Japan, and many of pathology technicians assist them in autopsies, biopsies, or cytologies. It is likely that many personnel in the pathology divisions face a significant risk of exposure to Mycobacterium tuberculosis at autopsy and at the time of frozen section diagnosis. Our preliminary study using frozen non-pathogenic bacterial colonies with a special antibiotic resistance has shown that, during the preparation of cryostat sections, the bacteria were detected in various work areas, particularly after use of a cryospray to freeze the material (8). The presence of Mycobacterium tuberculosis in the occupational environment of pathology divisions should also be confirmed by a study using air samplers, particularly during autopsy of active tuberculosis cadavers.

These findings strongly suggest that specific environmental condition in pathology divisions and departments represent an occupational hazard in Japan, particularly during autopsy of active tuberculosis cadavers, although the infection might be contracted from other hospital staff.

REFERENCES

1. Health and Welfare Statistics Association (1987) J Health Welfare Statist (monthly) {Kosei no Shihyo} 34(9-s): 145-150 (in Japanese)

2. Woolf B (1955) Ann Human Genet 19: 251-253

3. Mantel N, Haenszel W (1959) J Nat Cancer Inst 22: 719-748

4. Hannan J, Harkness WL (1963) Ann Math Statist 34: 1593-1595

5. Breslow NE, Day NE (1980) In: Davis W (eds) Statistical methods in cancer research: Vol. 1, The analysis of case-control studies. No.32, International Agency for Research on Cancer (IARC) Scientific Publications, Lyon, pp.122-159

6. Yates F (1934) Suppl T R Statiat Soc 1: 217

7. Sugita M, Tsutsumi Y, Suchi M, Kasuga H (1989): High incidence of pulmonary tuberculosis in pathologists of Tokai University Hospital: An epidemiological study, Tokai J Exp Clin Med 14: (in press)

8. Sugita M, Tsutsumi Y, Ishiko T, Suchi M, Kasuga H: Pulmonary Tuberculosis: An Occupational Hazard for Pathologists and Pathology Technicians in Japan (to be published)

HAZARDS ASSOCIATED WITH ASBESTOS, ORGANIC SOLVENTS AND OTHERS

Asbestos and MMMF

Occupational Epidemiology. H. Sakurai et al., editors

BIOLOGICAL EFFECTS OF MINERAL FIBRES: APPARENT INCONSISTENCIES BETWEEN EXPERIMENTAL DATA AND EPIDEMIOLOGICAL OBSERVATIONS

JACQUES DUNNIGAN
University of Sherbrooke, Sherbrooke, Québec, CANADA J1K 2R1

Human experience of exposure to different asbestos fibre types has shown an impressive difference in pathological potency between asbestos fibre types, chrysotile being much less fibrogenic and carcinogenic, and having very little mesothelioma-producing potential (if at all), compared to amphiboles. Recently, Wagner and co-workers pointed out: "We believe therefore that chrysotile is the least harmful form of asbestos in every respect and that more emphasis should be laid on different biological effects of amphibole and serpentine asbestos fibre."(1). Recently, man-made mineral fibres, especially rock/slag wools, have been positively correlated with excess incidence of lung cancer in production workers at low exposure levels(2), indeed at exposure levels (~1 f/ml) where chrysotile has been shown to produce no excess lung cancer(3). However, experimental data published from IN VITRO and IN VIVO assays have often resulted in inconsistencies with observations from epidemiological studies. In the recent years development of sophisticated techniques for tissue mineral analysis has led to possible explanations of the inconsistencies between animal experimental data and epidemiological evidence, pointing differences in durability of mineral fibres in the lung, and their different relative lifespan persistence between laboratory animals and man.

We wish to submit that another explanation may also reside in the basis for reporting the observed effects, i.e., per equal mass vs equal number of fibres.

Careful examination of the great majority of IN VITRO and IN VIVO experimental protocols to assess the biological effects of mineral fibres reveals that comparison of the effects (IN VITRO cytotoxicity in cellular and tissue systems, fibrogenicity and tumour yield in animal assays) has traditionally been based on a gravimetric dose basis, i.e., comparing the effects produced by equal mass of tested minerals (for example: 50 $\mu g/10^5$ cells; 20 mg dose by intraperitoneal injection; 20 mg/M^3 by inhalation, etc.).

Some attempts to transform retrospectively gravimetric doses into fibre number-doses have indicated that if based on <u>fibre number</u>, pathogenicity data showed that "fibre for fibre", chrysotile would be seen as less potent than the other asbestos fibre types, and possibly less than some other man-made mineral fibres as well. For instance, in a 1978 publication by Davis et al., the authors report that rats submitted to dust clouds of chrysotile, crocidolite and amosite showed more lung fibrosis and tumours after inhalation of chrysotile, than with either amphiboles. But, they state: "...it was found that the chrysotile dust clouds used in this study contained many more fibres longer than 20 microns than either of the amphibole dust clouds"(4).

Using animal data from Wagner JC(5), an analysis was made of effects per fibre rather than per unit mass relevant to the comparison of asbestos and man-made mineral fibres in the induction of pulmonary tumours by inhalation. The data reported show that while a similar mass dose (10 mg/M^3) of chrysotile produced a larger incidence of tumours than some man-made mineral fibres, the tumours yield per unit fibre dose (tumours per 100 f/cc X hours) was the following: UICC chrysotile: 1.8; rock wool: 5.1; glass wool with resin: 1.8; glass wool resin-free: 2.4(6).

In 1986, Goldsmith JR indicated that "based on fibre or particle counts, man-made mineral fibres appear to be more potent than asbestos with regard to chronic pulmonary disease"(7).

With regard to differences in potency between some natural mineral fibres, IN VITRO studies published recently show that when data are reported on a fibre number basis, chrysotile emerges as the least potent, when compared to crocidolite and erionite. Thus, the cytotoxic response of Chinese hamster lung V79 cells was studied, using sized fibres ($L \geq 8$ μ; $D \leq 0.25$ μ). Data show that while chrysotile appears to be more cytotoxic than crocidolite when the LD_{50} values (colony survival) is given per unit mass dose, they also indicate that the number of chrysotile fiber per unit mass is far greater than the number of crocidolite fibers(8). Broadly speaking, the same effect (LD_{50} cytotoxicity towards V79 cells) was produced by 1 erionite fibre, or 6 crocidolite fibres, or 350 chrysotile fibres. The same authors(9) had observed a similar ordering in relative potency in inducing mesothelioma in animal experiments. With erionite fibre taken as an index set at 100, crocidolite fibres showed an index of 23.5, and chrysotile showed an index of 0.3 (number of tumours/number of fibres ≥ 8 μ X ≤ 0.25 μ).

The following figure illustrates the difference in number of sized fibres per unit mass between three natural fibrous materials.

Number of Fibres ($X10^6$) per Milligram		CHRYSOTILE	CROCIDOLITE	ERIONITE
L: ⩾5 μ	D: ⩽0.1 μ	13,300	983	152
L: ⩾8 μ	D: ⩽025 μ	1,090	8.6	3.31

Data from PM Cook, US EPA, as reported by Coffin et al(9)

The following comparison of fibre number per unit mass of two different materials illustrates the importance of comparing biological potency on the basis of fibre numbers. Inhalation of aramid (Kevlar®) fibres at 18 mg/M^3 for 2 weeks has been reported to produce fibrosis in rats. The authors state that this mass dose is equivalent to 2,000 f/ml(10). An equivalent mass dose (18 mg/M^3) of UICC chrysotile will certainly produce fibrosis. But it must be realized that this mass dose of chrysotile is equivalent to ~240,000 f/ml.

Another report(11) by the same group mentions that chronic inhalation exposure to 100 f/ml of aramid has induced tumours and fibrosis. Using the authors' data (18 mg/M^3 = 2,000 f/ml), 100 f/ml of aramid would be equivalent to 0.9 mg/M^3; one might question if chrysotile, at a mass inhalation dose of 0.9 mg/M^3, would produce tumour!

It is interesting to note that in spite of the human data, some regulatory agencies such as U.S. EPA (1988), still maintain that chrysotile has the same potential as the other asbestos fibre types, and that man-made mineral fibres have lower pathogenic potential, BASED ON ANIMAL EXPERIMENTS USING EQUAL MASS DOSES.

Presently, TLVs for asbestos fibre types are in fibre numbers almost everywhere, whereas gravimetric standards (from ~5 to 10 mg/M^3) are still the current rule for man-made mineral fibres in many countries, although some national regulatory authorities have recently adopted standards in fibre numbers. Thus it will be interesting to follow the developments, and to watch how TLVs for man-made mineral fibres will eventually compare with each asbestos fibre type.

In the meantime, carefully planned animal experimentation, where doses are measured in fibre numbers, and where results are expressed in effects/fibre number, would certainly help to resolve the apparent inconsistencies between experimental and epidemiological data. In the meantime, presently available data seen to support the view that if natural mineral fibres such as chrysotile must be controlled to low levels such as 1 f/ml, so must man-made mineral fibres be controlled at the same levels, and possibly lower levels in the case of rock wool. These man-made mineral fibres, as well as the refractory (ceramic) fibres, are used/proposed as asbestos substitutes in a large number of applications such as: friction materials, thermal insulation, fibre-reinforced plastics and resins, gaskets and joints, etc.

REFERENCES

1. Wagner JC, Newhouse ML, Corrin B, Rossiter CER, Griffiths DM (1988) Brit J Ind Med 45:305-308

2. Doll R (1987) Ann Occup Hyg 31:805-819

3. Davis JMG, McDonald JC (1988) Brit J Ind Med 45:505-508

4. Davis JMG, Beckett ST, Bolton RE, Collings P, Middleton AP (1978) Brit J Cancer 37:673-688

5. Wagner JC (1982) In: Can Asb Inf C (ed) World Symposium on Asbestos, Montreal, pp. 244-266

6. Peto J (1989) In: Bignon J, Peto J, Saracci R (eds) Non-Occupational Exposure to Mineral Fibres, IARC Sc. Pub. No 90, Lyon, pp. 457-470

7. Goldsmith JR (1986) Amer J Ind Med 10:543-552

8. Palekar LD, Most BM, Coffin DL (1988) Environ Res 46:142-152

9. Coffin DL, Palekar LD, Cook PM, Creason JP (1988) In: Wehner AP, Felton D-L (eds) Biological Interaction of Inhaled Mineral Fibers and Cigarette Smoke, Battelle Press, Columbus Ohio, pp. 347-354

10. Lee KP, Kelly DP, Kennedy GL Jr. (1983) In: Toxicology and Applied Pharmacology 71:242-253

11. Lee KP, Kelly DP, O'Neal FO, Stadler JC, Kennedy GL Jr. (1988) In: Fundamental and Applied Toxicology 11:1-20

Occupational Epidemiology. H. Sakurai et al., editors

EFFECT OF INTENSITY IN ASBESTOS COHORT EXPOSURE-RESPONSE ANALYSES

PAMELA M. VACEK* AND J. CORBETT MCDONALD

Department of Clinical Epidemiology, National Heart and Lung Institute, Brompton Hospital, Fulham Road, London SW3 6HP (UK)

INTRODUCTION

The importance of exposure-response relationships for environmental hazards cannot easily be overstated. They allow scientifically based control limits to be set in the workplace and the magnitude of risks for the general population to be assessed. With the possible exception of ionizing radiation no environmental agent has been investigated more extensively than asbestos; even so, there are only about a dozen longitudinal studies in which both duration and intensity of exposure have been recorded. The analyses have usually been based on "accumulated exposure" ie the product of these two components, the individual contributions of which have not been adequately separated. As there is no biological reason to assume any simple equivalence between intensity and duration, especially when inevitably complicated by such related factors as short and long term variations in intensity and questions of residence time, extrapolation outside the range of actual observations could be seriously incorrect. This is especially a problem in estimating environmental risk for the general population where levels of exposure are usually far below those observed in occupational cohorts. These problems are generally ignored by legislators and others who accept uncritically the body of evidence which suggests that, at least for lung cancer, risk is directly related, and without threshold, to accumulated asbestos exposure (see McDonald & McDonald [1]). At least one possible explanation of the straight line relationships of varying slope which have been observed, is that the linearity is mainly determined by duration and the slope by various other factors including intensity, too poorly measured to affect the predominant pattern.

To explore these issues further, one of us (PMV) has adopted a new statistical approach to occupational cohort analysis. Available for this purpose were the data from five cohort studies conducted by our group, one very large in Quebec chrysotile miners and millers [2], three fairly large in American factory workers [3,4,5], and one quite small in Montana vermiculite miners exposed to fibrous tremolite [6]. Except for the friction products plant where there was little evidence of excess risk [5], the remaining studies yielded essentially linear exposure-response relationships for cumulative

*Present address: Medical Biostatistics, College of Medicine, The University of Vermont, Burlington, VT, 05405, (USA).

TABLE I

SUMMARY OF EXPOSURE DATA

Variable	Range of Dust Values (mpcf)	Time Weighted Average Dust Values	Years Spent at Level: Cases Mean	Total	%	Controls Mean	Total	%
Level 1	.00 (work gaps)	.00	2.7	615	16	2.2	46390	18
Level 2	.01 to .99	.60	0.5	110	3	0.8	15806	6
Level 3	1.00 to 2.99	2.17	3.3	767	21	2.9	60819	23
Level 4	3.00 to 9.99	5.43	3.4	783	20	2.6	55311	21
Level 5	10.00 to 24.99	15.30	2.7	630	16	1.8	38693	15
Level 6	25.00 to 49.99	35.89	1.9	443	11	0.9	19374	7
Level 7	50.00 or more	104.96	2.4	541	14	1.2	25980	10

	Cases Mean	Cases S.D.	Controls Mean	Controls S.D.
Net years of exposure	14.2	14.9	10.2	11.3
Gross years of exposure (including gaps)	16.8	16.1	12.4	12.9
Years since first employment	42.0	8.6	36.8	11.0
Cumulative exposure	400.4	658.2	210.7	434.9
Proportion who have smoked	91.7%		77.0%	

TABLE II

ESTIMATES OF MODEL PARAMETERS

Variable	b_i	S.E.	p-value
Years at Level 1: 0 exposure (gaps)	-.0007	.0139	.960
Years at Level 2: 0 to 1 mpcf	-.0341	.0284	.230
Years at Level 3: 1 to 3 mpcf	.0133	.0123	.279
Years at Level 4: 3 to 10 mpcf	.0015	.0144	.917
Years at Level 5: 10 to 25 mpcf	.0232	.0154	.132
Years at Level 6: 25 to 50 mpcf	.0704	.0189	<.001
Years at Level 7: >50 mpcf	.0519	.0153	<.001
Smoking (1 = ever, 0 = never)	1.4531	.2451	<.001
Years since first exposure	0320	.0104	.002

TABLE III

RISK ESTIMATES PER ANNUM (b_i) BY APPROXIMATE EXPOSURE LEVEL IN FIVE COHORTS

Intensity Level + (mpcf)	Miners & Millers: Chrysotile(2)	Tremolite(6)	Factory Workers: Textile(3)	Textile(4)	Friction(5)
0	.00	-	.05	.07	-.04
<5	-.03	-.05	.00	.02	-.01
.5, <1			-.11	.05	-.04
1, <3	.01	.14	.04*	.03	.00
3, <5	.00	.26	-.01	.09	-.07
5, <10			.11*	.24*	-.06
10, <25	.02	.13*	-	-	-
25, <50	.07*		-	-	-
50	.05*		-	-	-

\+ the levels shown are approximate; those for tremolite have been converted from fibre concentrations.

* $p = < 0.05$

exposure. Most workers, however, were exposed at several different dust intensities for varying durations during the course of their employment. Also, many workers had gaps in exposure, when they were not employed in the industry. We have used these details of exposure history to estimate risk for specific exposure intensities. In this paper, we shall deal primarily with our analysis of the Quebec cohort, although essentially the same approach was taken with the other four groups.

METHOD

All male lung cancer deaths occurring after 1950 and at least 20 years after first employment were grouped by year of birth, year of death and one of two main mining areas. The 230 lung cancer deaths formed 195 strata based on these variables. For each stratum controls were selected by two methods (a) all male workers born in the same year, employed in the same area and alive at the end of the year of death for each case or (b) four controls randomly selected from the 17 to 214 available who met the above criteria. Cases from other strata were eligible as controls. Only results obtained by the first method are presented below.

For each case and control, the intensity of dust exposure for each year of employment, expressed as millions of particles per cubic foot (mpcf) was categorized into one of seven exposure levels, as shown in Table 1. The number of years spent working at each level was obtained by summing the durations at each level up to nine years before year of death of the case. As in previous analyses, exposures less than nine years before death were not considered causative.

Conditional logistic regression was then used to fit the following multiplicative model for relative risk (RR):

$$RR = \exp\left(\sum_{i=1}^{9} b_i x_i\right)$$

The independant variables (x_i) represent smoking status, years since first employment and years spent at each of the seven exposure levels. The b_i parameters were estimated by an iterative procedure as described by Breslow etal [7] to maximize the conditional likelihood.

RESULTS

The results obtained by fitting the model to the cohort of 10,814 Quebec miners and millers using all possible controls are summarized in Table 2. With four controls per case, the findings were similar. The value for b_i represents the lung cancer risk, in terms of logarithm of relative risk, attributable to each year spent working at that dust level, after allowing for exposure at any other level, smoking and time since first exposure. Of the seven dust levels, only the coefficients for the two highest intensity categories were significantly different from zero. The coefficient for Level 7 was lower than that for Level 6, although the two are not significantly different from each other. This suggests that risk may level off at high intensities, rather than continue to increase as would be expected if it were simply a function of cumulative exposure.

The fact that the coefficients for dust intensities below 25 mpcf are not significantly different from zero does not, of course, mean that there is no lung cancer risk at these exposure levels. However, we must consider this a possibility, since our data provide no evidence to the contrary.

Similar analyses of the other four cohorts gave analagous results. In the two cohorts of asbestos textile workers [3,4] there was, again, no significant departure of the b_i value from zero until exposure intensity 4 (1.00-2.99 mpcf). On the other hand, the risk was highest in the highest exposure category (≥5.00 mpcf). These exposure levels were much lower than for the Quebec miners, whose risk of lung cancer in relation to cumulative exposure (mpcf.y) was many times lower than in the textile workers. Analysis of data for the small cohort of Montana miners and millers exposed to fibrous tremolite gave results similar in pattern to those for the Quebec cohort but at much lower levels of exposure. Analysis of data from the cohort of friction product workers gave no evidence of increased risk of lung cancer at any exposure intensity - much as had been found with accumulated exposure [5]. Although the exposure levels used for these analyses differed somewhat in the five cohorts, a simplified comparison of the findings is presented in Table 3.

COMMENT

It would be preferable to assess the risks associated with differing intensities by studying subjects at constant levels of exposure. Even without such data, it is possible to obtain valid estimates of risk for specific dust levels by using the approach described above. The risk estimates we obtained are not as precise as we would like, particularly at low exposure levels, where any effect would be small. However, we believe our approach to be a more sensible one for examining the exposure-response relationship than those which extrapolate the risk for different intensities from cumulative exposure results. The latter assume that all exposure levels carry a risk and that intensity and duration affect risk equally. Our results raise questions about the validity of these assumptions, suggesting that estimates based on cumulative exposure may contain bias, in addition to the imprecision inherent in any estimation procedure. A further advantage of the method described is that it could be used equally well for the analysis of categorical data - job titles for example - without need for knowledge of the exposure levels entailed.

REFERENCES

1. McDonald JC, McDonald AD (1987) In: Antman K, Aisner J (eds) Asbestos-related malignancy. Grune & Stratton, Orlando, pp 57-79.

2. McDonald JC, McDonald AD, Gibbs GW, Eyssen GE (1980). Brit J Ind Med; 37: 11-24.

3. McDonald AD, Fry JS, Woolley AJ, McDonald JC (1983). Brit J Ind Med; 40: 361-367.

4. McDonald AD, Fry JS, Woolley AJ, McDonald JC (1983). Brit J Ind Med; 40: 368-374.

5. McDonald AD, Fry JS, Woolley AJ, McDonald JC (1984). Brit J Ind Med; 41: 151-157.

6. McDonald JC, McDonald AD, Armstrong B, Sébastien P. (1986). Brit J Ind Med; 43: 436-444.

7. Breslow NE, Lubin JH, Marek P, Langholz B (1983). J Am Stat Assoc; 78: 1-12.

Organic solvents

© 1990 Elsevier Science Publishers B.V. (Biomedical Division)
Occupational Epidemiology. H. Sakurai et al., editors

MONITORING STYRENE NEUROTOXICITY WITH ^{3}H-SPIPERONE BINDING IN LYMPHOCYTES

HARVEY CHECKOWAY,[1] LUCIO G. COSTA,[1] TERESA COCCINI,[1] STEPHEN RAPPAPORT,[2] LUIGI MANZO[3]
[1]Department of Environmental Health, School of Public Health and Community Medicine, University of Washington, Seattle, Washington, USA
[2]Department of Biomedical and Environmental Health Sciences, School of Public Health, University of California, Berkeley, California, USA
[3]Institute of Pharmacology, University of Pavia Medical School, Pavia, Italy

INTRODUCTION

Toxicity to the central nervous system (CNS) has been the most convincingly demonstrated health effect of occupational styrene exposure. Workers exposed to concentrations in excess of 100 ppm exhibit the so called "prenarcotic syndrome" characterized by nausea, dizziness, and feelings of drunkenness (1) as well as neurobehavioral deficits (2). CNS effects at levels below 50 ppm are less well documented.

The mechanism of styrene-induced CNS toxicity is unknown, although there are provocative experimental data indicating that dopamine depletion by styrene or one of its metabolites may play a significant pathogenetic role. Increases in dopamine receptors, assessed by ^{3}H-spiperone (^{3}H-SP) binding, in brain striatum and striatal dopamine depletion have been reported in styrene-treated rats (3) and rabbits (4), respectively. Also, an increase in ^{3}H-SP binding has been detected in platelets of styrene-treated rats (5).

The objective of the present study was to evaluate the utility of monitoring ^{3}H-SP binding in lymphocytes of workers exposed to styrene as a marker of neurotoxicity. If the dopamine depletion hypothesis of styrene neurotoxic effect applies, then it would be predicted that ^{3}H-SP binding would be increased among exposed workers relative to non-exposed subjects, and binding would correlate with the extent of exposure. Of course, this argument requires that binding in lymphocytes mirrors effects in the CNS.

MATERIALS AND METHODS

Study Subjects

The study population consisted of 38 workers (18 males and 20 females; age range 22 to 63 years) from a plant that manufactures luxury yachts. A reference group of 17 non-exposed blood donors (10 males and 7 females; age range 27 to 40 years) was identified from among laboratory and professional staff at the University of Washington. The reference group provided an estimate of the expected range of values for ^{3}H-SP binding, whereas the main comparisons were made between worker subgroups classified according to styrene exposure levels.

Exposure Measurements

Between July, 1987 and June, 1988 there were seven exposure monitoring surveys conducted at the plant at roughly 6-week intervals. At each survey shift-long personal samples were collected with passive monitors (SKC Model 530); the samples were analyzed by gas chromatography (6). Eight-hour time-weighted exposures at the plant ranged from <1 to 91 ppm.

Blood samples were collected for measurement of styrene concentrations at the first, third, fifth and seventh survey. The blood styrene analysis was performed by the headspace technique using the method of standard addition. Three 1-mL aliquots from each worker were placed in 4-mL vials. Two microliters of DMSO, containing 0, 0.25, or 1.00 μg of styrene were injected into each aliquot of blood. The vials were placed in a heated block at 37 °C with periodic agitation for a minimum of 1 hour, whereupon 200 mL of headspace were injected into a gas chromatograph. The coefficient of variation of the method was estimated to be 0.20, based upon a repeated analysis of 5 samples.

^{3}H-Spiperone Analysis

An additional sample of blood was collected from each worker at the seventh survey. Blood samples containing volumes of 3-7 mL were collected in EDTA-treated vials. The samples were delivered to the laboratory for analysis of ^{3}H-SP binding within 24 hours of collection. Volunteers donated 10-mL samples of venous blood. Previous experimental work by two of us (TC and LGC) indicated that ^{3}H-SP binding was not detectable in circulating platelets, but could be detected in lymphocytes. Consequently, the assays were performed on study subjects' lymphocytes. The blood samples were layered on 3 mL of Histopaque (specific gravity 1.077) for separation of lymphocytes according to the method of Boyum (7). Binding of ^{3}H-SP in lymphocytes was determined by incubating 1 x 10^6 cells at 37 °C in 1 mL of Hank's solution with 3 nM of ^{3}H-SP in the presence (non-specific binding) or absence (total binding) of 10 μM haldoperidol (8). After incubation for 30 minutes, the samples were filtered through Whatman GF/C filters, which were washed with PBS buffer, air-dried, and counted for radioactivity. Results are expressed as fmol ^{3}H-SP specifically bound per 10^6 lymphocytes.

RESULTS

The median ^{3}H-SP binding was greater among the workers than volunteers: 67 vs. 57 fmol/10^6 lymphocytes. The ranges of values for the two groups overlapped; the ranges were 13 to 161 among workers and 42-86 for volunteers. However, inspection of the two distributions (Fig. 1) suggests a possible exposure-related difference.

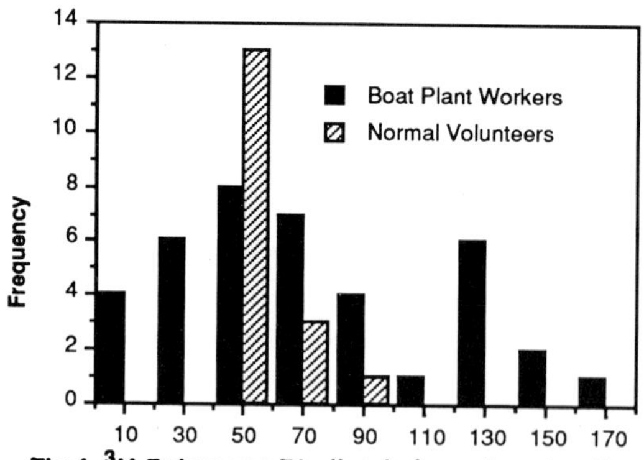

Fig 1. ^{3}H-Spiperone Binding in Lymphocytes (fmol/10^6 cells)

Comparisons between workers, classified by styrene exposure level, are given separately for males and females in Table I. Workers' styrene exposures were averaged over all surveys during the year in order to provide exposure estimates. In addition, the ^{3}H-SP data were adjusted by covariance analysis for effects due to age and cigarette smoking (current smokers vs. non- and ex-smokers). There is no discernible trend among males. However, among female workers, ^{3}H-SP binding increased according to exposure level: the median values are: 55.7, 75.0, and 107.0 for exposure categories <2, 2-19, and ≥20 ppm, respectively. Analyses with respect to exposure concentrations at the most recent survey when blood samples were obtained yielded similar patterns.

TABLE I: ^{3}H-Spiperone binding in lymphocytes (fmol/10^6 cells) adjusted for age and smoking status, by styrene exposure level averaged over one year.

	Exposure category (ppm)		
	<2	2-19	≥ 20
		Males	
No. subjects	8	2	8
Mean (SD)*	70.5 (37.8)	89.2 (58.7)	68.6 (36.1)
Median	58.1	89.2	58.4
		Females	
No. Subjects	7	8	5
Mean (SD)	47.4 (28.0)	89.1 (38.4)	79.6 (54.5)
Median	55.7	75.0	107.0

* Standard deviation

Comparisons of ^{3}H-SP, adjusted for age and smoking differences, were made with respect to blood concentrations of styrene averaged over the year (Table II). A slightly negative trend was noted for male workers, whereas the gradient among females is consistent with the data in Table I for exposure concentrations. Analysis by duration of employment did not reveal any consistent trends (data not shown).

TABLE II: ^{3}H-Spiperone binding in lymphocytes fmol/10^6 cells), adjusted for age and smoking status, by blood styrene concentration averaged over one year

	Blood styrene concentration (µg/L)	
	< 0.1	≥ 0.1
	Males	
No. subjects	8	10
Mean (SD)*	78.4 (43.2)	66.6 (32.5)
Median	64.0	58.4
	Females	
No. subjects	8	12
Mean (SD)	48.7 (26.0)	87.7 (44.4)
Median	56.7	91.9

* Standard deviation

DISCUSSION

Determinations of the neurotoxic properties of styrene among occupational groups customarily rely on reports of clinical symptoms, neurobehavioral testing, or neurophysiological function measurement. It would be of great benefit if a relatively simple, non-invasive technique could be developed to monitor for early signs of neurotoxicity. ^{3}H-SP binding in lymphocytes would appear to offer promise in this regard.

The results from this preliminary application of the ^{3}H-SP assay are not fully consistent with an exposure-response relationship, although there are suggestions of an effect among females. The small number of subjects studied and the great variability in the ^{3}H-SP binding data are important limitations of this investigation, however.

Recent experimental work strongly suggests that ^{3}H-SP may, in fact, label sigma receptors, rather than dopamine receptors (8). Sigma receptors have been implicated pharmacologically in the pathogenesis of psychosis (9), although a clear physiological role remains to be elucidated. Work in progress focuses on a larger scale application of lymphocyte assays using ligands, such as ^{3}H (+)-1,3, di-o-toluylguanidine, that are more specific than ^{3}H-SP for sigma receptors. These assays will be assessed in relation to styrene exposure concentrations, urine metabolite levels, and clinical symptoms of neurotoxicity.

ACKNOWLEDGMENTS

This work was supported in part by grants from NIEHS [ES-04696, ES-04705], NIOSH [OH-02620], and Fondazione Clinica del Lavoro. The authors are grateful to Martha Finley and Melinda Fujiwara for manuscript preparation.

REFERENCES

1. Lorimer WV, Lilis R, Fischbein A et al. (1978) Scand J Work Environ Health 4 Suppl 2:220-226

2. Gamberle F (1985) Scand J Work Environ Health 11 Suppl 1:65-74

3. Argawal AK, Srivastava SP, Seth PK et al. (1982) Bull Contam Toxicol 29:400-403

4. Mutti A, Romanelli A, Falzoi M et al. (1985) Arch Toxicol Suppl 8:447-450

5. Khanna AS, Argawal AK, Seth PK (1987) Biochem Arch 3:307-316

6. Rudling J (1987) Appl Ind Hyg 2:170-175

7. Boyum A (1967) Scand J Clin Lab Suppl 97:77-89

8. Coccini T, Checkoway H, Rappaport SM et al. (1989) Paper presented at the Second International Conference on Neurotoxicology, Barcelona, Spain

9. Deutsch SI, Weizman A, Goldman ME, Morhisi JM (1988) Clin Neuropharmacol 11:105-119

Occupational Epidemiology. H. Sakurai et al., editors

APPLICATION OF PHYSIOLOGICALLY-BASED PHARMACOKINETIC MODELING TO EXPOSURE ASSESSMENT IN OCCUPATIONAL SETTINGS

Akio Koizumi, Yasuhiko Wada, Sigetosi Kamiyama

Department of Hygiene, School of Medicine, Akita University Akita 010, JAPAN

INTRODUCTION

Physiologically based pharmacokinetic modeling (PPM) enables us to describe kinetic aspects of various chemicals in many species. Consequently, dose-response relationships obtained in various species by various routes of exposure can be rearranged in a common dose-response relationship on the basis of "internally achieved dose". Thus PPM appears to be useful for the exposure assessment under various scenarios (1,2).

The aim of the present study is to apply PPM to exposure assessment to trichloroethylene (TRI) and tetrachloroethylene (TETRA) in occupational settings. Using PPM, biological permissible values were simulated. In addition, effects of fluctuation of concentration on those values were also investigated.

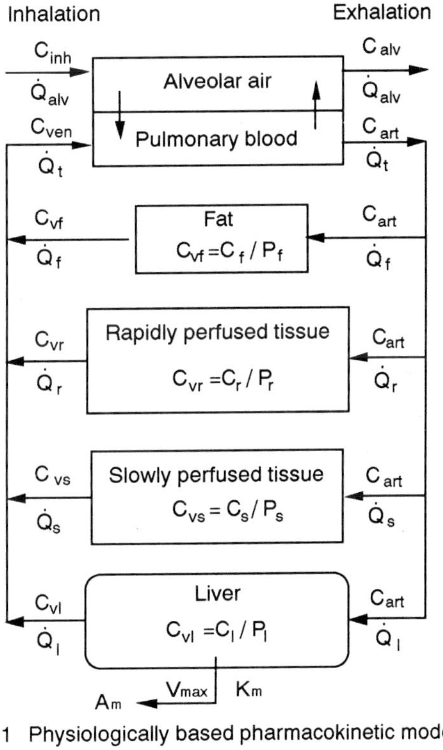

Fig. 1 Physiologically based pharmacokinetic model.

MATERIALS AND METHODS

Physiologically based pharmacokinetic model

A physiologically pharmacokinetic model composed of five tissue groups (1) was used throughout this study (Fig.1). The model was originally developed in rats and then was scaled up to the human. Physiological parameters used in the present study were obtained as described previously (2). Parameters for TRI and TETRA used in the study were obtained from the previous study (2). We assumed that a 70-kg man works for 8 hr a day and is exposed to those chemicals at the TLV (Threshold Limit Value) concentration.

Computer simulation

Simulation of differential equations describing the kinetics of TRI and TETRA were formulated as a computer program as outlined by Ramsey and Andersen (1) and Koizumi et al (3). Simulations were conducted with a basic-written program and were run on Macintosh computer.

RESULTS

PPM, which was originally developed in rats, was applied to simulate the biologically permissible value of exhaled air concentration and blood concentration of the two compounds for monitoring exposure intensities in occupational settings. The simulated maximum permissible values showed good agreement with those obtained by field surveys (Table).

TABLE

BIOLOGICAL PERMISSIBLE VALUES FOR TRI AND TETRA DETERMINED BY FIELD STUDIES AND SIMULATION

		Permissible values obtained by field studies & [simulation]	
Solvent	TLV	Solvent in Blood	Solvent in expired air
TRI	50 ppm x 8hr	0.9 mg/L [0.8]	50-80 mg/m^3 [50]
TETRA	50 ppm x 8hr	2.3 mg/L [1.8]	160 mg/m^3 [120]

It is well known that concentrations of chemicals in occupational settings are stochastic in nature and their intensities follow log-normal distribution. On the other hand it is also known that kinetic behaviors of chemicals have profound influences on correlation

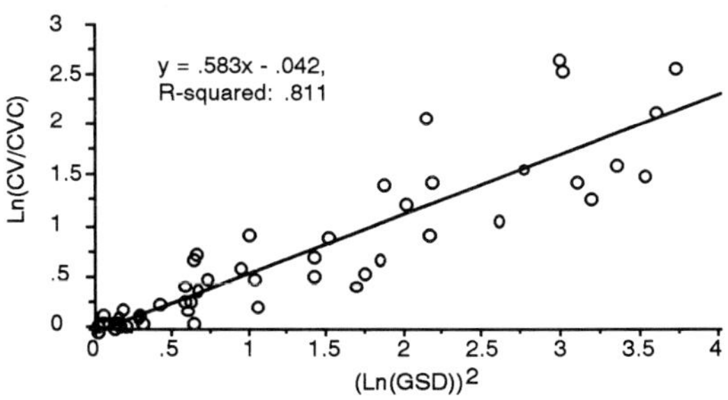

Fig. 2 Effect of GSD on CV/CVC.

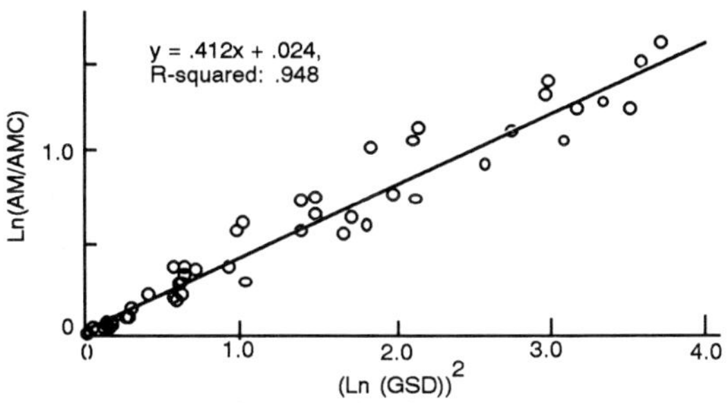

Fig. 3 Effect of GSD on AM/AMC.

between exposure intensities as indicated by the time-weighted average (TWA) and so called "body burden" (4). Namely, shorter the biological half life, the poorer the correlation between the above two values becomes in the two compartment model (4,5). However the effects of fluctuation of the exposure concentrations on biomonitoring values in complex systems remains unknown. Thus using PPM, we simulated the situations where the exposure concentration of TRI fluctuated. The concentrations fluctuated in a manner to follow a log-normal distribution of which geometrical standard deviations (GSD) are in a range between 1.0 to 7.4 with a fixed geometrical mean (GM) of 50 ppm. The simulation indicated that both of the blood concentration (CV) at the end of the work shift and amount metabolized (AM) within 24 hr after exposure (selected as a representative biomarker for "internally achieved dose") became larger than those values after the exposure at 50 ppm without fluctuation (abbreviated as CVC and AMC) as the GSD became larger. The ratio of CV over CVC increased as a function of GSD. Likewise, the ratio of AM over AMC increased as a function of GSD. On the other hand, both CV and AM were in proportion to TWA averages of fluctuated concentrations. The above relationships were theoretically predicted :

$$\mathrm{Ln(CV\ or\ AM)} \propto \mathrm{Ln(TWA)} \qquad \text{(Ln: Natural Logarithm)}$$

therefore, $\mathrm{Ln\ (CV\ or\ AM)} \propto \mathrm{Ln(GM)} + 0.5 \times (\mathrm{Ln\ (GSD)})^2$ ----- (Eq-1)

because $\mathrm{Ln(TWA)} = \mathrm{Ln(GM)} + 0.5 \times (\mathrm{Ln(GSD)})^2$

In fact, CV/CVC or AM/AMC were expressed as a function of GSD as shown in Fig. 2 and 3, respectively. Furthermore simulation revealed that AM were saturated above the CV=4mg/L (Fig. 4), which is equal to the value after exposure at 250ppm.

DISCUSSION

PPM has a potential to construct an unified pharmacokinetic model in several species. Thus if a PPM is constructed in animals, we can predict the fate of chemicals in humans by simply scaling up the model as shown in the present study. In addition, we can predict the " internally achieved dose " under exposure at various situations by simulation. This means that many biomonitoring standard values can be *a priori* predicted without accumulating historical data, if a reasonable PPM is constructed. Superiority of this simple approach to the traditional way is obvious.

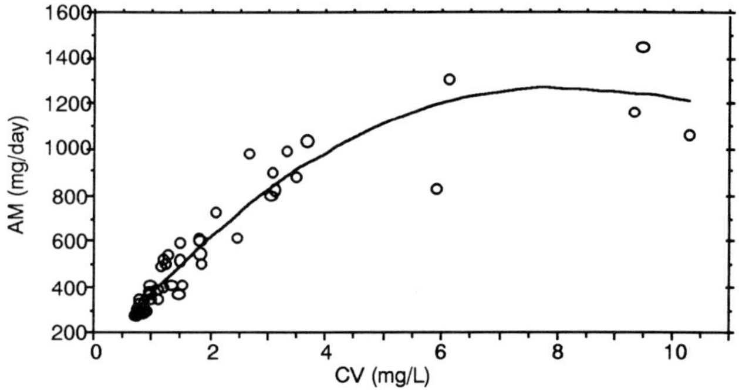

Fig. 4 Relationship between CV and AM.

We demonstrated that the biomonitoring values for TRI exposure, blood concentration (CV) and amount metabolized (AM) were well predicted by the equation (Eq-1). This indicates that both of the GM and GSD should be taken into account to assess the "internally achieved dose". Furthermore the blood concentration of TRI showed a good correlation ($r=0.953$ $p<0.01$) with the amount metabolized and thus the former parameters can be a good biomarker of the latter value unless metabolic saturation occurs.

In conclusion, the use of PPM seems promising in various areas ; those include risk assessment and exposure assessment under various situations. This approach will enable us to assess the toxicity of chemicals in workers by compiling diverse dose-response relations in animals and in humans.

REFERENCES

1. Ramsey JC, Andersen ME (1984) Toxicol Appl Pharmacol 73 : 159
2. Koizumi A (1989) Brit J Ind Med 46 : 239
3. Koizumi A, Ikeda M(1981) Am Ind Hyg Assoc J 42 :417
4. Roach SA (1977) Ann Occp Hyg 20 : 65
5. Koizumi A, Sekiguchi T, Konno M, Ikeda M (1980) Am Ind Hyg Assoc J 41 : 693

Occupational Epidemiology. H. Sakurai et al., editors

CLINICAL AND NEUROPHYSIOLOGICAL RESIDUAL ALTERATIONS OF SHOE-MAKER'S NEUROPATHY (N-HEXANE POLYNEUROPATHY) AT LEAST TEN YEARS AFTER THE ORIGINAL DIAGNOSIS

GIACOMO MUZI*, GIUSEPPE ABBRITTI*, MARCO DELL'OMO*, M. PATRIZIA ACCATTOLI*, GIANFRANCO PERTICONI**, TERESA A. CANTISANI**, RICCARDO URCIUOLI**

* Institute of Occupational Medicine, University of Perugia, ** Neurophysiopathology Unit, Regional Hospital, Perugia (Italy)

INTRODUCTION

Shoe-maker's polyneuropathy was a very frequently observed disease during the '70s both in Italy and other countries where shoe and leather industries were widespread (1-3). At present severe clinical pictures are rare; however, slighter forms are still possible where work is carried out in small artisan workshops or at home. A large number of studies have contributed to specifying the aetiology, which is presently attributed to n-hexane, the epidemiology and clinical aspects of the disease (1,4). In regard to the possible residual lesions of the neuropathy, there is not a great amount of information in the literature (5). For these reasons a clinical and neurophysiological study has been carried out to evaluate late residual alterations in shoe-maker's polyneuropathy, at least ten years after the first diagnosis.

MATERIAL AND METHODS

The study was carried out in shoe-makers of both sexes in whom polyneuropathy from solvents had been diagnosed between 1972 and 1978. Subjects with concomitant factors that cause peripheral neuropathy (occupational, pharmacological, alcohol abuse, etc.) or systemic diseases involving the nervous system were excluded from the study. The motor nerve conduction velocity (MNCV) of the peroneal nerve (PN) obtained at least 10 years before, at the time of the first diagnosis, was used as a reference parameter (4) to subdivide the patients into two groups: severe polyneuropathy (SPN) - subjects who at the first examination showed MNCV lower than 44 m/s as well as electromyographic alterations; mild polyneuropathy (MPN) - subjects with only electromyographic alterations. A questionnaire was used to collect the family and occupational history, concomitant diseases and present symptoms. The subjects affected by polyneuropathy and a control group underwent a neurological examination and an electrophysiological study of the peripheral nervous system (PNS). The following parameters were studied : 1. maximum motor nerve conduction velocity (MNCV) of the right (R) median, R ulnar, R and left (L) peroneal nerves. 2. the maximum sensory conduction velocity (SCV) of the R median, R ulnar and R sural nerves; 3. the distal latency (DL), duration (D) and amplitude (A) of the M response (Mr) evoked by

TABLE I
SYMPTOMS AND SIGNS MORE FREQUENTLY RECORDED IN SUBJECTS WHO HAD SUFFERED FROM MILD (MNP) OR SEVERE (SNP) SHOE-MAKER'S POLYNEUROPATHY AND IN CONTROLS

	Controls (n=31)		MNP (n=14)		SNP (n=24)	
	N	%	N	%	N	%
SYMPTOMS						
MUSCLE WEAKNESS						
upper limbs	1*≠	3.2	4≠	28.6	8*	33.3
lower limbs	0*°	0	5°	35.7	18	75.0
NUMBNESS OR TINGLING						
hands	0≠	0	1	7.1	4≠	16.7
feet	0*≠	0	3≠	21.4	8*	33.3
CRAMPING PAIN						
upper limbs	0	0	1	7.1	1	4.2
lower limbs	0*°	0	5°	35.7	8*	33.3
SIGNS						
MUSCULAR HYPOTROPHY	0*	0	1	7.1	13*	54.2
REDUCED MUSCULAR STRENGTH	1*	3.2	3	21.4	11*	45.8
DEEP TENDON REFLEXES						
increased	0*	0	0	0	6*	25.0
reduced	3≠	9.7	5	35.7	10≠	41.7

*,°: p 0.01; ≠:p 0.05. (Comparisons were performed either by chi-square test or Fisher's exact test).

TABLE II
ELECTROMYOGRAPHIC FINDINGS (RECRUITMENT PATTERN OF THE MUPs) IN SUBJECTS WHO HAD SUFFERED FROM MILD (MNP) or SEVERE (SNP) SHOE-MAKER'S POLYNEUROPATHY AND IN CONTROLS

	Controls (n-30)			MNP (n=12)			SNP (n=24)		
	IP %	RIP %	SRIP %	IP %	RIP %	SRIP %	IP %	RIP %	SRIP %
MUSCLES									
R EDB	90.0	10.0	--	58.3	41.7	--	20.8	66.7	12.5
L EDB	86.7	10.0	3.3	66.7	33.3	--	21.7	65.2	13.0°
R TA	100	--	--	100	--	--	95.7	4.3	--°
L TA	100	--	--	91.7	8.3	--	79.2	20.8	
R AP	100	--	--	100	--	--	95.8	4.2	--
R OP	100	--	--	100	--	--	95.7	4.3	--°

IP=Interference Pattern; RIP=Reduced IP; SRIP=Severely Reduced IP
R (right), L (left); EDB=Extensor Digitorum Brevis; TA=Tibialis Anterior; AP=Adductor Pollicis; OP=Opponens Pollicis. °: n=23

stimulation of the R median, R ulnar, R and L peroneal nerves; 4. Recruitment pattern (RP) of the motor unit potentials (MUPs) of the following muscles: R and L extensor digitorum brevis, R and L tibialis anterior, R adductor and R opponens pollicis; 5) the presence of spontaneous activity (SA) of denervation in the same muscles mentioned in point 4. The data obtained were elaborated using the SPSS program (6).

RESULTS

This study involved 31 controls and 38 patients with a previous diagnosis of shoe-maker's polyneuropathy. Fourteen of the patients were classified as having had a mild form and 24 a severe form of the disease. The mean age was similar in the two groups, as well as in the controls. Most of the subjects had not been exposed to solvents for nearly 10 years and all of them for the last 5 years. The subjects affected by neuropathy showed a significantly higher frequency of signs and symptoms of PNS involvement in comparison to the controls (Table 1); they were on the whole of slight entity, more frequent in patients who had been affected by a more severe neuropathy, and localized with a net prevalence to the distal segments of the lower limbs.

Electroneurographic examination showed that MNCV and SNCV of all the examined nerves were within the normal limits of our laboratory. However, in the median nerves they were slightly lower in the SPN with respect to the control subjects (MNCV: 54.9 ± 4.7 vs 58.6 ± 4.5, $p < 0.05$; SNCV: 56.4 ± 3.4 vs 59.4 ± 4.7, $p < 0.05$). Furthermore, the DL of the Mr was significantly reduced in both peroneal nerves in the SPN group ($p<0.05$) and in the ulnar ($p<0.05$) and L peroneal nerves ($p<0.01$) in the MPN group.

In regard to the electromyographic findings, spontaneous muscular activity of denervation was absent in all the cases. An alteration of the RP of the MUPs was evident in patients who had been affected by neuropathy (Table 2). A slightly reduced interference pattern of MUPs was recorded in 30-40% of the subjects of the MNP group and in approximately 65% of the SPN subjects at extensor digitorum brevis level. It was less frequently seen at the level of tibialis anterior muscles. A more severe compromission (moderate-severe reduction of MUPs) at the level of extensor digitorum brevis was present in a small number of SPN cases.

DISCUSSION

This study, although not yet concluded, does confirm other reports (5,7) and agrees with late clinical and elctrophysiological pictures described in patients with a previous diagnosis of neuropathy due to various solvents (8,9).

In our population no irreversible damage of the myelin sheath seems to persist in any of the cases, even in the more severe forms of the disease. In contrast, the recovery of motor units appears to be impaired when the initial damage to the nerves was more pronounced, especially in the distal segments of the lower limbs. Unexpectantly, this alteration was associated with a homogenous trend to a reduction of the DL of the Mr. This finding, if confirmed, could suggest a relevant anatomic and functional modification of the distal portions of nerve fibres as a consequence of later regeneration processes.

The neurological signs and symptoms, mostly localized in the distal segments of the lower limbs, agree with the results of the electrophysiological examination. It is necessary to consider that many of the subjects studied were beneficiaries of an invalid pension; therefore, an influence on the symptomatology cannot be excluded. The increase in the osteo-tendon reflexes in the SPN group could be indicative of permanent damage to the central nervous system, as described by other authors (10) in subjects with n-hexane poisoning.

In conclusion, this study suggests that after 10 years from the onset of shoe-maker's polyneuropathy, and at least 5 years from the end of exposure, the signs of neurogenic damage persist and are more evident in subjects that had had more severe clinical and neurophysiological manifestations.

ACKNOWLEDGEMENTS

This study was supported in part by a grant from the Ministry of Labour. The authors gratefully acknowledge the linguistic and editorial assistance of G. Hoddle Stoppini.

REFERENCES

1. Abbritti G, Siracusa A, Cianchetti C, Curradi F, Perticoni GF, De Rosa F (1976) Br J Ind Med 33:92
2. Inoue T, Takeuchi Y, Takeuchi S et al (1970) Jap J Ind Health 12:73
3. Sobue I, Yamamura Y, Ando K, Iida M, Takayanagi T (1968) Clinical Neurology 8:393
4. Cianchetti C, Abbritti G, Perticoni GF, Siracusa A, Curradi F (1976)J Neurol Neurosurg Psychiatry 9:1151
5. Perticoni G, Cianchetti C (1976) Elletromyogr Clin Neurophysiol 16:493
6. Nie NH, Hull CH, Jenkins JG et al. (1975) SPSS: Statistical Package for Social Science, McGraw Hill Book Company, New York
7. Passero S, Battistini N, Cioni R, Giannini F, Paradiso C, Battista F, Carboncini F, Sartorelli E (1983) Ital J Neurol Sci 4:463
8. Seppalainen AM, Antti-Poika M (1983) Scand J Work Environ Health 9:15
9. Corsi G, Maestrelli P, Picotti G, Manzoni S, Negrin P (1983) Br J Ind Med 40:209
10. Chang YC (1987) J Neurol Neurosurg Psychiatry 50:269

© 1990 Elsevier Science Publishers B.V. (Biomedical Division)
Occupational Epidemiology. H. Sakurai et al., editors

CHRONIC NEUROBEHAVIOURAL CHANGES IN PAINTERS

A. SPURGEON, C.N. GRAY and J. SIMS

Institute of Occupational Health, University of Birmingham, Unviersity Road West, P.O.Box 363, Birmingham, B15 2TT, UK

INTRODUCTION

A variety of organic solvents such as toluene, xylene and styrene, are used in many industrial processes ranging from painting, varnishing, carpet laying, paint manufacture and boat making. The acute neurotoxic effects of such solvents, for example fatigue and dizziness, have been known for a long time. However, less is known about chronic neurological effects which have been investigated only comparatively recently.

The controversial claims by Scandinavian researchers (e.g. Mikkelsen et al, 1988) and others of adverse neuropsychiatric effects of chronic exposure have been well publicised. However, a variety of methodological criticisms have been made of the Scandinavian work (Grasso et el 1984) and both the existence and nature of chronic effects remains a matter of dispute.

The present study represents the first phase of a large scale investigation carried out in the UK into the possible chronic neuropsychological effects of long term exposure to paint solvents.

METHOD

The investigation was a cross sectional study involving psychological assessment of brush painters and matched controls.

Subjects

After exclusion for specified health conditions (5 subjects) 90 painters employed by the West Midlands Regional Health Service in the UK acted as subjects. This volunteer study population represented 67% of all painters employed in the Regional Health Service. Ninety age-matched controls were randomly selected from a pool of manual workers employed on the same sites, in specified occupations involving either no solvent exposure or very little. All participants were male. The age range was 25-65 years.

Procedure

All participants completed a set of questionnaires under the supervision of an interviewer, following which they completed a battery of computer-administered psychological tests. Testing was carried out under standardised conditions in a mobile laboratory driven on site. It was carried out during mornings only to standardise time-of-day effects on test performance and following an exposure-free period of at least 12 hours to minimise any short term effects. Sixty-three per cent of subjects had been free of exposure for at least 48 hours.

Questionnaires

(i) A medical history questionnaire identified exclusion factors and information about possible confounders e.g. alcohol consumption.

(ii) The General Health Questionnaire (GHQ) (Goldberg 1970), a standardised measure of psychiatric morbidity.

(iii) The Cognitive Failures Questionnaire (CFQ) (Broadbent 1982), a measure of behavioural memory.

(iv) The Orebo Questionnaire-16 (Hogstedt-16), a measure of the frequency of symptoms reported to be associated with solvent exposure.

(v) An occupational history questionnaire.

(vi) A pre-test questionnaire relating to immediate factors which might affect test performance e.g. recent sleep loss.

(vii) A two factor mood scale, the Stress Arousal Checklist (SACL) (Mackay et al 1978), was completed before and after testing to assess initial mood and mood changes during the procedure.

Cognitive Tests

Five tests were selected from the Neurobehavioural Evaluation System (NES) (Baker et al 1985). This test battery was designed for use in epidemiological studies to assess the effects of exposure to neurotoxicants on a range of cognitive functions. The tests are self-administered using a Compaq portable computer. Interviewer-involvement is minimal so that standardisation of administration and scoring is enhanced. This also facilities comparision of results with other studies using the same system. The specific tests selected were Symbol-Digit Substitution, Serial Digit Learning, Pattern Memory and Continuous Performance (CPT). In addition vocabulary was included as a surrogate measure of pre-morbid ability.

Exposure

Age and years of painting were highly correlated ($r = 0.86$) therefore age was taken as a surrogate measure of exposure and subjects were grouped accordingly (4 groups).

RESULTS

Scores relating to the major outcome variables were compared using paired t-tests. These are summarised in Table 1.

These initial comparisons indicated a significant difference between the groups in the Symbol-Digit substitution test. Subsequent division into 4 age groups indicated that, as expected, response time increased with age in both painters and controls. Painters showed consistently longer response times than controls although a significant difference between means was only apparent in the oldest age-group (age range 56-65, $p = 0.02$)

TABLE 1

OUTCOME VARIABLES : COMPARISON OF PAINTERS AND CONTROLS

	Painters (n=90) $\bar{X}\pm SD$	Controls (n=90) $\bar{X}\pm SD$	p value
G.H.Q. max score = 30	2.5± 4.5	1.9± 3.1	0.27
C.F.Q. max. score = 100	35.4±14.5	34.7±11.0	0.70
Questionnaire-16 max. score = 16	3.4± 3.1	3.1± 2.9	0.49
Symbol-Digit test Response time per trial in seconds	27.9± 9.1	25.3± 6.8	0.02
Serial Learning Derived score max. = 16	9.2± 4.6	8.1± 5.2	0.14
Pattern Memory No. correct max. = 14	12.3± 1.7	12.4± 1.7	0.60
C.P.T. Resp. time - m.secs.	449.6±46.4	443.7±41.3	0.33

A significant difference in vocabulary scores was evident between the exposed and control groups (p=0.01) as a whole but not in the highest age-range (p=0.68)

Mood

Both before and after testing the painters showed significantly higher levels of stress than the controls (p=0.04, p=0.009 respectively). There was no difference in the arousal level between the two groups prior to testing but following testing the arousal level of the controls was significantly higher that that of the painters (p=0.05)

DISCUSSION

The results gave no indication of a higher occurrence of mental health problems or of symptoms associated with solvent exposure. Painters, however, experienced higher levels of stress than controls in the testing situation. This may represent an increased vulnerability, although it may simply reflect an understandably greater anxiety among subjects about the results. The higher general level of alertness of the controls after testing would support suggestions that solvent exposure is associated with a lowered level of arousal and responsiveness.

Clearly high stress and low arousal may also impair test performance, although, if this was a strong influence, one would presumably observe an effect across all tests. However, a significant difference in the performance levels of the two groups was observed only in the symbol-digit substitution test. The expected slowing of response with age was slightly more marked in the painters and the difference was statistically significant in those over the age of 55. It seems unlikely that this is accounted for by a difference in pre-morbid ability since the vocabulary scores of painters and controls in this age-group did not differ.

Overall the results suggest that slight cognitive impairment may result after many years of solvent exposure. However, the test in question, although reputed to be a sensitive measure, involves a variety of skills. In addition the effect oberved represents only a slight slowing of response. The precise nature of the effect therefore and its significance for general quality of life is debatable. This question may be best addressed in the future by the use of tests designed specifically to assess particular aspects of cognitive performance.

ACKNOWLEDGEMENTS

The authors gratefully acknowlege the support ot the UK Health and Safety Executive in funding this investigation.

REFERENCES

1. Baker EL, Letz R, Fidler A. (1985) A computer-administered neurobehavioiural evaluation system for occupational and environmental epidemiology. J. Occupational Medicine 27:206-212

2. Broadbent DE, Cooper DF, Fitzgerald P, Parkes KR (1982) The Cognitive Failures Questionnaire (CFQ) and its correlates British J. Clinical Psychology 21:1-16

3. Grasso P, Sharrat M, Davies DM, Irvine D (1984) Neurophysiological and Psychological Disorders of Occupational Exposure to Organic Solvents. Food and Chemical Toxicology 22 No.10:819-852

4. Goldberg DP, Cooper B, Eastwood MR, Kedward HB, Shepherd M (1970) A standardised psychiatric interview for use in community surveys. British J. Preventive and Social Medicine 24:18-23

5. Mackay C, Cox T, Burrows G, Lazzerini T (1978) An inventory for the measurement of self-reported stress and arousal. British J. of Social and Clinical Psychology 17:283-84

6. Mikkelsen S, Jorgensen M, Browne E, Gyldensted C (1988) Mixed Solvent Exposure and organic Brain Damage. Acta Neurological Scandinavica. Supplement no 118 Vol 78

© 1990 Elsevier Science Publishers B.V. (Biomedical Division)
Occupational Epidemiology. H. Sakurai et al., editors

NEUROPSYCHIATRIC DISORDERS AMONG PAINTERS

C. VAN VLIET[1], G.M.H. SWAEN[1], A. VOLOVICS[2], J.J.M. SLANGEN[1], J.M.M. MEIJERS[1], TJ. DE BOORDER[1], F. STURMANS[3]

[1]Department of Occupational and Environmental Health and Toxicology, University of Limburg, PO Box 616, 6200 MD Maastricht (The Netherlands)
[2]Department of Biostatistics, University of Limburg (The Netherlands)
[3]Department of Epidemiology, University of Limburg (The Netherlands)

INTRODUCTION

Chronic neurotoxic effects in relation to long-term organic solvent exposure have received substantial scientific and public interest during the past fifteen years. Several articles thouroughly reviewing this issue have been published[1,2]. However, there is still no international agreement with respect to the existence and the nature of these effects[3].

From the nature of the syndromes supposed to be associated with long-term exposure to organic solvents, such as "presenile dementia and the psycho-organic syndrome" emerges the question whether the involved exposed workers are at higher risk for being prematurely disabled due to neuropsychiatric disorders.

So far the relationship between organic solvent exposure and premature disability due to neuropsychiatric disorders has been investigated in four Scandinavian[4-7] and one Swiss study[8]. All Scandinavian studies reveal positive relationships, whereas the study conducted outside Scandinavia does not show such clear positive relationships between organic solvent exposure and neuropsychiatric disorders. Recently a Dutch case-control study has been carried out investigating the same relationship. This case-control study will be discussed here.

MATERIAL AND METHODS

The first step at the start of a population based case-control study is to define the population from which cases and controls will be selected. The population base was taken from the Dutch Painters and Construction Workers Organizations. These organizations have been founded by employers and employees in order to execute a number of social laws, such as health care, unemployment and disability insurances for painters and construction workers. In The Netherlands the disability pension system has its legal basis in a specific disability act. According to this act payment of disability benefits starts after 52 weeks of illness. Local departments of social security physicians engaged in granting of disability benefits cover the members of both organizations. Members of the above mentioned organizations, receiving disability benefits, are centrally registered.

If only the members of the painters organization were included in the study, nearly all cases and controls would have been more or less exposed to organic solvents. In order to include non-exposed persons in the study population, one fifth of the construction workers organization was incorporated into the study. A selection was made by including only those members of the construction workers organization in our study population, who were born on day no. 06, 07, 16, 17, 26, 27 of any month in any year. From this combined population of about 74,000 persons, as registered in July 1985, cases and controls were selected.

Cases were defined as male persons receiving disability benefits for mental disorders as from a date between 1 July 1984 and 1 july 1986. Diagnoses of persons receiving disability benefits for neuropsychiatric disorders are awarded by social security physicians. These diagnoses were coded by expert nosologists according to a classification based on the 9th revision of the International Classification of Diseases. The control population consisted of a stratified random sample of male persons from the Dutch Painters and Construction Workers Organizations not receiving these benefits.

Cases and controls were approached by telephone. Participants received a questionnaire. Questions were asked about their occupational history, exposure to organic solvents and the presence of potential confounding factors, such as alcohol intake, age, education level and stress factors.

RESULTS

Odds Ratios

252 Cases (response 61.6%) and 822 controls (response 69.7%) participated in our study by returning questionnaires. All persons who worked or had worked as painter, car sprayer, road marker or carpet layer, as stated in the questionnaire, were classified as exposed to organic solvents, while all other persons were classified as non-exposed. The risk to receive disability benefits due to neuropsychiatric disorders was not increased for exposed workers, compared to non-exposed workers (OR = 1.01). Adjustment for a number of confounding factors increased the Odds Ratio (OR = 1.17), but not to a level indicating a statistical significant association between occupational organic solvent exposure and neuropsychiatric disorders leading to long term disability.

A subdivision of the main group neuropsychiatric disorders in different diagnostic categories revealed a statistically significant increased risk among exposed workers to receive disability benefits due to neurotic disorders (OR = 2.30). However, other diagnoses that may be not easily distinguishable from neurotic disorders (e.g. ICD-309: adjustment reactions) were more often awarded to non-exposed persons. A combination of these diagnoses did not show an increased risk for painters. Therefore it can not be excluded that the detected association between organic solvent exposure and disability due to neurotic disorders was the result of classification bias.

Dose-response relationships

Our study did not show a relationship between exposure dose, expressed in duration of exposure (years) and the risk of premature disability due to neuropsychiatric disorders. However, the translation of exposure dose into the number of working years is a crude estimate of exposure. Not every painter will be exposed to the same level of organic solvents. In the analysis of our data an attempt has been made to quantify this individual variation by the introduction of the painters index. This painters index is based on information from the questionnaires about painters activities assumed to be associated with high exposure to organic solvents (paint spraying, using alkyd paints and paint removers).

Not only painters, but also other construction workers may regularly work with organic solvents or organic solvent containing products (such as glues). Therefore a "general" exposure index, taking into account these exposures, was constructed. With regard to the painters index a positive dose-response relationship was detected. A higher value of this exposure index appeared to be associated with a higher risk of receiving disability benefits due to neuropsychiatric disorders. Strikingly, a positive dose-response relationship of the general exposure index could be demonstrated for painters, but not for other construction workers. Possibly the exposure of painters to organic solvents is, even at the same level of this general exposure index, more intensive than among construction workers.

Further analysis into the contributing elements of the painters index elucidated that the increased risk to be prematurely disabled due to neuropsychiatric disorders was mainly connected to "working with the paintspray" and "working with paintremovers". Some other painting activities were also associated with elevated odds ratios, particularly working in poorly ventilated rooms.

CONCLUSION

To conclude, it must be stated that the existence of a small increased risk among painters to be prematurely disabled due to neuropsychiatric disorders can not be excluded. The increased risk applies especially to painters who are exposed to high concentrations of organic solvents during their work. However, the detected associations are weaker than emerging from the Scandinavian studies.

ACKNOWLEDGEMENTS

This study was supported by a grant from the Dutch Organization for the Improvement of Working Conditions in the Construction Industry (Stichting Arbouw).

REFERENCES

1. Grasso P, Sharrat M, Davies DM, Irvine D (1984) Neurophysiological and psychological disorders and occupational exposure to organic solvents (Review section). Fd Chem Toxic 22;10:819-852

2. Baker EL, Smith TJ, Landrigan PJ (1985) The Neurotoxicity of Industrial Solvents: A Review of the Literature. Am J Ind Med 8:207-217

3. Waldron HA (1986) Solvents and the brain (Editorial) Br J Ind Med 43:73-74

4. Axelson O, Hane M, Hogstedt C (1976) A case-referent study on neuropsychiatric disorders among workers exposed to solvents. Scand J Work Environ Health 2:14-20

5. Lindström K, Riihimäki H, Hänninen K (1984) Occupational solvent exposure and neuropsychiatric disorders. Scand J Work Environ Health 10:321-323

6. Mikkelsen S (1980) A Cohort Study of Disability Pension and Death among Painters with special Regard to disabling presenile Dementia as an occupational Disease. Scand J Soc Med 16;34-43

7. Olsen J, Sabroe S (1980) A Case-Reference Study of Neuropsychiatric Disorders among Workers Exposed to Solvents in the Danish Wood and Furniture Industry. Scand J Soc Med 16:44-49

8. Gubéron E, Usel M, Raymond L, Tissot R, Sweetnam PM (1989) disability, mortality and incidence of cancer among Geneva painters and electricians: a historical prospective study. Br J Ind Med 46:16-23.

Other chemicals

Occupational Epidemiology. H. Sakurai et al., editors

549430

AN EPIDEMIOLOGICAL STUDY ON OCCUPATIONAL ACUTE PYRETHROIDS POISONING IN COTTON FARMERS

S. CHEN* P. YAO* Z. ZHANG* J. SUN** Y. WU* F. HE* Y. LI* L. LIU* Q. LI* X. ZHANG*

ABSTRACT:

A cross sectional survey on the prevalence of acute pyrethroids poisoning in cotton farmers was conducted in Gaocheng county, Hebei province from June to August in 1987 and 1988. Totally 3113 sprayers were followed up. 834 (26.8%) were clinically affected. Only 10 of them developed significant systemic symptoms, including listlessness and mascular fasciculation.

The highest exposure level in the breathing zone was 0.53ug/hr for deltamethrin (DM) and 1.19 ug/hr for fenvalerate (F). The exposure duration was about 4 hrs per day (1-3 days). The urine samples, samples from gauze pad and skin were measured for DM and F by GC. A metabolite of DM, dibromovinyl-dimethycyclopropane carboxylic acid (Br_2A), was measured by HPLC. The dermal contamination (0.02-1.56mg/hr for DM and 1.25-6.42mg/hr for F) is the main exposure route for cotton growers.

INTRODUCTION

Pyrethroids have been introduced and extensively used in the cotton growing area of China since 1982. Animal experiments showed acute poisoning in mice and rats manifested as choreoathetosis and convulsion[1]. Except irritation effects on skin there were no clinical data about acute pyrethroids poisoning in occupationally exposed subjects until several outbreaks of acute intoxication due to pyrethroids exposure occured among the spraymen in the cotton growing areas in China in 1982 [2,3].

SUBJECTS AND METHODS

A cross sectional survey was conducted in 8 villages of Gaochen County, Hebei Province from June to August 1987 and 1988 on 3113 persons from 3053 families. 3004 subjects who used pyrethroids were interviewed with the questionnaire and followed up for 72 hrs. The WHO procedures had been followed [4]. The field work was conducted by the project team and 18 field enumerators. Training of all field staff in data collection techniques was provided prior to the starting of survey. The completed form of questionnaires were checked up by the project personnel every day. All new cases of acute pyrethroid poisoning in the survey were identified by at least two project personnel based on the diagnostic criteria being established.

---

* The Institute of Occupational Medicine, Chinese Academy of Preventive Medicine

** Institute of Occupational Health of Hebei Province

The air samples, urine samples and samples taken from gauze pad and skin were measured for deltamethrin and fenvalerate by GC. A metabolite of deltamethrin, dibromovingl-dimethycyclopropane carboxylic acid (Br_2A), was measured by HPLC.

RESULTS

Exposure levels

The consumption of pyrethroids emulsion (2.5% deltamethrin, 20% Fenvalerate and 10% cypermethrin) was about 40 ml (4-5 hrs per day, 1-3 days) for most spraymen (68.4%). The estimated respiratory exposure at the breathing zone was 0.53ug/hr for deltamethrin (0.01-0.89ug/m^3) and 1.19ug/hr for fenvalerate(0.06-1.98ug/m^3). In totally 143 gauze pads for 18 subjects per day obtained in 1987 the dermal exposure estimated on nude skin was 0.02-1.56mg/hr for deltamethrin and 1.25-6.42mg/hr for fenvalerate.

Biological monitoring

Urine samples were collected from subjects (12 with deltamethrin, 16 with fenvalerate) at 0,3,6,9,12,24,48,72 hr. respectively after beginning of the spraying. The highest contents of pyrethroids in urine detected were 0.3 ug/l for deltamethrin, 0.4 ug/l for deltamethrin-organophosphate and 0.33 ug/l for fenvalerate. The deltamathrin and fenvalerate in urine decreased rapidly after spraying. The deltamethrin metabolite, Br_2A, was detected in 9 of 12 spraymen urine samples, ranged from 9 to 140 ug/l of urine[5]. The measurement of Br_2A in 10 spraymen urine was repeated in July, 1989. The exposure was 3 days and 4hrs spraying per day. Br_2A was detected in all spraymen. The concentration range was 0.1-3ug/l, much lower than it was in 1987[6].

Current effects of pyrethroids on cotton farmers:

In the studied group of 3113 spraymen 834 (26.8%) had various symptoms(Tab. 1). Among

TABLE 1 SYMPTOMS AND SIGNS ON 3113 PYRETHROIDS SPRAYMEN

Symptoms	No.	%	Symptoms	No.	%
Abnormal sensations	768	92.1	Blurred vision	23	2.8
Dizziness	121	4.5	Chest Tightness	18	2.2
Headache	99	11.9	Listlessness	10	1.2
Fatigue	91	10.9	Skin papules	1	0.1
Nausea	68	8.2	Muscular fasciculation	1	0.1
Anorexia	44	5.3	Others	25	3.0
General malaise	33	5.3			

them 696 sprayed pure pyrethroids, 138 sprayed pyrethroids-organophosphates. Most of them complained of abnormal facial sensations, including burning and tingling sensations, which emerged as initial symptoms, which developed within 4 hours and readily disappeared within 24 hours. Systemic symptoms, such as dizziness, headache, fatigue, nausea, anorexia, were more frequently seen, and ten spraymen who developed significant systemic symptoms were diagnosed as mild acute pyrethroid poisoning. Among them, there were four cases of acute deltamethrin poisoning, four fenvalerate poisoning, and two deltamethrin-DDVP mixture poisoning with normal blood cholinesterase activity, and all recovered within 2-4 days.

Effects of Previous Exposure to Pyrethroid

There were 2131 cotton grower in this study who were exposed to pyrethroids previously between 1982-1988 and experienced abnormal facial sensation or dizziness, headache, nausea after spraying, but all recovered satisfactorily in two days. No sequelae were found. There were 697 spraymen who had the related symptoms, of them 58.8% was found to have similar symptoms during previous exposure. In 1434 spraymen who never had any symptoms, only 9.5% of them developed related symptoms. The difference between two groups is significant ($P < 0.01$).

Causal Factors:

In this study the results shows that there are more frequent related symptoms appeared in the young men. The longer spraying duration, the more pyrethroid consumtion in field, the heavier exposure, then the more related symptoms. Moreover, the spraymen using sprayers with leakage or stoppage during operating had more frequent related symptoms. There were a significant statistical difference between the compared groups.

DISCUSSION:

The results of the survey showed that a total of 834 subjects among 3113 spraymen were clinically affected, 696 (22.4%) and 138 (4.4%) with pure pyrethroids and pyrethroid-organophosphate exposures respectively. The abnormal facial sensations are thought to be specific manifestation of increased excitability of facial sensory nerve ending (7) and readily disappear within 24 hours. Systemic symptoms resulted from pyrethroid exposure indicate an involvement of nervous system which was generally mild in the majority of exposed subjects. This is in accordance with the diagnostic criteria of acute pyrethroid poisoning being used in this epidemiological study.

Out of 3113 spraymen, only ten who were diagnosed as mild occupational acute pyrethroid poisoning with a prevalence at 0.31% in pure pyrethroids exposed subjects and 0.38% in subjects with pyrethroid-organophosphate exposures. It has been known that the toxicity of pyrethroids in mammals is lower than that of organophosphates (8). The prevalence of acute pyrethroid poisoning of cotton farmers in this study is also obviously lower than that of acute organophosphates poisoning in the cotton areas of China, which was reported to be 0.11-

0.16% (9). On the other hand, it has been reported that the organophosphates could inhibit the degradation of pyrethroids and consequently increase the toxicity of pyrethroids (10). However, no significant difference was found between the prevalence of pyrethroid poisoning and the pyrethroid-organophosphate poisoning in this study.

Synthetic pyrethroids metabolize and excrete rapidly (3). The retrospective survey done in this study on cotton growers showed no evidence of long standing effects. This result indicates that pyrethroids seem to be unlikely to have chronic toxicity in man. However, the different clinical effects of pyrethroids on the two groups of spraymen with or without symptoms after spraying during 1982-1987 indicates the different individual sensibility of the population.

There are a number of causal factors related to the occurrence of acute pyrethroid poisoning. Sloppy handling during spraying leading to heavy skin contamination is the most improtant reason for the occurrence of acute intoxication. Assessment of exposure for each cotton farmer in the study shows that the dermal route had about 2900 fold of excess risk in comparison with respiratory route for deltamethrin and about 5400 fold for fenvalerate. Hence, minimizing the dermal exposure during spraying should be the priority in the prevention of acute pyrethroids poisoning in cotton farmers. The biological monitoring of the deltamethrin metabolite Br_2A in the spraymen urine showed that the training courses of field staff and education about the knowledge and correct usage of pyrethroids had the positive results. The Br_2A levels in the urine samples were about 40 times less in 1989 than before. It means that the strategies of education for improving the knowledge, attitude and practice of pyrethroid usage in cotton farmers as well as the promulgation of regulations and precautionary guidelines for safe handling of pesticides are obviously very important and necessary.

Acknowledgements:

This work was carried out with the aid of a grant from the International Development Research Centre, Ottawa, Canada.

References

1. Sun J, Z Chen, S. Wang, L. Liu, F.He (1986): Chinese J Hyg Res 15(5): 42-45.
2. He F, S. Wang, L. Liu, S. Chen, Z. Zhang, J. Sun (1989): Arch Toxicol 63:54-58.
3. Zhang Z, P Yao, J. Sun, S. Chen, Q. Li, F. He: To be published.
4. Pesticide Development and Safe Use Unit Divison of Vector Biology Control (WHO,1982) Field surveys of exposure to pesticides standard protocol. VBC/82.1.
5. Yao P, Y. Li, X .Zhang, F. He (1989): Chinese J Hyg Res. 16, (in press).
6. Yao P, Y. Li, Y. Ding, Z. Zhang, F. He: Unpublished Data.
7. Le Quesne PM, Maxwell CI (1980): Neurotoxicology 2:1-11.
8. Roussel Uclaf (Translated by Waldren B V de G) (1982): Deltamethrin Monograph.
9. Shih J, Z. Wu, Y. Wang, S. Xue, X. Gu : Scand J Work Evniron Health 11: Suppl 4, 49-54.
10. Houston DH (1979): in Bridges J W et al (ed) Progress in drug metabolism. PP. 224-255. John Wiky & Sous. Chichester.

Occupational Epidemiology. H. Sakurai et al., editors

THE EFFECT OF MAINTENANCE FREE RESPIRATOR ON THE PREVENTION OF LEAD ABSORPTION IN LEAD USING WORKERS OF KOREA

B.K. LEE, K.D. AHN, T.S. NAM

Institute of Industrial Medicine School of Medicine, Soonchunhyang University, Chonan, Choongnam, Korea

ABSTRACT

One year field study of 400 lead workers on the effect of maintenance free respirator (MFR) to alleviate the lead burden revealed that MFR protection program with biological monitoring with simple measurement of ZPP could be applied as an interim method to prevent lead workers from lead burden even in fairly bad working condition until fundamental environmental control will be taken in Korea.

INTRODUCTION

Lead poisoning in lead using industries of Korea are still prevalent due to relatively bad working condition, absence of proper health education and lack of on-going medical surveillance and low wearing rate of respirators[1]. The best way to prevent lead poisoning would be to eliminate the lead from the air at workplace, but this is not always practical or possible even in developed countries.

Even though control of lead in air at workplace is mandatory in Korea, the working conditions of many lead using industries are not well controlled to meet the government lead standard (0.15 mg/m^3)[2].

Furthermore the working condition of lead industries whose size are small or medium can not be expected to be improved to compile government lead standard within a year or so.

To reduce the number of cases of lead poisoning and to alleviate lead burden of lead workers whose working condition is fairly bad, the effect of maintenance free respirator (MFR) were studied.

SUBJECTS & METHODS

A total of 400 lead workers in 10 lead using industries were investigated.

Zinc protoporphyrin (ZPP) was selected as an index of biological monitoring of lead workers and checked regularly 5 times per year on the spot. Blood lead (PbB) & delta-aminolevulinic acid in urine (ALAU) were also measured on ad hoc basis.

Five lead using industries provided maintenance free respirators (3M Model No. 8710^R) to the workers and 2 lead using industries provided half face respirators and remaining industries didn't provide any type of respirators.

Other selected variables for this study were environmental condition of workplace (ENV), level of health education (HE), general sanitary condition of industry (SC).

RESULTS

Changes of mean ZPP of lead workers by type of respirator and grouping of their working condition are in figure 1 & 2.

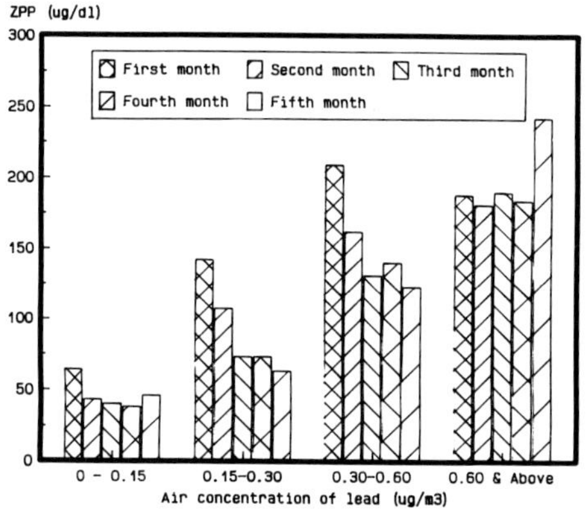

Fig. 1. Mean ZPP of workers (MFR) by their working condition

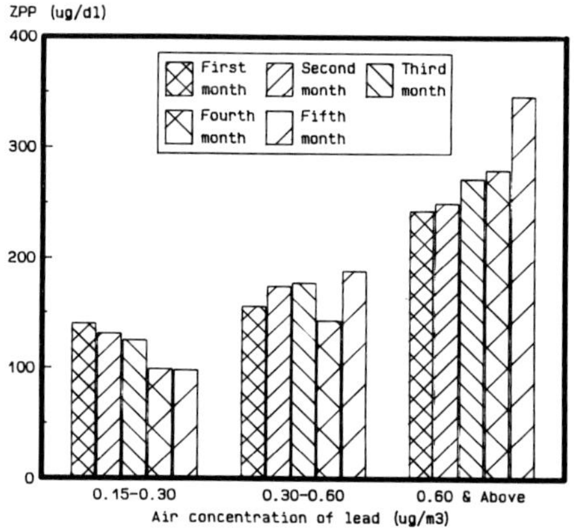

Fig. 2. Mean ZPP of workers (Non-MFR) by their working condition

To observe the effect of respirator and other selected variables on the changes of ZPP between first measurement & third measurement, stepwise multiple regression analysis were applied to 3 groups which were categorized by their initial ZPP levels (Table 1).

TABLE I

Summary of stepwise miltiple regression for dependent variable DIFF (difference of ZPP in whole blood for 5 months) on selected variables (RESP, ENV, HE, SC) by grouping of workers of their initial ZPP level).

Initial ZPP	Variable entered	Number In	Partial R^2	Model R^2	F-Statistics	P-value
below 100 ug/dl	ENV	1	0.059	0.059	10.14	0.0017
100-149 ug/dl	ENV	1	0.233	0.233	17.26	0.0001
	RESP	2	0.045	0.278	3.45	0.068
150 and above ug/dl	RESP	1	0.152	0.152	25.54	0.0001
	ENV	2	0.033	0.184	5.78	0.017
	HE	3	0.013	0.201	2.89	0.091
	SC	4	0.029	0.221	3.61	0.059

In group whose initial ZPP was below 100 ug/dl, only environmental condition played significant role on the difference of ZPP.

While environmental condition still played most significant role to the difference of ZPP in group whose initial ZPP was between 100-149 ug/dl, type of respirator played most significant role to make the difference of ZPP in group whose initial ZPP were above 150 ug/dl, and environmental condition, level of health education and sanitary condition in order attributed to the changes of ZPP.

To observe the effect of respirator and other variables with repeated time effect on blood ZPP of lead workers during one year observation, repeated measure method of analysis of variance statistics were applied (Table 2).

TABLE II

Repeated measure analysis of variance of ZPP on selected variables (RESP ENV, HE, SC)

Effect	F-Statistics	Degree of Freedom	P-value
Between Subjects			
RESP	1.42	2.390	.2426
ENV	13.76	2.390	.0001
HE	20.67	1.390	.0001
SC	1.20	2.390	.3034
Within Subjects			
TIME	11.48	4.1560	.0001
TIME * RESP	6.03	8.1560	.0001
TIME * ENV	5.54	8.1560	.0001
TIME * HE	8.30	4.1560	.0001
TIME * SC	1.47	8.1560	.1615

While the effect of the variable ENV & HE were significant both between and within subjects, respirator effect were not significant between subjects but were significant within subjects.

Correlation analysis revealed that blood lead was better correlated with LOGZPP (natural logarithm transformation of ZPP) & LOGALAU (natural logarithm transformation of ALAU) than with ZPP & ALAU.

The regression equation of LOGZPP and LOGALAU on blood lead are as follows:

LOGZPP = 0.0335 PbB + 2.432 (r=0.78)

LOGALAU = 0.0284 PbB + 0.116 (r=0.72)

DISCUSSION

Respiratory protection is often regarded as a last method to apply for protecting workers' health in occupational health service, but frequently it is the only protective method to keep the lead workers from lead poisoning.

The significant decreases of mean ZPP of lead workers with MFR indicated that MFR could reduce lead burden of workers whose working condition were relatively bad.

The differences of change rate of mean ZPP of lead workers between MFR & non-MFR workers could be attributed to the protection effect of respirator itself & high wearing rate of MFR than non-MFR.

The other advantage of wearing MFR is the effect of health education by wearing them. Each workers could compare the difference of respiratory protection observing the dusty adsorption of lead on outside of white MFR within a day. Another effect of MFR is to make the lead workers to realize the hazard of lead and the seriousness of lead poisoning by knowing the strong committment of employer to spend 10 times more cost to provide MFR to lead workers even in bad bussiness condition.

Lilis, et.al.[3] (1977) claimed that ZPP measurement had several advantages over direct measurement of blood lead. Those are as follows: ZPP levels are indicative of lead exposure averaged over 3-4 months and do not reflect day-to day variation of lead absorption. And measurement of ZPP is quick, cheap, reproducible & portable to carry out test on the spot.
Moreover, ZPP in blood has still close correlation with blood lead[4].

Current study revealed that the correlation between ZPP & blood lead was highly correlated. But the logarithm transformation of ZPP was better correlated with blood lead. This result supports the curvilinear relationship between ZPP and blood lead claimed by many authors[4].

Thus ZPP measurement with logarithm transformation could be used as an indirect measurement of blood lead.

REFERENCES

1. Lee BK (1982) Occupational lead exposure of storage battery workers in Korea. Brit. J. Ind. Med. 39:283-289

2. Lee BK, Ahn KD & Lee KM (1986) The effect of occupational health service on the improvement of worker's health in lead using industries. Korean J. Occup. Health 26:63-72

3. Lilis R.,et. al. (1977) Prevalence of lead disease among secondary lead smelters & biological indicators of lead exposure. Environmental Research 14:255-285

4. WHO (1980) Recommended health-based limits in occupational exposure to heavy metals WHO Tech Report. Ser 647

An Analysis of Encephalic Biocurrent in Workers Exposed to Organic Fluoride

Li Shihui, Guo Jianhua, and Sheng Qiang
Shanghai Institute of Occupational
Health of Chemical Industry
Shanghai, People's Republic of China

In order to investigate the effects of prolonged exposure to organic fluoride on central nervous system (CNS), electroencephalograms (EEG) of 34 workers employed in manufacturing polytetrafluoroethylene were recorded and analyzed.

Materials and methods

1. Study subjects: Thirty-four workers employed in manufacturing polytetrafluoroethylene in a chemical works and an institute in Shanghai were randomly selected as exposed group, 25 males and nine females aged 27 to 58 with an average of 41.1 years. Duration of their employment in exposed environment averaged 18.2 years, seven with 11 to 15 years, 20 with 16 to 20 years, and another seven with more than 20 years. In order to eliminate the difference in EEG patterns between the subjects with various ages and living conditions, 41 healthy and non-directly-exposed workers, 31 males and nine females aged 29 to 57 with an average of 40.0 years, were selected as controls from the same chemical works and institute as the exposed group done. Duration of their employment averaged 17.3 years. All the subjects were chosen with medical histories and physical examinations, exclusive of those with neurological disorder or severe medical illness. None of them had a history of acute organic fluoride poisoning.

2. Electroencephalography: EEGs were recorded in examinees' sitting position by Electroencephalograph ND-82B. Electrodes were put according to international 10-20 system. Activation was challenged by twice-repeated eyes open-closed test and three-minute hyperventilation.

3. Analysis of EEG:

(1) Frequencies and amplitudes were measured for three minutes, and their averages were calculated. Alpha rhythm was recorded by unipolar lead in occipital area. Fast and slow waves were analyzed in the cerebral areas where the most noticeable EEG was recorded.

(2) Alpha index was defined as the proportion of length of alpha rhythm in 100-centimeter-length waves of EEG.

(3) Amplitude modulation of alpha rhythm was evaluated in terms of appearance of spindle form in EEG, i.e., presence of regular, or incomplete spindle form, or absence of spindle form were regarded as good, fair, or poor modulation respectively.

(4) Inhibition of visual reaction was classified into no, partial, or complete based on the extent of inhibition of alpha rhythm in eyes open-closed test. Visual reaction time and recovery time were also measured. EEG waves were categorized into no, partial (appearance of more theta waves), or complete (appearance of more delta waves) change, according to EEG frequencies after hyperventilation.

(5) Each EEG was read with masking method by three physicians independently, and evaluated as normal, borderline, mild, moderate, or severe abnormal, based on adult EEG diagnostic criteria(1).

Results

1. Table 1 shows there was a very significant difference of EEG abnormality rates between exposed and control groups.

Table 1. Comparison of EEG Abnormality between Two Groups

Groups	No. Subject	No. Normal	No. Abnormal	% Abnormal	X^2	P
Exposed	34	15	19	55.9	7.11	<.01
Control	41	31	10	24.4		

Among 19 cases with abnormal EEG in exposed group, 15 were classified as borderline abnormal, and four mild, and among 10 cases in control group, six classified as borderline, and four mild abnormal.

Table 2 shows a tendency that EEG abnormality rates increased with duration of employment.

Table 2. EEG Abnormality of Exposed Workers with Different Durations of Employment

Duration of Employment (years)	No. Subject	No. Normal	No. Abnormal	% Abnormal
11-	7	4	3	42.9
16-	20	9	11	55.0
21-	7	2	5	71.4

2. Changes of frequency, amplitude, and index of alpha rhythm: There were no significant differences of frequency and amplitude modulation between exposed and control groups ($P > .05$). The differences of average amplitude and frequency of alpha rhythm in both cerebral hemispheres between the two groups did not reach significant levels ($P > .05$).

3. Abnormal EEG changes: Main manifestation of abnormal EEGs was the increase of theta waves, and delta waves were very seldom seen. Amplitude of theta waves averaged 26.88 microvolts within the range of low amplitude. The most pro-

minet theta waves were seen in the central frontal area, usually as scattered slow activities in a short interval. The difference of average indices of theta waves between the two groups did not reach a significant level ($P > .05$).

4. There was no significant difference in EEG changes with challenge.

Discussion

1. Effects of prolonged exposure to organic fluoride on CNS have not been reported abroad. Recently, dynamic observations on health status of workers employed in organic fluoride industry were carried out at home. The results showed a few workers long-term exposed to organic fluoride suffered from neurosis syndrome and dysfunction of autonomic nervous system, and the prevalence of neurosis syndrome increased with duration of employment. Also, some researchers made EEG observations on workers exposed to organic fluoride and found that the proportion of abnormal EEGs in long-term exposed workers was higher than what normal persons could have, and the characteristic of their EEG changes was intermittent low-amplitude slow activities. The results of this paper showed the difference of EEG abnormality rates between exposed and control groups reached a very significant level. Main abnormal EEG changes in our study was increase of theta waves which was regarded as a pathological reaction reflecting inhibition of CNS. Our results also suggested the longer the exposure to organic fluoride, the more effects on the function of cerebral cortex. So it could be seen that prolonged exposure to organic fluoride did cause effects on the function of cortex.

2. The extent of cerebral affliction can be expected based on the changes of EEG waves. Usually, it is believed that mild cerebral affliction only shows slow activity, or decrease of cycles in EEG, and nearly no increase of amplitude. Our results also indicated the proportion of borderline abnormal was significantly higher than that of mild abnormal in 19 cases with abnormal EEG in exposed group. All those mentioned above showed the effects of prolonged exposure to organic fluoride on cerebral cortex were only mild affliction. Therefore, it is recommended that employees exposed to organic fluoride be followed up earlier as their EEGs showing borderline abnormal. In consideration of EEG being a non-invasive and objective indicator for identification of CNS function, it is suggested that EEG be used as a routine in health surveillance for employees exposed to organic fluoride.

References

(1) Feng Yingkun. Clinical Electroencephalography, 2nd ed. Beijing: People's Health Publishing House. 1979:61.

Occupational Epidemiology. H. Sakurai et al., editors

THYROID VOLUME AND FUNCTION AND PHYSICAL FITNESS AMONG WOMEN OCCUPATIONALLY EXPOSED TO COBALT BLUE DYES

EVA PRESCOTT[1)], BO NETTERSTRØM[1)], JENS FABER[2)], LAZLO HEGEDÜS[2)].

1) Clinic of Occupational Medicine, University Hospital of Copenhagen, Denmark.
2) Department of Endocrinology and The Ultrasonic Laboratory, Herlev University Hospital, Denmark.

The purpose of the study was to examine if exposure to cobalt in the porcelain industry had effects on the thyroid gland and the heart. Such effects have been reported from other kinds of exposure to cobalt.

The study group consisted of plate painters from two Danish porcelain factories. Sixteen women who were exposed to cobaltsilicat (Co_2SiO_4), 36 women to cobaltaluminat ($CoAl_2O_4$)and 48 age matched women, who had never been exposed to cobalt occupationally underwent clinical examination. The following measurements were made. Ultrasonic measurement of the volume of the thyreoid gland, analysis of the levels of T_4, T_3, TSH, cholesterol, hemoglobin and red cell morfology in the blood, cobalt excretion in urine, measurements of blood pressure, EKG and submaximal oxygen uptake a.m. Åstrand.

Exposure data showed cobalt values around TLV, 0.05 mg/m^3 in the workingplaces, where cobaltsilicat was used and half the TLV where cobaltaluminat was used.

The cobalt excretion was found to be 5-10 times higher in the cobaltsilicat exposed group than in the two other groups. This group had significantly higher serum T_4, free thyroxine and blood pressure than other groups. The submaximal oxygen uptake was lower. There were, however, no differences between the groups regarding other variables, including Body Mass Index.

The results indicate that cobaltsilicat stimulates thyroid function. The study will be extended to a larger group of women exposed to cobaltsilicat.

TABLE I

PARACLINICAL DATA ON TWO COBALT EXPOSED GROUPS OF WOMEN AND A CONTROL GROUP

	EXPOSED		CONTROLS
	Co_2SiO_4	$CoAl_2O_4$	
Urine-Co/creatinine (µg/mmol)	1.02***	0.19	0.13
Thyreoid volume (ml)	15.5	18.4	18.8
TSH (U/l)	1.9	1.6	1.9
T_4 (nmol/l)	111.4***	96.7	93.6
T_3 (nmol/l)	2.1	2.2	2.1
V O_2 (ml/kg/min)	31.0**	34.9	34.5

** p 0.01

*** p 0.001

Occupational Epidemiology. H. Sakurai et al., editors

EVALUATION OF URINARY β_2-MICROGLOBULIN, N-ACETYL-β-GLUCOSAMINIDASE, AND METALLOTHIONEIN AT A LOW LEVEL EXPOSURE TO CADMIUM PIGMENT DUST

SHOSUKE SUZUKI*, HIROSHI KOYAMA*, TOMOYUKI KAWADA*, TAKAO NAKURA*, IDA FARIDA RIVAI*, CHIHARU TOHYAMA** AND MASATAKA MURAKAMI**

*Department of Public Health, Gunma Univ. School of Med., Showa 3, Maebashi 371 (Japan) **Environmental Health Science Division, National Institute for Environmental Studies, Onogawa, Tsukuba 305 (Japan)

INTRODUCTION

Urinary metallothionein (MT) and N-acetyl-beta-D-glucosaminidase (NAG) have been found to be better biological indicators of cadmium (Cd) exposure than beta-2-microglobulin (BMG) in urine at lower Cd exposure[1]. Biological significance of NAG has not yet been known in terms of Cd absorption and the health effect[2], although that of BMG has been well-informed[3,4].

We studied the health examination data of Cd pigment workers and tried to clarify characteristics of indicators of Cd exposure, NAG, MT and BMG, with a special reference to their age, cigarettes smoking, years of employment and levels of Cd in urine (Cd-U) and of Cd in blood (Cd-B).

SUBJECTS AND METHODS

Subjects. Health examinations of 79 and 129 workers at a Cd pigment manufacturing factory were carried out in 1987 and 1988, respectively. The factory is the same as that in our earlier reports[1,5]. Cd workers were exposed to CdS and CdSe dust for about 10 years in average. Nine workers were exposed to a maximum concentration of 350 μgCd/m^3, and a time-weighted average concentration of 3.0 μgCd/m^3 (8 hrs TWA)[1]. The next highest exposure group of 17 workers, was exposed to 0.18 μgCd/m^3 (8 hrs TWA). These two groups of workers were combined and considered as an exposure group. The rest of the workers were not exposed substantially to Cd, and used as a control group.

Methods. Spot urine samples were collected in the morning and analyzed for Cd-U, BMG and NAG according to the methods cited earlier[1]. MT in urine was determined by a single-antibody radio-immunoassay after the dialysis[6]. All of their concentrations were corrected by urinary creatinine concentration[1]. Whole blood drawn from antecubital vein was analyzed for cadmium (Cd-B)[1].

RESULTS

Geometric means of Cd-B and Cd-U of the exposed group were significantly higher than those of the control group, but no significant difference was observed between the two groups of the other parameters of Cd exposure or, NAG, BMG and MT (TABLE I). The highest Cd-U level found in the exposed group was less than 10 μg/g cr both in 1987 and 1988 (Fig.1).

TABLE II shows relationships of Cd-B and Cd-U with age, years of employment, and cigarettes smoking. Cd-B is closely related to a number of cigarettes smoked per day although Cd-U is related more to age and years of employment.

TABLE I .

GEOMETRIC MEANS AND THE STANDARD DEVIATIONS OF THE FIVE Cd EXPOSURE PARAMETERS OF NON-EXPOSED AND EXPOSED WORKERS EXAMINED IN 1988.

Parameters	Non-Exposed			Exposed			t-test
	N	Mean	SD	N	Mean	SD	
Age (years old)	103	29.6[1]	6.2[1]	26	35.0[1]	8.3[1]	**
Cd-B (μg/ℓ)	101	1.05	1.73	22	1.39	1.52	*
Cd-U (μg/g cr)	103	0.96	1.89	26	1.54	2.11	**
NAG (U/g cr)	102	2.11	1.65	26	2.50	1.77	
BMG (μg/g cr)	101	60.45	3.56	26	50.91	3.39	
MT (μg/g cr)	103	36.30	1.68	26	38.21	2.05	

[1]) Arithmetic mean ± its SD. N: Number of workers examined.
* & ** indicate significance level at 0.05 & 0.01, respectively.

TABLE II .

COEFFICIENTS OF CORRELATION BETWEEN EITHER LEVEL OF Cd-B AND Cd-U, AND AGE, YEARS OF EMPLOYMENT, AND A NUMBER OF CIGARETTES SMOKED PER DAY OF NON-EXPOSED AND EXPOSED WORKERS EXAMINED IN 1988.

	Cd-B		Cd-U	
	Non-Exposed	Exposed	Non-Exposed	Exposed
Age	0.072	0.228	0.314**	0.523**
Years of employment	-	0.361	-	0.706**
Cigarettes per day	0.390**	0.083	0.239*	0.174

*: $p < 0.05$, **: $p < 0.01$

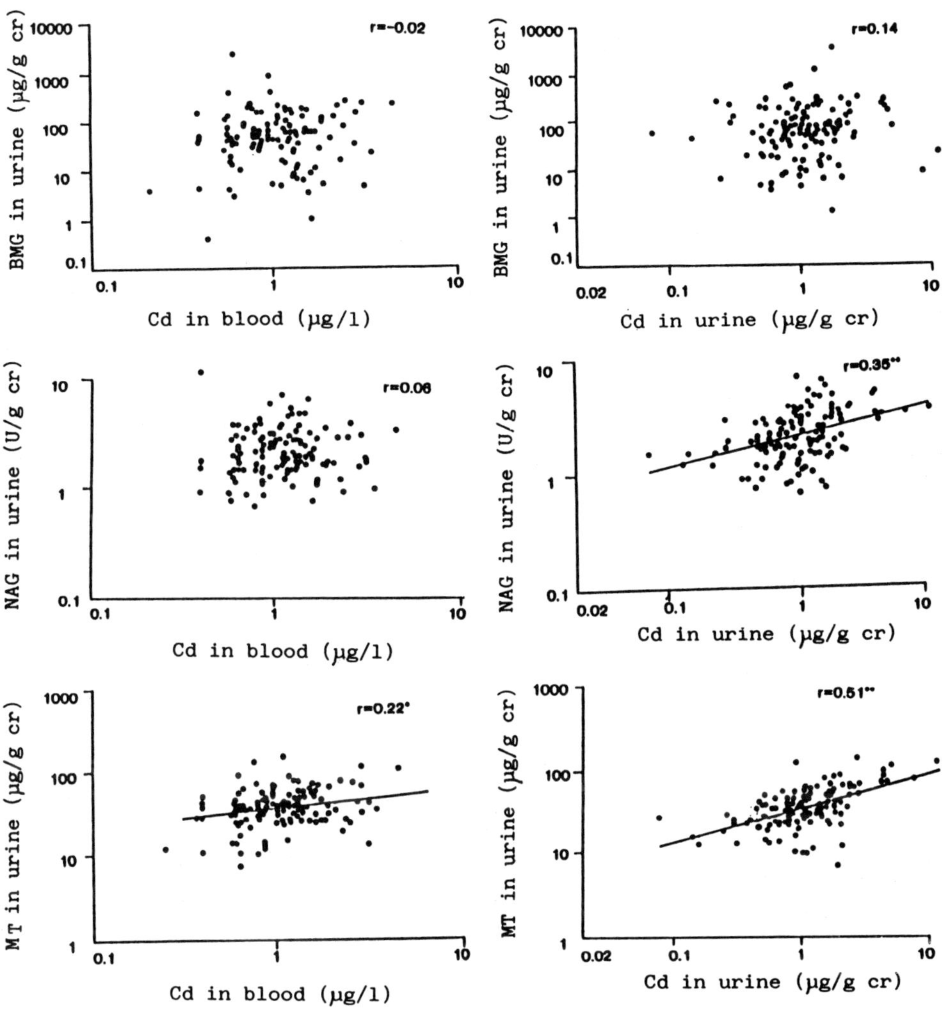

Fig. 1. Relationships of Cd-B (left) and Cd-U (right) with BMG, NAG, and MT in Cd workers examined in 1988.

Table III summarizes relationships of either level of Cd-B and Cd-U with urinary levels of BMG, NAG and MT, and between levels of Cd-B and Cd-U. BMG had no correlation both with Cd-B and Cd-U. MT showed the highest correlation both with Cd-B and Cd-U, and NAG showed the next highest correlation with Cd-U and had little (1988) or smaller (1987) correlation with Cd-B (TABLE III and Fig.1).

Increased excretion level of BMG in urine is known to be one of the earliest signs of renal mal-absorption caused by Cd accumulated in kidney. The increased excretion of BMG was not observed in the present study (TABLE I). And no correlation of BMG was observed with neither Cd-B nor Cd-U. In the present study NAG correlated with Cd-U only, however, MT showed the closest relationship both with Cd-B and Cd-U (TABLE Ⅲ & Fig. 1).

TABLE Ⅲ.

COEFFICIENTS OF CORRELATION BETWEEN EITHER LEVEL OF Cd-B AND Cd-U, AND BMG, NAG AND MT IN Cd EXPOSED AND NON-EXPOSED WORKERS EXAMINED IN 1987 AND 1988.

Cd-B vs.:	1987 (N=79)	1988 (N=122)	Cd-U vs.:	1987 (N=79)	1988 (N=122)
BMG	-0.07	-0.02	BMG	0.05	0.14
NAG	0.21*	0.06	NAG	0.45**	0.35**
MT	0.40*	0.22*	MT	0.62**	0.51**
Cd-U	0.40*	0.42**	Cd-B	0.40*	0.42**

N: Number of workers examined.
* & ** indicate significance level at 0.05 & 0.01, respectively.

<u>Conclusion</u>. The present result suggests that Cd-B reflects a relatively recent exposure to Cd since Cd-B level was found to be related to a number of cigarettes smoked per day, and that Cd-U indicates the accumulation of Cd in the kidney[7]. MT correlates with both Cd-B and Cd-U, whereas NAG correlates closely with Cd-U only. A possible explanation is that the biosynthesis of MT in liver is accelerated upon absorption of Cd, and MT produced in the liver is released to circulation and then to the kidney. On the other hand, NAG in urine has closer relation to Cd accumulated in kidney, suggesting a release of this lysosomal enzyme due to damadge of renal epithelium. BMG will be increased later when impairment of renal reabsorption occurs. MT may be used as a most sensitive indicator for Cd exposure and accumulation. NAG in urine may be used as a sensitive indicator of not only Cd accumulation but also a slight damage of renal epithelium when the exposure level to Cd is relatively low, Cd-U level lower than 10 μg/g cr.

REFERENCES

1. Kawada T, Koyama H, Suzuki S (1989) Brit J Industr Med 46:52-55
2. Bernard A, Lauwerys R (1989) Brit J Industr Med 46:679-680
3. Tsuchiya K, Iwao S, Sugita M, Sakurai H (1979) Environ Health Perspect 28:147-53
4. Bernard A, Buchet JP, Roels H, Masson P, Lauwerys R (1979) Enr J Clin Invest 9:11-22
5. Kawada T, Koyama H, Suzuki S (1987) Jpn J Ind Health 29:214-215
6. Tohyama C, Shaikh ZA (1981) Fundam Appl Toxicol 1:1-7
7. Suzuki S, Taguchi T (1980) J Toxicol Environ Health 6:783-796

MUSCULOSKELETAL AND VIBRATION-INDUCED DISORDERS

Occupational Epidemiology. H. Sakurai et al., editors
549431

SENSITIVITY AND SPECIFICITY OF SIGNS AND SYMPTOMS IN FIELD STUDIES OF OCCUPATIONALLY-RELATED CARPAL TUNNEL SYNDROME

S. BARNHART, P. DEMERS, M. MILLER, W. LONGSTRETH, L. ROSENSTOCK
University of Washington. Occupational Medicine Program,
Seattle, WA. 98195

INTRODUCTION

Carpal tunnel syndrome (CTS) is a common disorder of the upper extremities characterized by pain, dysesthesias and weakness resulting from compression of the median nerve as it crosses the wrist. CTS has been associated with several risk factors including female gender, diabetes, acromegaly, hypothyroidism, rheumatoid arthritis, narrow carpal tunnel, and occupation (1-3).

Studies of the epidemiology of carpal tunnel syndrome (CTS) are compromised by a lack of an accepted "gold standard" for CTS and lack of knowledge of the sensitivity and specificity of signs, symptoms and electrodiagnostic tests for CTS. To evaluate the sensitivity and specificity of tests for CTS we formulated a "gold standard" for CTS to include each of the following: 1) abnormal electrodiagnostic study; 2) ever having (one or more) hand pain, paresthesias, or nocturnal symptoms, and; 3) Phalen's and/or Tinel's sign.

METHODS

The study was conducted at a local ski assembly plant which employed approximately 400 workers. The study sample was recruited after the jobs in the facility had been classified as repetitive or non-repetitive with respect to stress on the wrist by one of the authors (PD). Criteria for repetitive jobs entailed repeated and/or sustained activities that involved: 1. flexion, extension or ulnar deviation of the wrist by 45 degrees; 2. radial deviation of more than 30 degrees; or 3. use of a pinch type grip. Non-repetitive jobs included those that did not meet the criteria for repetitive jobs. There were 257 subjects who met the criteria for repetitive and non-repetitive jobs who were recruited for the study. Following data collection, but before any analyses were performed subjects in either group were excluded if they did not meet all of the following eligibility criteria: employed in any job by the company for at least 6 months prior to their evaluation; in the job used for this study within the past two weeks; employed in this job for a minimum of ten weeks; and not employed in the other risk category in the past 6 months.

Data were collected after obtaining written informed consent. Information included a self-administered questionnaire, directed physical examination and electrophysiologic testing (4).

Case definitions for CTS are below:

"Gold Standard"	Presence of each: 1) abnormal electrophysiologic test, and 2) ever having hand pain, numbness or nocturnal symptoms, and 3) Phalen's and or Tinel's signs.
Case Definition I:	Electrophysiologic Criterion: Median nerve distal sensory latency (Msl) minus Ulnar nerve distal sensory latency $\geq$ 0.5 milliseconds
Case Definition II:	Electrophysiologic Criterion and Signs: Presence of the electrophysiologic criterion and Phalen's sign or Tinel's sign
Case Definition III:	Electrophysiologic Criterion and Either Signs and/or Symptoms Presence of electrophysiologic criterion and signs and/or ever having hand pain tingling, numbness and nocturnal hand pain.

RESULTS

Among the approximately 400 employees at the plant, 152 were classified as having repetitive jobs and 105 employees as having non-repetitive jobs. Of these, 80 of those with repetitive jobs and 53 of those with non-repetitive jobs fulfilled the criteria of being eligible, participated, and returned the self-administered questionnaire for participation rates of .53 and .50 respectively. Of the 133, 68 were males and 65 females. The mean age was 39 years for males and 36 years for females.

The prevalence of CTS among the entire cohort was; right hand 7(51%), left hand 4(31%), and either or both hands 8(6%). All of the cases of CTS, as defined by the "Gold Standard" were among those with repetitive jobs.

The sensitivity and specificity of signs, symptoms and CTS case definitions are shown in Table I.

TABLE I

Sensitivity and specificity of sign, symptom, and case definitions for CTS:

	Sensitivity		Specificity	
	Right	Left	Right	Left
Signs & Symptoms				
Hand Pain	86	75	21	21
Parasthesias	100	100	25	27
Nocturnal Pain	100	75	47	46
Phalen's Sign	57	50	82	82
Tinel's Sign	43	50	96	87
CTS Case Definition				
Case Definition I	100	100	80	86
Case Definition II	100	100	99	99
Case Definition III	100	100	81	87

DISCUSSION

The choice of appropriate case definitions for carpal tunnel syndrome for use in field studies remains problematic. From our data it is evident that symptoms such as hand pain, paresthesias, and nocturnal pain are quite sensitive but not very specific. Phalen's and Tinel's signs are not very sensitive, but are much more specific. Given these limitations, case definitions which rely solely on a sign or symptom risk misclassifying subjects in surveys of CTS prevalence.

Focusing on case definitions for carpal tunnel syndrome, three separate case definitions were compared to the gold standard case definition for carpal tunnel syndrome. Case Definition I used an abnormal electrodiagnostic study as the necessary and sufficient criterion and had (by definition) a sensitivity of 100% but a specificity of 80% and 86% for the right and left hand. Case Definition III, which required an abnormal electrodiagnostic study and the presence of signs and/or symptoms demonstrated a similar level of specificity. Case Definition II, which required the presence of an abnormal electrodiagnostic study and the presence of Tinel's and/or Phelan's Signs had a specificity of 99% for both the right and the left wrists.

Despite limitations in determining the validity of the gold standard, we conclude that among symptoms, nocturnal pain had the greatest sensitivity and specificity when compared to hand pain or paresthesias. In addition, while not very sensitive indicators of CTS, Phalen's and Tinel's signs were more specific than any of the symptoms examined. Given these findings caution should be applied in the construction of case definitions to assure adequate sensitivity and specificity and to avoid misclassifying subjects. Further investigations should focus on the validity of case definitions for CTS.

REFERENCES

1. Stevens J, Sun S, Beard C. Carpal tunnel syndrome in Rochester, Minnesota, 1961-1980. Neurology 1988; 38:134-138

2. Barnhart S, Rosenstock L. Carpel tunnel syndrome in grocery checkers: A cluster of work-related illness. West J Med 1987; 147:37-40

3. Armstrong T, Chaffin D. The carpal tunnel syndrome and selected personal attributes. J. Occup Med 1979; 21:481-486

4. Felsenthal G. Median and Ulnar distal motor and sensory latencies in the same normal subject. Arch Phys Med Rehabil 1977; 58:297-302

ASSESSING PREVALENCE RATES AND ASSOCIATION OF OCCUPATIONAL MUSCULOSKELETAL DISORDERS: EXAMINATION OF TOTAL SAMPLE VERSUS QUESTIONNAIRE POSITIVES

MATS HAGBERG
Division of Work and Environmental Physiology, National Institute of Occupational Health, S-171 84 Solna, Sweden, and Department of Occupational Medicine, Karolinska Hospital, S-104 01 Stockholm, Sweden.

INTRODUCTION

It would be efficient in occupational health surveillance if musculoskeletal disorders/diseases could be assessed by questionnaire. In some investigations of occupational musculoskeletal disorders questionnaires have been used as a screening instrument to reduce the number of physical examinations that has to be performed. When using questionnaire as a screening instrument one has to be aware of two problems: 1. If the sensitivity of the questionnaire is less than 100% there will be an underestimation of prevalence rates. 2. If the sensitivity of the questionnaire is not the same in the exposed and the referent group, the association (e.g. relative risk) will be misjudged (under or overestimated). The aim of the present investigation was to study the magnitude of the described two problems in a study base of male industrial workers.

STUDY BASE AND METHODS

The study base consisted of 90 male platers, 70 male assemblers at a truck assembly line, and 61 male office workers. Immediately prior to a physical examination according to a prewritten protocol all the 221 workers answered a questionnaire. The outcome of the questionnaire was compared to the outcome of the physical examination. This was done by computing the point-prevalence rates and rate ratios of four musculoskeletal diseases/disorders for both a. the total sample examination and b. the situation if only the questionnaire screening positives had been examined. For *Carpal tunnel syndrome (CTS)* platers and office workers were compared. Assemblers were compared to office workers concerning *Tension neck syndrome, Shoulder tendinites and Lumbar insufficiency.* The screening question for *Carpal tunnel syndrome* was *"Do you have tingling or numbness in hand/fingers at night?"* The criteria for *CTS* at the physical examination was a positive Phalens test and symptoms of tingling at night. The three screening questions for *Tension neck, Shoulder tendinitis and Lumbar insufficiency* was *"Do you have complaints (discomfort, stiffness, pain etc) in the neck/shoulder joint - upper arm/low-back?"* The criteria for *Tension neck* was tenderness over the upper part of the trapezius muscle and symptoms of discomfort from the neck. For *Shoulder tendinitis (rotator cuff and biceps tendinitis)* the criteria were pain at isometric contraction of muscle, tenderness at insertions and symptoms of shoulder joint pain. *Lumbar insufficiency* criteria were paravertebral tenderness in the lumbar region and symptoms of pain or discomfort from the low-back.

Confidence intervals for rates were computed as confidence intervals for proportions (1). Test base confidence intervals were computed for the age standardized (Mantel-Haenszel) rate ratios (1). In tables with zero cells .5 was added to each of the cells in the table.

RESULTS

The point-prevalence rates were underestimated for all four disorders among the exposed if just the questionnaire positives were examined (Table). Among the referents an underestimation of point-prevalence rate of *Shoulder tendinitis* would have happened if only the questionnaire positives were examined (Table). Except for *Shoulder tendinitis* an underestimation of the rate ratio had occurred if just the screening positives had been examined (Table).

TABLE

POINT-PREVALENCES IN PER CENT (%) AND AGE STANDARDIZED RATE RATIOS (SRR) FOR THE FOUR STUDIED MUSCULOSKELETAL DISORDERS

The 95 per cent confidence intervals are given within parantheses. Total represents the result of examination of all exposed and referents. Q-pos represents the result if only the screening positives had been examined.

	Point-prevalence rate %		SRR
	Exposed	Referents	
CTS			
Total	12.2 (5.5-19.0)	1.6 (0-4.8)	7.8 (1.1-57)
Q-pos	7.8 (2.2-13.3)	1.6 (0-4.8)	5.1 (0.7-38)
Tension neck			
Total	11.4 (4.0-18.9)	0	4.8 (0.9-25)
Q-pos	4.3 (0-9.0)	0	3.0 (0.5-18)
Shoulder tendinitis			
Total	10.0 (3.0-17.0)	1.6 (0-4.8)	2.3 (0.5-13)
Q-pos	4.3 (0-9.0)	0	2.6 (0.4-15)
Lumbar insufficiency			
Total	24.3 (14.2-34.3)	1.6 (0-4.8)	4.2 (0.8-24)
Q-pos	18.6 (9.5-27.7)	1.6 (0-4.8)	3.6 (0.7-19)

DISCUSSION

The sensitivity of the questionnaire was different in the exposed group compared to the referent group. If only the screening positives had been examined then the risk of musculoskeletal disease associated with exposure might have been misjudged. If your inference was soley based upon significance you would have concluded that *Carpal tunnel syndrome* was associated with exposure when all exposed and referents were examined but not if you only had examined the questionnaire screening positives. One would have expected that the subjects with symptoms had reported those in the questionnaire, since symptoms were admitted during physical examination. When confronting some of the subjects with the fact that they admitted to have *tingling of hand and fingers during night* after the physician found a positive Phalens test but had failed to report that in the screening questionnaire, a common reply was that *"I didn't think it was important"*. The major shortcoming of this study is the small studybase resulting in wide confidence intervals. The criteria of the studied musculoskeletal disorders may have been too generous. It is possible that the sensitivity of the questionnaire may have been increased if the questions had involved period-prevalences. This study supports that for true prevalence measures of musculoskeletal disorders the total population of exposed and referents has to be examined. The use of screening questionnaire as selection to physical examination may lead to underestimation of rates and misjudgement of the risk of musculoskeletal disease associated with exposure.

REFERENCE

1. Sullivan KM, Foster DA (1983). dEPID A program for stratified and standardized analysis. Version 2.11. Division of Nutrition, Centers for Disease Control, 1600 Clifton Road, Atlanta, GA 30333.

Occupational Epidemiology. H. Sakurai et al., editors

549432

CUMULATIVE TRAUMA DISORDERS IN A MEATPACKING PLANT, UNITED STATES

Thomas Hales, Lawerence Fine, Daniel Habes, Richard Horning, James Boiano

National Institute for Occupational Safety and Health, Cincinnati, Ohio

ABSTRACT

On March 3, 1988, the National Institute for Occupational Safety and Health (NIOSH) received a request from the Occupational Safety and Health Administration (OSHA) for technical assistance in evaluating cumulative trauma disorders (CTDs) among employees of a large meatpacking plant. The study's objectives were to describe the incidence, prevalence, and pattern of upper extremity (UE) CTDs within this plant. Using the company maintained records (OSHA 200 Logs), this plant's upper extremity CTD incidence rate was 41.7 per 100 full-time workers per year compared to 6.7 reported for the meatpacking industry [Rate Ratio (RR)=6.24, 95% Confidence Interval (CI) 5.8, 6.7], or 0.1 per 100 full-time workers per year reported for all US industries in 1987 (RR=417.1, 95% CI 390.0, 455.6). Two hundred of the plant's 2000 employees (10%) were selected to participate in the prevalence study. One hundred and forty of the 200 selected workers had UE CTDs determined by questionnaire for a 1-year period prevalence of 70%. One hundred of the 200 selected workers had current UE CTDs by questionnaire and physical examination, for a point prevalence of 50%. From the incidence data, hands and wrists were the most frequently affected areas (52% and 29%, respectively), followed by elbows (10%), shoulders (7%), and neck (2%). Tendonitis, strains, and carpal tunnel syndrome were the most common diagnoses, (35%, 25%, and 14%, respectively.) This study found a high incidence rate and prevalence of UE CTDs within this meatpacking plant.

INTRODUCTION

In the early 1980's several studies reported the association of employment in the meatpacking industry and cumulative trauma disorders (CTDs).[1-5] This association continued in 1987, where 52,000 of the 135,000 employees (39%) in the meatpacking industry [Standard Industrial Classification (SIC) # 2011] suffered a work-related injury or illness, making it the second most dangerous industry in America.[6] CTDs make-up 83% of all illness, and 17% of combined injuries and illnesses within the meatpacking industry.[6] Despite this recognition and awareness, the incidence of CTDs within the industry increased 85% from 1984 to 1987.[7] In March 1988, the Occupational Safety and Health Administration (OSHA) requested technical assistance from the National Institute for Occupational Safety and Health (NIOSH) to evaluate the incidence, prevalence, and pattern of upper extremity (UE) CTDs within a specific meatpacking plant.

METHODS

Process Description

This plant began operation in 1909 producing beef and pork products for wholesale distribution. The slaughtering processes for cattle and hogs are similar. The animals are killed and suspended by their hind limbs from an overhead chain conveyor. The chain conveyor line moves at a pre-determined speed while workers positioned along the lines eviscerate and dissect the animal. The workers performing the evisceration and dissection are equipped with saws, straight knives, whizard knives (electric powered hand knife with a rotating cutting blade), hydraulic clippers, and hooks. In addition to whole meat products, the plant also produces processed meat including sausages, weiners, liverwurst, and canned hams. Although work in these departments (Smoke Meat Pack, Sausage Cooler, Sausage Manufacture, Curing, and Canning) sometimes involves knife use, most jobs involve operating machines which produce and package the processed meat.

Incidence Rates

Incidence rates for UE CTDs were calculated for the whole plant and specific departments using OSHA 200 logs for the one-year period 5/1/87 to 4/30/88. This time period was used because a union strike at the plant resulted in a replacement workforce starting on 5/1/87. OSHA 200 Logs are records maintained by the employer listing all employees injured on the job or employees with a work-related illness as mandated by the Occupational Safety and Health Act. All work-related deaths and illness are recordable, while work-related injuries are recordable if they involve one or more of the following: loss of consciousness, restriction of work or motion, transfer to another job, or medical treatment other than first aid.[8] OSHA log entries of CTDs are typically listed in the "7f" column of the illness section titled "disorders associated with repeated trauma." The total number of CTDs entered onto the OSHA 200 log was divided by the total number of employee hours worked for the whole plant (or for the specific departments being evaluated) from 5/1/87 to 4/30/88. This type of incidence rate, using employee hours worked, is used by the Bureau of Labor Statistics (BLS).[6]

All OSHA 200 Log entries were reviewed for their appropriateness to be included as an UE CTD. We defined UE CTDs as disorders caused, aggravated, or precipitated by repeated motion, vibration, or pressure to the neck, shoulders, elbows, wrists, or hands. All sprains, fractures, lacerations, and contusions were excluded. In addition, medical conditions involving the back, chest wall, and lower extremities were excluded. The specific medical diagnoses are included in Table 1.[9-11] Each worker entered onto the log could be diagnosed with one or more conditions, and affect one or more joint areas. Thus, bilateral carpal tunnel syndrome was recorded as one entry affecting the left and right wrists and hands. We defined an "arm" entry as one affecting the shoulder, elbow, and wrist joint areas, and a "forearm" entry as one affecting the elbow, and wrist joint areas.

Period Prevalence

Period prevalence rates for the 12 months prior to NIOSH's study were calculated from standardized questionnaires administered to current employees. The questionnaires elicited demographic information, work history information including months/years on the job, prior health history information including chronic diseases and prior upper extremity injuries, and information on the type and time spent on various recreational activities. The remainder of the questions addressed upper extremity pain or discomfort experienced within the previous year. If the workers had experienced recurring difficulty in one or more parts of the upper extremity, more detailed information was sought regarding the subject's complaint including location, duration, onset, aggravating factors, and treatment.

Selection Criteria

All departments listed on the OSHA request were observed during a walk-through survey. Two departments were selected as apparently having lower exposure to repetitive and forceful hand-wrist motions than the other departments listed on the OSHA request. These two departments, Smoke Meat Pack and Sausage Cooler, will be referred to as the lower exposure departments (LED). All employees working the day-shift from the LED were invited to participate in NIOSH's study.

From the other departments listed on the OSHA request, 40 jobs in five departments were selected based on a) apparently higher exposure to repetitive and forceful hand-wrist motion based on observations during the walk-through survey, and b) jobs which employed the largest numbers of workers. These five departments (Hog Kill/Pork By-Products, Pork Cut, Pork Trim, Ham Bone, and Beef Fabrication) will be referred to as the higher exposure departments (HED). All day-shift employees working any of these 40 jobs were invited to participate in the study.

Case Definition

A case of UE CTD was defined as one or more symptoms (pain, numbness, tingling, aching, stiffness, or burning) in one of the 5 upper extremity joint areas (neck, shoulder, elbow, wrist, or hand) which satisfied the following criteria:

a. No previous accident or sudden trauma to the joint; and

b. Symptoms began after employment at the plant; and

c. Symptoms occurred within the past year; and

d. Symptoms lasted more than one week, or occurred more than 3 times in the previous year.

Comparisons of all UE and hand-wrist CTDs one-year period prevalences between the HED and LED are reported as prevalence ratios (PR) (HED/LED) with 95% 2-tailed Confidence Intervals (95% CI).

Point Prevalence

All employees completing the questionnaire described above had a physical examination performed by physicians trained in internal and occupational medicine blinded to the questionnaire results. These exams were limited to evaluation of the neck and UE, and were designed to detect UE CTDs. The examinations included inspection, palpation, range of motion (active, passive and resisted), and various maneuvers. Endpoint diagnoses included tendon related disorders (bicipital tendonitis, rotator cuff tendonitis, epicondylitis, tenosynovitis, trigger finger, DeQuervain's disease), peripheral nerve entrapments (carpal tunnel syndrome, Guyon tunnel syndrome), muscular disorders (tension neck syndrome), and localized osteoarthritis (wrist and proximal interphalange joint). An UE CTD case was defined as a worker who satisfied the questionnaire case definition (criteria listed in the preceding section) and the presence of a UE CTD on physical examination affecting the same specific symptomatic joint area mentioned on the questionnaire.

Comparisons of all UE and hand-wrist CTDs point prevalences between the HED and LED are reported as prevalence ratios (PR) (HED/LED) with 95% CI.

RESULTS

Incidence Rates

For the one year study period, 880 OSHA 200 Log entries satisfied our case definition of UE CTD for an incidence rate of 41.7 per 200,000 work hours [100 full-time workers (ftw) per year]. One-hundred-thirty-three cases of carpal tunnel syndrome (cts) were entered on the logs for an incidence rate of 6.3 per 100 (ftw) per year.

Hands and wrists were the most frequently affected areas (52% and 29%, respectively), followed by elbows (10%), shoulders (7%), and neck (2%). Tendonitis, strains, and carpal tunnel syndrome were the most common diagnoses (Table 1).

Period Prevalence

One hundred and forty-nine day-shift workers were employed in the 40 jobs selected from the HED. Five (3%) of these 149 workers refused participation, and 12 selected employees were not made available to NIOSH researcher because, it was explained, their absence would disrupt the production line. Ninety-three day-shift workers were employed in the two LED. Twenty-five (27%) of these 93 employees refused participation. Fourteen of these 25 refusals did not care to participate because they stated they lacked UE problems while the remaining 11 did not clearly state why they refused participation.

Our study group thus consisted of 200 employees: 68 from LED, and 132 from HED. One hundred and forty of the 200 workers had UE CTDs determined by questionnaire for an overall one-year period prevalence of 70%. Employees in the HED had an UE CTD one-year period prevalence of 80%, while the LED employees had an upper extremity CTD period prevalence of 50% (PR=1.61, 95% CI = 1.25, 2.07). (Table 3) The one-year period prevalence of hand-wrist CTDs for the HED was 74% compared to 41% in the LED (PR=1.80, 95% CI 1.33, 2.44).

TABLE 1

MEDICAL CONDITIONS DEFINED AS
UPPER EXTREMITY CTDs REPORTED ON THE OSHA 200 LOGS

	#	(%)
Tendonitis	369	34.2%
Strain	265	24.6%
Probable carpal tunnel syndrome	133	12.3%
Possible carpal tunnel syndrome	17	1.6%
Stenosing tenosynovitis (trigger finger)	92	8.5%
Stenosing tenosynovitis (deQuervain's)	26	2.4%
Tennis Elbow, Epicondylitis	47	4.4%
Tenosynovitis	38	3.5%
Myalgia, Myositis	19	1.8%
Neuralgia, Neuritis	16	1.5%
Synovitis	15	1.4%
Bursitis	13	1.2%
Ganglion Cyst	12	1.1%
Miscellaneous+	14	1.3%
	1079++	100.2%**

\+ Miscellaneous diagnoses include costochondritis, irritation, rotator cuff, torticollis, fingernail avulsion, arthritis, overuse syndrome

++ Number is greater than 880 (the number of entries) because more than one diagnosis could be listed for each entry

** Due to rounding errors

Point Prevalences

One hundred of the 200 workers had current UE CTDs by questionnaire and physical examination, for an overall point prevalence of 50%. Employees in the HED had an UE CTD point prevalence of 62%, while the LED employees had a UE CTD point prevalence of 27% (PR=2.35, 95% CI = 1.55, 3.56). (Table 3) The point prevalence of hand-wrist CTDs for the HED was 57% compared to 21% in the LED (PR=2.76, 95% CI 1.69, 4.50).

DISCUSSION

Incidence Rates

The plant had an upper extremity CTD incidence rate of 41.7 per 100 ftw per year compared to 6.7 reported for the meatpacking industry [Rate Ratio (RR)=6.24, 95% CI 5.8, 6.7] or 0.1 reported for all US industries in 1987 (RR=417.1, 95% CI 390.0, 455.6).[7] Several biases can influence the CTD incidence rates between meatpacking plants. These include differing: 1) access to the first aid department for symptomatic employees (reporting bias), 2) criteria for CTD diagnosis (misclassification bias), and 3) criteria for a work-related injury and/or illness being "recordable" onto the OSHA 200 Logs (recording bias). These biases could account for some of the observed differences of the CTD incidence rate at this meatpacking plant compared to the meatpacking industry's rate. This investigation did not address the extent of these biases among other meatpacking plants, nor the magnitude of its effect on the meatpacking industry's CTD incidence rate.

TABLE 2

OVERALL and HAND-WRIST CTD CASES BY DEPARTMENTS

	Number of Workers	Questionnaire (Q) # (%)	Q and PE* # (%)
HIGH EXPOSURE DEPARTMENTS			
Hog Kill/By Products	(12)		
Overall cases		10 (83%)	8 (67%)
Hand-Wrist cases		8 (67%)	7 (58%)
Pork Cut/Conversion	(20)		
Overall cases		16 (80%)	10 (50%)
Hand-Wrist cases		15 (75%)	9 (45%)
Pork Trim	(18)		
Overall cases		16 (89%)	14 (78%)
Hand-Wrist cases		15 (83%)	13 (72%)
Ham Bone	(41)		
Overall cases		36 (88%)	34 (83%)
Hand-Wrist cases		36 (88%)	33 (81%)
Beef Fabrication	(41)		
Overall cases		28 (68%)	16 (39%)
Hand-Wrist cases		24 (59%)	13 (32%)
Subtotal:	(132)		
Overall cases		106 (80%)	82 (62%)
Hand-Wrist cases		98 (74%)	75 (57%)
LOWER EXPOSURE DEPARTMENTS			
Smoke Meat Pack	(40)		
Overall Cases		21 (53%)	12 (30%)
Hand-Wrist Cases		20 (50%)	9 (23%)
Sausage Cooler	(28)		
Overall Cases		13 (46%)	6 (21%)
Hand-Wrist Cases		8 (29%)	5 (18%)
Subtotal:	(68)		
Overall Cases		34 (50%)	18 (27%)
Hand-Wrist Cases		28 (41%)	14 (21%)
ALL DEPARTMENTS TOTAL:	(200)		
Overall cases		140 (70%)	100 (50%)
Hand-Wrist cases		126 (63%)	89 (45%)

* PE = Physical Examination

The plant's cts incidence rate was 6.3 per 100 ftw per year. Using a age-and sex-adjusted cts incidence rate of 0.105 as the referent, this plant's rate ratio for developing cts would be 60.0 (95% CI 50.3, 71.1).[12] The plant's cts incidence rate could not be adjusted for age and gender because the OSHA 200 Logs do not contain age or sex information and we did not obtain it from other sources. Advancing age and female gender are two risk factors for developing cts, but this plant's workforce is composed mainly of of young men.[12] Adjusting the plant's cts incidence rate for age and sex would most likely increase the rate ratio. The methods to identify cts cases in this working population (OSHA 200 Logs) were very different from the methods used to identify cts cases in the population based study (medical records) used as the referent. It is not possible to predict the direction in which the rate ratio would be affected by this bias, but with an estimated rate ratio of 60.0, the association of employment at this plant and cts is not from bias in identifying cts cases on the OSHA 200 log.

Calculating UE CTD incidence rates for specific jobs was not undertaken for two reasons. First, the employees frequently used vernacular job terms not recognized by the foremen, supervisors, or nursing personnel, therefore the job title listed on the OSHA 200 Log was inaccurate. Second, the number of employee hours worked for specific jobs was not available.

Period and Point Prevalence

The departments with the highest incidence rates for UE CTDs also had the highest prevalence of UE CTDs determined from the questionnaires and physical examinations. The OSHA 200 Logs indicate other high risk jobs and departments exist, but were not studied due to resource and time constraints. The lower exposure departments (LED), Smoke Meat Pack and Sausage Cooler, have point prevalences for UE CTDs of 30% and 21%, respectively. Selection bias may have contributed to these two departments' high point prevalences. Twenty-five of the 93 selected employees in the LED refused participation (27%). Fourteen of these 25 stated that they did not care to participate because they lacked upper extremity problems. The lower participation rate most likely resulted in over-estimates of the period prevalences of upper extremity CTDs within these two departments. If all employees refusing study participation lacked UE CTDs, the point prevalences for Smoke Meat Pack would be 25%, and 13% for Sausage Cooler. A point prevalence of 25% or 13%, however, is still high compared to true low risk working environments, which are estimated to have UE CTD point prevalences of less than 1%.[13] The high prevalence of CTDs in these two LEDs is confirmed by the OSHA 200 Log data. The Smoke Meat Pack department had an upper extremity CTD incidence rate of 47.9 per 100 ftw per year, while the Sausage Cooler department had an upper extremity incidence rate 15.4. Both these rates are above the average for the meatpacking industry (6.7 per 100 ftw per year in 1987).[7]

During the period 5/1/87 to 4/30/88 employee turnover was reported to be between 200 and 400%. This high rate of employee turnover suggests that survivor bias may be a substantial problem in our investigation. "Survivors" are usually healthier (that is, lacking illness or injury that would interfere with work) than those who have left employment. This "healthy worker" or "survivor effect" has been described in studies of the meatpacking and other industries, and is an inherent bias of this study's cross-sectional design.[1] Neither of these selection biases, however, invalidate the basic conclusion of this study: all departments studied with questionnaires and physical examinations had substantially elevated rates of upper extremity CTDs.

CONCLUSION

This study found a high incidence rate of UE CTDs and carpal tunnel syndrome among workers at this meatpacking plant for the one-year period 5/1/87 to 4/30/88. In addition, a high prevalence of upper extremity CTDs and hand-wrist CTDs was found among current workers.

ACKNOWLEDGMENT

The authors would like to acknowledge Micheal Goldman and Susan Stock for their contribution to this report.

REFERENCES

1 Viikari-Juntura, Eira. Neck and upper limb disorder among slaughterhouse workers; an epidemiologic and clinical study. Scand J Work Envir Health 1983;9:283-90.

2 Findel ML: The effects of repeated mechanical trauma in the meat industry. Am J Ind Med 1985; 8:375-79.

3 Falck B, Aaenio P: Left-sided carpal tunnel syndrome in butchers. Scand J Work Environ Health 1983; 9:291-97.

4 Masear VR, Hayes JA, Hyde A: Industrial causes of carpal tunnel syndrome. J Hand Surg 1986; 11A:222-27.

5 Streib EW, Sun SF. Distal ulnar neuropathy in meat packers: an occupational disease? JOM 1984;26:842-43.

6 Occupational injuries and illnesses in the United States by industry, 1987. USDOL, Bureau of Labor Statistics, May 1989.

7 Chin Ling Wang, Bureau of Labor Statistics, personal communication, 7/18/88.

8 U.S. Department of Labor, Bureau of Labor Statistics: Recordkeeping Guidelines for Occupational Injuries and Illnesses - September 1986 - page 59. O.M.B. No. 1220-0029.

9 Silverstein, B. Surveillance in Cumulative Trauma Control Program. Presented at the Occupational Disorders of the Upper Extremities Course, June 27-29, 1988, Chicago, IL.

10 Putz-Anderson, V. Cumulative Trauma Disorders: A manual for musculoskeletal diseases of the upper limbs. Taylor and Francis LTD. March 1988.

11 Travers, PH. Soft tissue disorders of the upper extremities. In Occupational Medicine: State of the Art Review, Worker Fitness and Risk Evaluations. Himmelstein JS, Pransky GS Editors. Vol 3, No 2, April-June 1988. Janley and Belfus Inc., Philadelphia.

12 Stevens JC, Sun MD, Beard CM, O'Fallon WM, Kurland LT. Carpal tunnel syndrome in Rochester, Minnesota, 1961 to 1980. Neurology 1988; 38:134-138.

13 Silverstein BA, Fine LJ, Armstrong TJ: Hand wrist cumulative trauma disorders in industry. Br J Ind Med 1986; 43:779-784.

Occupational Epidemiology. H. Sakurai et al., editors

SELF REPORTED MUSCULOSKELETAL SYMPTOMS AMONG OFFICE VIDEO DISPLAY TERMINAL OPERATORS

NICHOLAS HEYER, HARVEY CHECKOWAY, WILLIAM DANIELL, SANFORD HORSTMAN, JANICE CAMP

Department of Environmental Health, School of Public Health and Community Medicine, University of Washington, Seattle, Washington, USA

INTRODUCTION

In the past ten years, concern about possible health effects associated with working with video display terminals (VDTs) has grown. The most widely recognized standards in the U.S. for work with VDTs have been put forward by the American National Standards Institute,[1] including standards for screen characteristics, lighting and illumination, work station design, task design, and general office environment. Health effects associated with VDT use have been reviewed by Bergqvist.[2] This review concluded that there was some evidence for visual and musculoskeletal symptoms associated with VDT use. Visual effects were thought to be associated with screen display and lighting characteristics. Constraint of posture and task design were considered important factors in the reporting of musculoskeletal symptoms. More recently, a Massachusetts study[3] found increased reporting of visual and musculoskeletal complaints among 1,545 VDT operators in six industries. The frequency of these complaints increased with the number of hours spent working with a VDT.

METHODS

The present study was designed to 1) estimate the prevalence of vision and musculoskeletal complaints among VDT operators in the Puget Sound area of Washington State; and 2) evaluate the association between VDT work station design and/or job task, and the prevalence of reported symptoms. Participation was requested from employers in various industries which were expected to have intensive VDT use. Employees were defined as VDT operators if they worked at VDTs for four hours or more per day. A comparison group of non-VDT employees was defined as working two hours or less per day at a VDT. Each participating VDT operator and non-VDT employee completed a self administered questionnaire. The data collected included job title, duration of employment, hours of VDT work per day, job satisfaction, VDT training, adjustability of equipment, quality of video image, and reported symptoms.

Additional data on the working environment of VDT operators were collected by 'work units', which were defined as workers located within a well defined area and sharing the same supervisory structure. The information was collected by direct worker observations and by supervisor interviews. Ten to fifteen minute observations were conducted on a 20 percent sample of workers in each work unit. These observations included measurements of noise and illumination levels, determination of the percentage of time spent keying into the computer, and evaluation of work station design, video image, and VDT operator posture. Supervisor interviews were used to evaluate work schedule policies and employee-employer relations, and to define job tasks by job title.

Reported symptoms were collected within categories. Vision symptoms included irritation, tiredness and blurred vision. Musculoskeletal symptoms included numbness, tingling, weakness, stiffness or cramping of the back, neck, and upper and lower extremities. Comparisons of symptom prevalence were made between subgroups of workers classified by job task, hours of VDT work per day, and work station characteristics. Prevalence ratios and 95 percent confidence limits were computed to estimate effects of exposure variables.[4]

RESULTS

Only four of the twenty-one companies invited to participate were included in this study. Most refused to participate, while one did not meet our study requirements. The employers participating included a small communications company, an airline reservations facility, a large communications company, and a department of state government. A total of 894 VDT operators agreed to participate in the study. This represents approximately 63 percent of the almost 1400 employees estimated to be eligible. In addition, 105 non-VDT employees were recruited as a comparison group. Final analysis was restricted to the 702 female VDT operators in 19 work units, and 52 female non-VDT employees who met all study criteria.

Table I: Prevalence of Symptoms - VDT Operators vs. Non-VDT

Symptom	VDT % Sx	Non-VDT % Sx	Prevalence Ratio	95% Confidence Interval
Head	64	58	1.10	0.76-1.59
Eye	68	42	1.61	1.05-2.47
Back	55	46	1.20	0.79-1.81
Neck	53	37	1.42	0.89-2.24
Arm	16	8	2.04	0.75-5.54
Hand	31	13	2.32	1.09-4.92
Leg	36	33	1.11	0.68-1.82

Table II: Prevalence of Symptoms - By Hours Worked at a VDT (>6 vs. 4-6)

Symptom	>6 hrs. % Sx	4-6 hrs. % Sx	Prevalence Ratio	95% Confidence Interval
Head	65	59	1.09	0.87-1.37
Eye	70	64	1.10	0.88-1.36
Back	55	55	1.00	0.79-1.27
Neck	54	49	1.10	0.86-1.41
Arm	15	17	0.87	0.57-1.34
Hand	31	32	0.96	0.71-1.32
Leg	36	37	0.99	0.74-1.32

Possibly due to the self selection of employers willing to participate, variability for many of the factors measured or observed in this study was small. All work units had adjustable chairs, but minimally adjustable tables. Employee satisfaction was generally high, and work schedules and break policies were similar among employers. There was only minimal training available for working with VDTs, and virtually all VDT screens were observed to have significant levels of glare.

Exposure factors for which there was sufficient variation among the study participants to allow analysis included VDT operator vs. non-VDT employee; number of hours worked at a VDT (4-6 hours vs. more than six hours); doing "entry" tasks (word processing and data entry) vs. interactive tasks (generally customer representative or sales work); and working in a unit where a majority of the VDT operators observed were working with their neck extended or flexed (up/down) as opposed to a neutral position. None of the associations analyzed was changed substantially by adjustment for age, level of education, job satisfaction, or years at current job; consequently, only crude prevalence comparisons are presented.

VDT operators had a generally higher prevalence of symptoms than non-VDT employees, with differences most pronounced for symptoms of the eyes, neck, arm and hand (Table I). However, there was no association observed with the number of hours worked at a VDT (Table II). VDT operators doing entry tasks had increased symptoms of the back, neck, arm and hand compared to those doing interactive tasks (Table III). This pattern was also observed for operators with non-neutral neck angle (Table IV). There was a high correlation between doing entry tasks and working with a non-neutral neck angle.

Table III: Prevalence of Symptoms - By VDT Task (Entry vs. Interactive)

Symptom	Entry % Sx	Interactive % Sx	Prevalence Ratio	95% Confidence Interval
Head	71	62	1.14	0.88-1.48
Eye	77	67	1.16	0.90-1.48
Back	77	52	1.49	1.16-1.92
Neck	70	50	1.40	1.08-1.83
Arm	30	13	2.23	1.46-3.40
Hand	54	28	1.94	1.42-2.65
Leg	47	35	1.37	1.00-1.89

Table IV: Prevalence of Symptoms - By Neck Angle (Neutral vs Non-Neutral)

Symptom	Non-Neutral % Sx	Neutral % Sx	Prevalence Ratio	95% Confidence Interval
Head	67	63	1.05	0.83-1.34
Eye	78	66	1.17	0.93-1.47
Back	76	51	1.50	1.18-1.89
Neck	74	49	1.51	1.19-1.93
Arm	31	13	2.48	1.67-3.68
Hand	52	27	1.91	1.42-2.56
Leg	47	35	1.35	1.00-1.82

DISCUSSION

This study confirmed previous observations that VDT operators experience more vision and musculoskeletal symptoms then other office workers. In addition, job task was observed to be an important factor in the reporting of symptoms. In particular, entry tasks, requiring higher levels of keying and more restrained postures, resulted in increased symptoms of the upper body and extremities. Working with a non-neutral neck angle was associated both with doing entry type tasks and increased reported symptoms. It is possible that interactions between work station design and job tasks are responsible for the observed increases in reported symptoms. Structuring work to reduce highly repetitive tasks and offering frequent work breaks may reduce the number of reported symptoms among VDT operators.

BIBLIOGRAPHY

1. ANSI (1986) American National Standards for Human Factors Engineering of Visual Display Terminal Work Stations. American National Standards Institute
2. Bergqvist UOV (1984) Video display terminals and health. Scand J Work Environ Health 10:suppl 2
3. Rossignol AM, Morse EP, Summers VM, Pagnotto LD (1987) Video display terminal use and reported health symptoms among Massachusetts clerical workers. J Occup Med 29(2):112-118
4. Rothman KJ (1986) Modern Epidemiology. Little-Brown, Boston

Occupational Epidemiology. H. Sakurai et al., editors

RAYNAUD'S PHENOMENON IN THE LOWER EXTREMITIES AND OCCUPATIONAL VIBRATION-EXPOSURE

AKINORI HISASHIGE, NOBUHUMI YASUDA, MIKI TOKUHIRO, HIROSHI OHARA
Dept. of Public Health, Kochi Medical School, Nankoku, Kochi, 781-51 JAPAN

INTRODUCTION

The intermittent blanching of the fingers or hands (Raynaud's phenomenon) is the most prominent symptom resulting from occupational vibration-exposure to the hand-arm transmitted vibration. The causal relationship between Raynaud's phenomenon and vibration exposure transmitted to the hand-arm has been established, although the etiology of this phenomenon has not been fully elucidated (1-3).

Recently, Raynaud's phenomenon in the lower extremities (eg., toes or feet) among workers using vibrating tools has recieved much attention. However, there were only a few case-reports (4-6) and its cause and mechanism had not been examined yet. To examine the relationship between occupational vibration-exposure transmitted to extremities and Raynaud's phenomenon in the lower extremities, a case-control study was conducted.

SUBJECTS AND METHOD

The study subjects were 1,247 chain saw operators among forestry workers who took a specific examination for vibration-disease at K hospial, which is the only special hospital for occupational disease in Kochi Prefecture and which has been carrying out this examination among almost all forestry workers in this area.

Cases consisted of 34 forestry workers who have experienced Raynaud's phenomenon in the lower extremities. Two controls of the same number were selected from forestry workers who had never experienced Raynaud's phenomenon in the lower extremities; the first control group (control A) consited of workers with experience of Raynaud's phenomenon in the upper extremities. The second control group (control B) consited of workers without experience of Raynaud's phenomenon in any extremities. They were matched to cases by age (± 5 years), area, type of employment (eg., private or National) and period of first examination (± 5 years).

To identify cases and controls, medical charts and health examination records from the first visit to the present were used, and interviews and consultations were carried out by medical doctors. The information on general demographic characteristics, working conditions, vibration-exposure and occupational histories was derived in the same way. Raynaud's phenomenon was observed and confirmed by medical doctors and/or nurses except in several cases where Raynaud's phenomenon was relatively mild.

There are two kinds of occupational vibration-exposures suspected of causing Raynaud's phenomenon in the lower extremities; one is vibration-exposure to the hand-arm which was substituted by the total operating time (hours) of vibrating

Table 1. Characteristics of Raynaud's phenomenon in the lower extremities

Items	N=34
Season	(%)
only in winter	27 (79.4)
Frequency (in cold seasons)	
several times/month	30 (88.2)
Range	
over 5 toes	22 (64.7)

Table 2. Characteristics of Raynaud's phenomenon in the upper extremities

Items	cases (N=34)	control A (N=34)
Season	(%)	(%)
not only in winter	23 (67.7)	22 (64.7)
Frequency (in cold seasons)		
almost everyday	26 (76.5)	16 (47.1)*
Range		
exceeds fingers	6 (17.6)	4 (11.7)

* P=0.02, Fisher's exact metod (both sided)

tools. The other is vibration-exposure to the lower extremities transmitted by supporting chain saws with thighs and legs. However, it is very difficult to estimate. Therefore, the proportion of working time associated with vibration-exposure to the lower extremities, to total working time was estimated by each worker and used as the index.

Diseases suspected to cause Raynaud's phenomenon in the lower extremities, such as arteriosclerosis, collagen diseases, hematological diseases and so on, were ruled out among all cases by clinical findings, clinical courses and results of laboratory tests (eg., BSR, CRP, immuno globlin , RA).

The average age (± S.D.) at present among the cases is 60.7 ± 5.8 years. The main type of employment was the National forestry (58.8%). The main period of the first examination was from 1975 to 1979 (76.5%). There were no statistically significant differences in these items between cases and controls, since they were matched in the selection.

The characteristics of Raynaud's phenomenon in the lower extremities among the cases are shown in Table 1. This phenomenon occured usually in winter and its frequency was usually several times per month. The range of Raynaud's phenomenon exceeded 5 toes in total among over half of the cases. In the most sever case, it reached the upper part of legs. Raynaud's phenomenon in the hand preceded those in the lower extremities in all cases. Table 2 shows Raynaud's phenomenon in fingers and hands among cases and control A. Its grade was so severe that it occurred not only in winter and its range exceeded fingers among over 10 % of subjects. Moreover, in terms of frequency, proportion of occurrence almost everyday among cases was significantly higher than that among control A.

RUSULTS

Table 3 shows the odds ratios for Raynaud's phenomenon in the lower extremities with total vibration-exposure time transmitted to the hand-arm and the lower extremities between cases and control B without any Raynaud's phenomenon. These odds ratios (95% C.I.) were 48.2 (11.0-211) and 20.0

(4.7-88.4) respectively. Altough they are statistically significant, odds ratio with vibration-eposure to the hand-arm was obviously higher than that to the lower extremities. Moreover, there was observed a dose-effect relationship for the vibration-exposure to the lower extremities.

Table 4 shows the odds ratios for Raynaud's phenomenon with total vibration-exposure to the hand-arm and the lower extremities between cases and control A with Raynaud's phenomenon in the fingers or hands. These odds ratios (95% C.I.) were 13.6 (2.7-68.1) and 5.5 (1.3-22.7). Also in this comparison, odds ratio with vibration-exposure to the hand-arm was higher than that to the lower extremities. A dose-effect relationship was observed for the exposure to the hand-arm rather than that to the lower extremities.

Table 3. Odds ratios, with 95% confidence limits for Raynaud's phenomenon in the lower extremities with vibration-exposure

Exposure	Cases (N=34)	Control B (N=34)	Odds ratios (95% CI)
Total exposure to hand-arm (hrs.)	(%)	(%)	
- 9999	3 (8.8)	28 (82.4)	
10000-	31 (91.2)	6 (17.6)	48.2 (11.0-211)
Total exposure to lower extremities (hrs.)	(%)	(%)	
- 999	5 (14.7)	21 (61.8)	
1000 -	10 (29.4)	9 (26.5)	4.7 (1.2-17.6)
2000 -	19 (55.8)	4 (11.7)	20.0 (4.7-88.4)

Table 4. Odds ratios, with 95% confidence limits for Raynaud's phenomenon in the lower extremities with vibration-exposure

Exposure	Cases (N=34)	Control A (N=34)	Odds ratios (95% CI)
Total exposure to hand-arm (hrs.)	(%)	(%)	
- 9999	3 (8.8)	17 (50.0)	
10000-	19 (55.9)	12 (35.3)	9.0 (2.2-37.3)
15000-	12 (35.3)	5 (14.7)	13.6 (2.7-68.1)
Total exposure to lower extremities (hrs.)	(%)	(%)	
- 999	5 (14.7)	15 (44.2)	
1000 -	10 (29.4)	6 (17.6)	5.0 (1.2-20.9)
2000 -	8 (23.5)	7 (20.6)	3.4 (0.8-14.4)
5000 -	11 (32.3)	6 (17.6)	5.5 (1.3-22.7)

DISCUSSION

This study showed the extremely high odds ratios for Raynaud's phenomenon in the lower extremities with occupational vibration-exposure, whether it was transimitted to the lower extremities or not. This result indicates that Raynaud's phenomenon in the lower extremities is strongly related to occupational vibration-exposure. Moreover, it was observed that odds ratio with vibration-exposure to the hand-arm was two or three times higher than that to the lower extremities, in comparing cases with not only control A but also control B. Moreover, the level of vibration-exposure to the hand-arm was considerablly higher than that to the lower extremities.

These findings suggest that vibration-exposure to the hand-arm plays a major part in Raynaud's phenomenon in the lower extremities compared with vibration-exposure to the lower extremities. However, althogh the level of vibration-exposrue to the lower extremities is not so high, it is vulnerable to the information (memory) bias. Therefore, in evaluating its relative risk correctly, further examination will be needed.

On the other hand, concerning the process of Raynaud's phenomenon in the lower extremities, it was observed to follow that in the fingers and hands. In addition, odds ratio with vibration-exposure between cases and control B was higher than that between cases and control A. These results imply that it occurs after the incidence of Raynaud's phenomenon in the fingers and hands by being exposed to vibration continuously.

The pathogenesis or etilogy of Raynaud's phenomenon in the fingers and hands of occupational origin (vibration induced white finger or VWF) has not been fully clarified yet. The over activity of sympathetic nervous system and/or local alterations in digital blood flow are considered to be the main pathophysiologic mechanisms for its development (7-10).

In Raynaud'phenomenon in the lower extremities, it is thought that the same mechanisms as in VWF operate. However, taking into consideration the results of this study, the sympathetic nervous system would play the dominant part. On the other hand, concerning the effect of vibrtion-exposure to the hand-arm to the lower extremities, an experimental study (11) showed that vibration-exposure to the hand yielded a significant decrease in skin temperature not only in hands but also toes. This does not necessarily explain the incidence of Raynaud's phenomenon in the lower extremities, but does confirm the role of the sympathetic nervous system.

REFERENCES

1. Taylor W (ed) (1974) The vibration syndrome, Academic Press, London
2. Brammer AJ, Taylor W (eds) (1982) Vibration effects on the hand and arm in industry, Jhon Wiley & Sons, New York
3. Futatsuka M, Sakurai T, Ariizumi M (1984) J Arch Occup Environ Health 54: 201-221
4. Suzuki Y et al (1966) Shikoku Igakku Zasshi 22:70-72
5. Gomibuchi K, Ohoi T (1967) Jpn J Traum Occup Med 15:177-182
6. Hashiguchi T et al (1988) Jpn J Traum Occup Med 36:651-656
7. Gemne G (1982) Scand J Work Environ Health 8:243-249
8. Pyyko I (1982) In: Brammer AJ, Taylor W (eds) Vibration effects on the hand and arm in industry, Jhon Wiley & Sons. New York, pp 13-24
9. Olsen N et al (1985) Br J Ind Med 42:272-275
10. Bovenzi M (1986) Eur J Appl Phisiol 55:381-389
11. Kondo T et al (1987) Ind Health 25:41-53

Occupational Epidemiology. H. Sakurai et al., editors

549434

AN EPIDEMIOLOGICAL STUDY ON THE EFFECT OF IMPROVED WORK CONDITIONS ON PREVENTION OF OCCUPATIONAL CERVICOBRACHIAL DISORDER

T. ITANI, M.GOTO, T.ISOJIMA, H.ONO AND H.AOYAMA

Department of Hygiene, Okayama University Medical School, Okayama, 700 JAPAN

INTRODUCTION

Occupational cervicobrachial disorder (OCD) is an occupational disease caused by work requiring repeated hand-arm movements or holding superior limbs in the same position. The main symptoms of the disorder are muscle fatigue in the cervicobrachial area[1] and disturbance of the autonomic nervous system. The first cases of this disorder were found in the 1960's among key punchers, the so-called "key puncher's disease"[2] in Japan. Since then, many other cases have been reported among various kinds of workers such as typists, supermarket cash register operators, telephone operators and assembly workers[3-4].

This research was carried out to clarify the importance of improving work conditions and upgrading health care systems as preventive measures of OCD.

MATERIAL AND METHODS

The following two work places were selected for investigation;

Case 1: Photo-film rolling workers in a photo-film production factory.

Case 2: Ticket sellers at a pari-mutuel ticket window.

Symptoms related to OCD were examined in both cases before and after improvements and the results were compared respectively. The symptoms were judged by a medical exam conforming with the Committee's Report[5] in cases 1. A questionnaire survey was taken about the symptoms of OCD in case 2. A medical exam was not carried out in case 2 because the cooperation of the company was not obtained.

Table 1. Work contents of photo-film rolling workers

Work Group	Group A	Group B	
Machines	Automatic winding and capping machine	Winding machine	Capping machine
Working operation	Take an automatically wound film in front Put the wound film into the film case Set the case to the capping machine (capped by the machine)	Take a film from the film stock box in front Set the film to a reel Set the reel to the rolling shaft and wind the film Put the wound film on the conveyer	Take a wound film from the conveyer Put the wound film into the film case Set the case to the capping machine (capped by the machine)
Cycle period	4-6 sec	6-8 sec	3-5 sec
Number of operations per day	ca. 5500	ca. 4000	ca. 6500

RESULTS

Case 1: Cervicobrachial Disorder in Photo-film Rolling Workers

There are two methods of photo film rolling performed in a darkroom. The work is detailed in table 1.

Improvement of Work Conditions. The work hours were shortened to 5 hours and 30 minutes from the previous 6 hours. The longest continuous work length was shortened from 100 minutes to 55 minutes. A work rotation system and a degree of workers' participation in production planning were introduced as work improvements. The winding machine and the machine that mounts caps on film cases were also improved so that the work movement, projecting the arm in the upper forward direction, was reduced. Furthermore, work chairs at each work place were replaced with chairs with an easily adjustable seat height and with a wide back rest.

Gymnastics to be performed during break times in the darkroom were developed to improve work place fitness. Sport facilities were also improved by extending volleyball courts and building a field athletic course to promote intra-company sport competition meets and exercise during lunch breaks.

Medical Examination, Health Consultation and Health Education. The medical exam and post exam health care such as health consultation and health education were enforced. An occupational health doctor and occupational health nurses were stationed to perform daily health care services, and to inspect and guide improvements of work conditions.

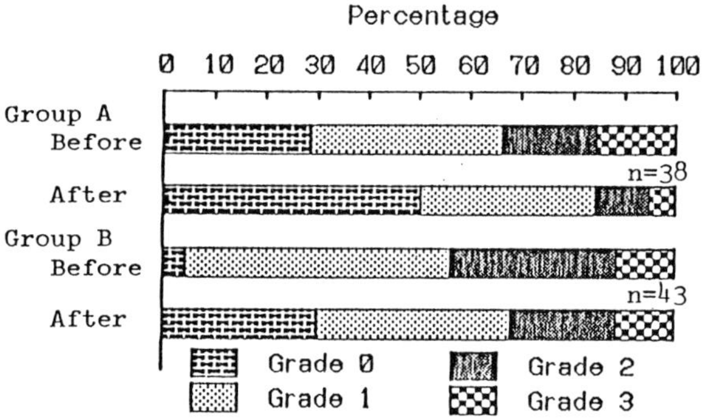

Fig.1 Changes of the clinical grades of OCD among photo-film rolling workers
Grade 0-3: Clinical grade of OCD proposed by the Committee on Cervicobrachial Syndrome

Evaluation of Health Care Activities. Figure 1 shows an analysis of the results of the medical exams of the workers received both exams before and after health care activities,

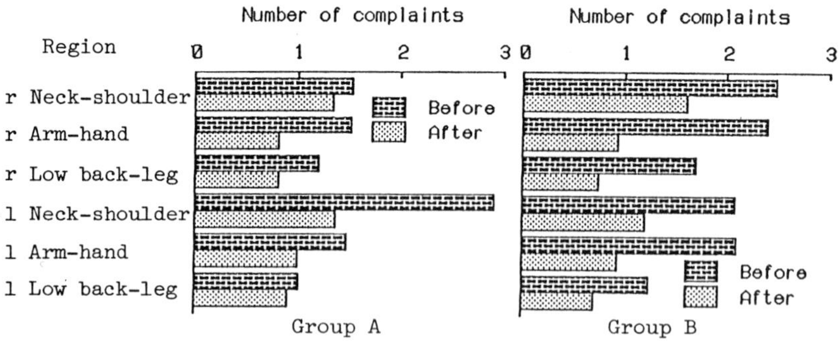

Fig.2 Average number of subjective symptoms for workers before and after the improvement .

and figure 2 shows changes in the workers' symptoms.

Case 2: Cervicobrachial Disorder in Off-track Pari-mutuel Cashiers

Off-track pari-mutuel cashier work consists of selling betting tickets for horse races held on weekends at places other than race tracks. An overall health care system could not be developed in this case, unlike the preceeding case. Improvements were made only to the machines.

Improvement of Work Conditions

The differences between the conventional ticketmachine and the new ticket machine are shown in table 2. The conventional ticket machine was operated by two workers, who had to keep standing during work. Each ticket machine issued one kind of ticket for each race. In contrast, the new ticket machine is operated by one worker sitting on a chair. The betting tickets are magnetic cards on which the machine can register up to ten bets for multiple races. The input information is shown on a visual display terminal in front of the worker. Along with the introduction of the new ticket machine, the method and content of ticketing were changed drastically. The results of the time study are given in Table 3, showing the changes of work content.

Table 2. Characteristics of the new and former type machines

	New type	Former type
Key board		
type of switch	electric	mechanical
length of stroke	short	long
inquired pressure	50g/cm	100g/cm
Display	on a ticket	VDT
Working posture		
standing	7.8%	74.3%
sitting	91.2%	23.1%

Table 3. Workload of the workers using new and former type machines

Amount of products	New type	Former type
customers/day/mach.	152	151
tickets/day/mach.	1702	6216
time/one customer		
less than 30 sec	40.2%	32.1%
120 sec or more	14.4%	9.0%
time for service	77.9%	52.1%
touches/day/mach.	26892	6838

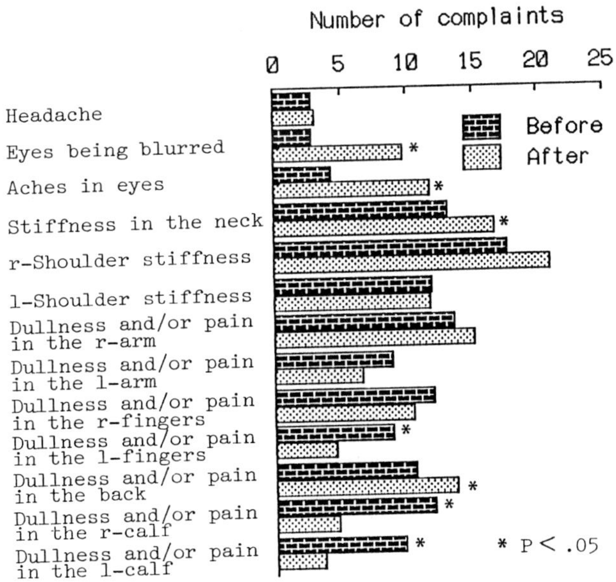

Fig.3 Changes of the rates of complaints after the introduction of new machines (n=547)

<u>Evaluation of Preventive Measures</u>. The prevalence of subjective symptoms among conventional and new ticket machine operators is shown in figure 3.

DISCUSSION

Cervicobrachial disorders are not caused by a single factor. It has been reported that preventive measures against not only OCD but also diseases caused by industrial fatigue should be overall measures to improve both the workers situation and environmental factors.

Present study made it clear that OCD can be prevented through health care activities such as medical exams and their follow-up, health consultation, and health education as well as through the improvement of work conditions such as shorter work hours, and improved work methods and machines. Which of these measures is the most effective item cannot be analyzed by the methods applied to this research. An overall preventive program based upon the improvement of working conditions is obviously useful for preventing OCD. Cervicobrachial disorders are thought to originate simultaneously from work load and poor working conditions. On the other hand, case 2 is an example of only improving machines. In this case, symptoms of the neck and shoulder were aggravated after carrying out the measures. Only maniphalanx and crusal symptoms were alleviated slightly. It is proved that OCD cannot be prevented effectively by only improving the work machine without implementing a health care program and upgrading other work conditions. The results of case 2 support the idea that preventive measures of OCD indispensably require upgrading the overall health care program in addition to the improvement of machines for reducing muscular load.

CONCLUSION

Preventive measures were applied to two work places in which the incidence of OCD among workers was a health problem. The effect of the measures was evaluated by comparing the symptoms of workers before and after the implementation.

The results show that only improving the machines as a preventive measure can not alleviate OCD, so that an overall preventive program consisting of a comprehensive improvement of work conditions such as work hours and work methods and the establishment of health care systems is necessary.

REFFERENCES

1. The Committee on Cervicobrachial Syndrome of Japanese Association of Industrial Health (1974) Jpn. J. Ind. Health 16: 160-164
2. Kubota, S. (1969) Occupational Diseases and their Prevention, Kouseisha, Tokyo, pp 563-596
3. Itani, T. (1976) J. Sci. Labour 52: 585-597
4. Ohara, H. et al. (1979) J. Human Ergol. 8: 39-45
5. The Committee on Cervicobrachial Syndrome of Japanese Association of Industrial Health (1973) Jpn. J. Ind. Health 15: 304-311

Occupational Epidemiology. H. Sakurai et al., editors

THE EFFECTS OF MENTAL STRESS AND SOCIAL SUPPORT ON THE DEVELOPMENT OF MUSCULOSKELETAL MORBIDITY IN THE ENGINEERING INDUSTRY

Päivi Leino[1], Anna-Liisa Lyyra[2]

[1]Department of Public Health, University of Tampere
[2]Department of Statistics, University of Jyväskylä (Finland)

INTRODUCTION

There is some evidence suggesting a role of psycho-social stress in the aetiology of musculoskeletal disorders[1-3]. Frese observed that psychological stress at work, as assessed at an individual and an aggregate level, predicted later musculoskeletal complaints[4]. Psychological work stress was associated with musculoskeletal morbidity in the Mini-Finland Study[5]. Leino has shown that psychophysiological symptoms of stress predict the occurrence of these disorders in the material of the present study[6].

Although the impact of supportive social relationships on health has been a popular research area in recent years[7-8], social support has not to date evoked much scientific interest in the study of musculoskeletal disorders. Cobb and Kasl[9] reported, however, that joint swelling under a stressful life circumstance was more frequent in workers with little support from spouse.

The purpose of this study was to investigate whether perceived psycho-social stress factors and social support are related with musculoskeletal morbidity in white-collar and blue-collar workers at an initial examination and prospectively.

MATERIALS AND METHODS

902 employees of three plants of the engineering industry in Finland were studied for perceived stress, social support and musculoskeletal morbidity by questionnaire and physical examination in 1973. A sampling stratified for age-group, gender and occupational class was used. 654 subjects were studied again in 1983, when 412 (80 white-collar women, 63 blue-collar women, 119 white-collar men and 150 blue-collar men) of them were still profitably employed. These 412 persons were taken into the longitudinal analyses.

Stress. With psycho-social stress we refer to a relationship between individual and environment that the subject appraises as adverse of taxing[10]. The score of perceived stress was a sum score of the following questionnaire items, all scored from 1 to 5: "Do you feel that you are overstrained by your work?", "Do work concerns bother you at home?", "How mentally strenuous do you consider your work to be?", "How much strain does pressed workpace put on you?" (very little, ..., very much); "I am countinuously afraid of making mistakes in my work", "I often feel uneasy about getting dismissed from work", "Financial problems are a continual burden for me", "Children and other relatives continuously cause trouble for me" (fully disagree, ..., fully agree); "Are you satisfied with how interesting or varied your work is?" (very satisfied, ..., very unsatisfied); "How much disagreement between personnel groups is there at your workplace?" (none, ..., very much). There were missing data in 1-3 items in 62 subjects. The score was weighted by the number of items with data.

Social support. Social support was understood as the quality of relationships at work, with friends, and in marriage, as perceived by the subject. The measure of support was constructed as a sum score of the following items, scored from 1 to 5: "How much mutual help do fellow employees give to one another at your workplace?" (not at all, ..., very much); "Is your foreperson or supervisor able to appreciate the difficulties of your work?" (very badly, ..., very well); "Does your foreperson or supervisor take your personal problems into consideration?" (never, ..., mostly); "I have no close friends to confide to", "I feel lonely at weekends" (fully agree, ..., fully disagree); "What things do you usually discuss with your spouse?" (only the most necessary matters, ..., all matters). The last item was not responded to by 186 unmarried subjects. Seven additional subjects had one item with missing data. The score was weighted with the amount of items with data. 21 persons with missing data in half of the items were left out of the analyses.

The internal consistency of the stress and support scores (the variance of the total scores obtained before weighting) was acceptable: the alpha coefficient of the stress score was 0.71 and that of the support score 0.69.

Musculoskeletal morbidity

Rheumatic symptoms. In the questionnaire an inquiry was made about the occurrence and frequency of aches and pains in different parts of the body: "Have you had ache, stiffness, sensitivity to movement, numbness or pain in joints or muscles in the below mentioned locations, and how often during the past year?" The list included the following items: shoulder, upper arm; elbow, forearm; wrist, hand, fingers; hip joint; thigh; knee; calf; ankle, foot; sole, toes; neck, cervical and occipital region; radiation of cervical pain to the arm; thoracic region; lumbosacral region; radiation of lumbosacral pain to the leg. Each item was scored from 1 (never) to 4 (often or continuously). The right and left side were scored separately. The rheumatic symptoms score is a sum score of all the items.

Musculoskeletal findings. Two trained physiotherapists performed the clinical examination of the musculoskeletal system. Pains in the muscles and joints were assessed by palpation, and restrictions in the movements of joints were measured. Ranges of movement of joints were generally measured in active motion, except in hips and ankles. The guidelines published by the American Association of Orthopaedic Surgeons[11] were used as follows: 0 = symptomless, 1 = pain in the movement of the joint and/or on palpation, 2 = range of movement restricted by less than 25 % of the normal range, 3 = restriction by 25 to 50 %, 4 = restriction by more than 50 %. In the cervical spine the fourth grade was: restriction by more than 60 degrees and positive compression or intervertebralis sign, and in the lumbosacral spine: marked inflexibility or neurologic signs in the lower extremities (positive Laseque's or Ely's test). Twenty-one variables based on the examination were summed to form the musculoskeletal findings score.

At baseline 54 persons went through a second examination by the same physiotherapist in a few days' to two weeks time after the first examination. The reliability of the score was r = .93 in men and r = .77 in women. At follow-up a second physiotherapist made an repeated examination for 54 subjects. The kappa-coefficients of the main items of the score were satisfactory (from .60 to .65), except for the low back (.40).

Statistical methods. Analyses were made separately in four gender-occupational class groups. Analysis of variance and covariance and linear multiple regression analysis (SPSS-X) were used. Because of multicollinearity problems in analyses of the interactive effects of stress and support ridge-type regression estimation was made[12].

RESULTS

The blue-collar workers had more stress, less social support, and more rheumatic symptoms and clinical musculoskeletal findings than the white-collar staff (figure).

The association of perceived stress with rheumatic symptoms and musculoskeletal findings at baseline was statistically significant in men (table). The association of social support with morbidity was meager, being, however, significant in relation to musculoskeletal findings in the blue-collar women.

Baseline stress level did not predict the development of rheumatic symptoms during the 10-year follow-up, but its effect on the change in musculoskeletal findings in the blue-collar groups was statistically significant (table). Baseline social support was consistently in a negative association with the development in the morbidity scores during follow-up.

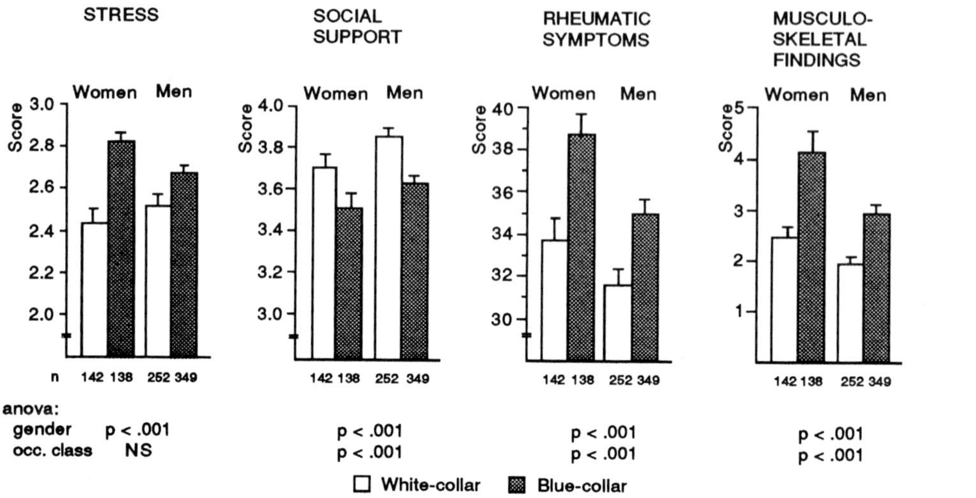

Figure: Means and standard errors of the stress, support and morbidity scores by gender and occupational class at baseline.

Table: Standardized multiple regression coefficients for the effects of stress and social support a) from models with stress / support and age as independent variables, b) from models with baseline stress / support scores, the relevant baseline morbidity score, and age as independent variables.

	a) Baseline		b) Follow-up	
	Rheumatic Symptoms '73	Musculoskeletal Findings '73	Rheumatic Symptoms '83	Musculoskeletal Findings '83
STRESS				
Women				
White-collar	.15	.10	-.01	.09
Blue-collar	.15	.08	.18	.18*
Men				
White-collar	.26***	.15*	.05	.05
Blue-collar	.24***	.12*	-.01	.23**
SOCIAL SUPPORT				
Women				
White-collar	-.10	-.03	-.14	-.06
Blue-collar	.05	-.18*	-.01	-.13
Men				
White-collar	-.09	-.01	-.02	-.08
Blue-collar	-.05	-.01	-.08	-.14

***p < .001, **p < .01, *p < .05

DISCUSSION

We found the appraisal of stressful loads in daily life to be associated with musculoskeletal morbidity in men in cross-sectional analyses and to predict the occurrence of clinical musculoskeletal findings in blue-collar workers during a 10-year follow-up period. Perceived social support was mostly non-significantly in a negative association with morbidity.

Many studies link lack of support with distress, disease, and increased mortality, but the strength of the evidence concerning its relationship to somatic diseases has also been questioned[13]. A debate is going on about the relative importance of support to well-being in its own right vs. as a moderator, or buffer, of stress.[14-15]

In this study the measures of stress and support did not interact in producing the associations with musculoskeletal morbidity. There were no significant linear interaction effects either at baseline or longitudinally. When interaction was studied by analysis of covariance (covariates age and, in the longitudinal analyses, baseline morbidity) with dichotomized stress and support scores, only one significant interaction effect was observed, but this was not as predicted by the stress buffering hypothesis.

The effect of stress on rheumatic symptoms in men was rather convincing in the cross-sectional analyses but non-existent in the longitudinal ones. Conversely, the effect of stress on musculoskeletal findings was stronger longitudinally than at baseline. It may be that rheumatic symptoms, being more variable than clinical findings, concurrently reflect a stress state. Clinical findings are slower to develop and not reversible to the same extent. They may thus be the result of a longer-lasting stress state.

Our results add to the evidence of an effect of mental stress on musculoskeletal disorders. The mechanism of the effect is obscure. The concept of somatization as it refers to a subject's misinterpretation of his or her psychological distress as somatic dysfunction[16] seems insufficient to account for our findings, while in our material both the perception of mental distress and clinically observable physical morbidity were present.

REFERENCES

1. Magora A. Investigation of the relation between low back pain and occupation. V. Psychological aspects. Scand J Rehab Med 1973;5:191-6.
2. Anderson KO, Bradley LA, Young LD, McDaniel LK, Wise CM. Rheumatoid arhritis: review of psychological factors related to etiology, effects, and treatment. Psychol Bull 1985;98:348-87.
3. Lichtenberg PA, Swensen CH, Skehan MW. Further investigation of the role of personality, lifestyle and arthritic severity in predicting pain. J Psychosom Res 1986;30:327-37.

4. Frese M: Stress at work, coping-strategies and musculoskeletal complaints. In Osterholz U, Karmaus W, Hullmann B, Ritz B, eds. Work-related musculo-skeletal disorders, Proceedings of an International Symposium. Bonn: Projektträger "Humanisierung des Arbeitslebens" 1987:121-39.
5. Sievers K, Mäkelä M, Klaukka T, Melkas T. Work stress and musculoskeletal disease (In Finnish with English summary). In Kalimo E, Kallio V, eds. Juhlakirja Jaakko Pajula II. Helsinki: Kansaneläkelaitos 1989:425-40.
6. Leino P. Symptoms of stress predict musculoskeletal disorders. J Epidemiol Community Health 1989;43:293-300.
7. Broadhead WE, Kaplan BH, James SA et al. The epidemiologic evidence for a relationship between social support and health. Am J Epidemiol 1983;117:521-37.
8. House JS, Landis KR, Umberson D. Social relationships and health. Science 1988;241:540-5.
9. Cobb S, Kasl SV. Termination: the concequencies of job loss. DHEW Publications, NIOSH 1977:77-224.
10. Lazarus RS, Folkman S. Stress, appraisal, and coping. New York: Springer 1984.
11. American Association of Orthopaedic Surgeons. Joint motion - a method of measuring and recording. Chicago: AAOS 1965.
12. Hoerl AE, Kennard RW. Ridge regression: biased estimation for nonorthogonal problems. Technometrics 1970;12:55-67.
13. Wallston BS, Alagna SW, DeVellis BME, DeVellis RF. Social support and physical health. Health Psychol 1983;2:367-91.
14. Thoits PA. Conceptual, methodological and theoretical problems in studying social support as a buffer against life stress. J Health Soc Behavior 1982;23:145-59.
15. Alloway R, Bebbington P. The buffer theory of social support - a review of the literature. Psychol Med 1987;17:91-108.
16. Lipowski ZJ. Somatization: the experience and communication of psychological distress as somatic symptoms. Psychoter Psychosom 1988;47:160-7.

Occupational Epidemiology. H. Sakurai et al., editors

549435

OCCUPATIONAL CERVICOBRACHIAL DISORDER AMONG INTERNATIONAL TELEPHONE OPERATORS

C.Y. PARK, K.H. CHO, S.H. LEE
Catholic Industrial Medical Center, Catholic University Medical College, Seoul, KOREA

INTRODUCTION

It is reported in industrialized countries that simple repetitive works in mechanized and automated workplaces caused a fairly large number of cevicobrachial disorders among typists, telephone operators, keypunchers, etc. and their major complaints consisted of musculoskeletal symptoms, such as muscle pain, stiffness, fatigue and tiredness, numbness, tenderness and so on.

Meanwhile, the diagnosis of this condition seems rather difficult, because current practice of diagnosis tends to depend mainly on the evaluation of working conditions and vague subjective symptoms rather than clearer objective signs and laboratory findings. In consequence, the prevalence of cervicobrachial disorders tends to show wide variations from one investigator to another, even though studies were performed on a similar group of workers. (1 - 3)

In view of the rapid mechanization and automation of offices and factories in Korea, we tried in this study to disclose the magnitude of occupational cervicobrachial disorder (OCD) problems among international telephone operators and to develop diagnostic procedures which are more specific and helpful in field examinations.

MATERIAL AND METHODS

Two hundred ninty female international telephone operators were studied with regard to their working conditions (workstation, work posture, work load and work environment), subjective complaints (pain, stiffness, tiredness numbness, tingling etc.), objective signs (muscle tenderness, swelling, joint mobility), including neurological findings (paresthesia, Adson's test, Morley test and Spurling test) and grip strength.

Of these workers, 33 subjects were selected through our screening criteria; namely more than 50% positive responses to questionaire (criteria 1), 40 to 50% positive responses to questionaire with any one of objective signs (critria 2), more than 2 of objective signs regardless of questionaire responses (criteria 3).

Twenty eight out of these 33 screened subjects were further examined in terms of rheumatoid factor, muscle enzymes such as creatine phosphokinase (CPK), aldolase and aspartate aminotransferase (AST), electromyography (EMG) and X ray findings.

RESULTS AND COMMENT

Table I showed the higher prevalence of musculoskeletal symptoms in the shoulder, the hands and fingers and the arms which were followed by the neck and the lower back. It was also found the back pain increased significantly, as the work duration extended over 5 years.

TABLE I

PREVALENCE OF MUSCULOSKELETAL COMPLAINTS BY WORK DURATION

(%)

Part of Body	Work Duration (yrs)				Total
	<5	5 - 9	10 - 14	15≦	
Neck	45.7	40.2	39.5	26.2	38.6
Shoulder	71.4	63.5	69.7	57.1	65.2
Arms	57.1	48.9	56.6	35.7	50.0
Hands & Fingers	42.9	56.2	65.8	38.1	54.5
Upper Back	11.4*	27.7	36.8	33.3	29.0
Lower Back	14.3*	38.0	42.1	38.1	36.2
Lower Limbs	37.1	21.9	25.0	23.8	24.8

Musculoskeletal complaints :
pain, stiffness, tiredness, numbness and tingling.
* $P < 0.05$ between group I and other groups each.

Among various parts of body, the prevalences of muscle tenderness on the shoulder and the arms were higher than the other parts of body. It was also noted that muscle tenderness on the shoulder and the arms significantly increased after work duration of 5 years (Table II).

TABLE II

PREVALENCE OF MUSCLE TENDERNESS BY WORK DURATION

(%)

Location	Work Duration (yrs)				Total
	<5	5 - 9	10 - 14	15≦	
Neck	5.7	4.4	5.2	7.1	5.2
Shoulder	5.7*	32.1	31.6	31.0	30.3
Arms & Forearms	14.3*	24.8	28.9	28.5	25.2
Hands & Fingers		0.7	5.2	7.1	2.8
Back	8.5	9.4	5.2	14.3	9.0
Lower limbs		1.5		2.4	1.0

* $P < 0.05$ between group I and other groups each.

In Table III, as a whole, about 28% of workers showed one or more positive findings in the neurological tests. The most common finding was paresthesia which was followed by positive Morley test.

TABLE III

PREVALENCE OF POSITIVE NEUROLOGIC SIGNS BY WORK DURATION

(%)

Item	Work Duration (yrs)				Total
	< 5	5 - 9	10 - 14	15≦	
Adson's Test	2.9	0.7	1.3		1.0
Spurling Test		0.7	2.6	7.1	2.1
Morley Test	11.4	8.0	11.8	19.0	11.0
Paresthesia	11.4	14.6	23.7	21.4	17.6
Any of the above	20.0	22.6	35.5	38.1	27.9

In general, symptoms and signs were mainly noted on the shoulder, the arms and the hands and fingers.

No association was noted between painful musculoskeletal complaints and work years, while the prevalence of muscle tenderness and neurological findings was higher among workers with longer work experiences.

There are conflicting reports concerning the relationship between duration of employment and onset of OCD and as yet no agreement has been reached (2,4). It does appear, however, the inexperience in performing tasks can lead to increased muscle tension (5).

Table IV shows that the percentage of workers with weaker grip strength of the major hand tended to be higher among myalgia patients than among non-myalgia patients.

TABLE IV

DISTRIBUTION OF GRIP STRENGTH OF MAJOR HAND IN MYALGIA SUBJECTS AND OTHERS

(%)

Subjects	Grip Strength (Kg)			
	less than 20	20 - 24	25 - 29	over 30
Myalgia (N=114)	19.3*	28.1	36.8	15.8*
Non myalgia (N=176)	10.2	26.1	33.0	30.7

* $P < 0.05$ between myalgia group and others

Serum CPK and AST showed significant linear association with positive questionaire responses (Fig. 2 and 3). It was also reported raised serum levels of muscle enzymes in some industrial workers with acute neck and shoulder disorders (6).

It was suggested that these muscle enzymes would be helpful in diagnosis for OCD.

Further work is needed to confirm or refute these findings.

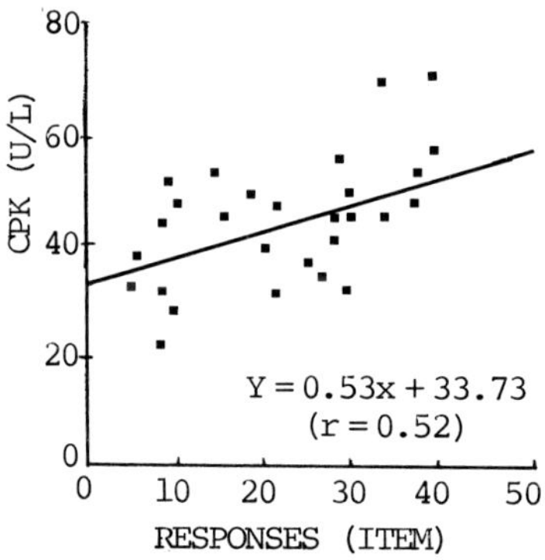

Fig 2. Relationship between serum creatine phosphokinase level and positive responses to questionaire

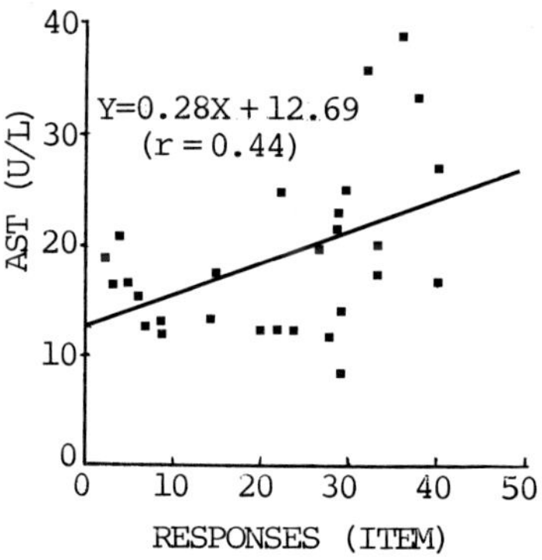

Fig 3. Relationship between serum aspartate aminotransfease level and positive responses to questionaire

REFERENCES

1. Ferguson D (1971) Brit J Industr Med 28: 280-285

2. Maeda M, Hünting W, Grandjean E (1980) J Occup Med 22: 810-816

3. Ohara H, Itani T, Aoyama H (1982) J Human Ergo (Tokyo) II : 55-63

4. Smith AB, Tanaka S, Halperin W, Richards RD (1982) Report of a cross sectional survey of video display terminal users at the Baltimore Sun. NIOSH, Center for Disease Control, Cincinnati, OH

5. Dalton S, Hazleman BL (1987) In : Raffle PAB, Lee WR, McCallum RI, Murray R (eds) Hunter's Disease of Occupations. Little, Brown, Boston/ Toronto, pp 620-633

6. Bjelle A, Hagberg M, Michaelsson G (1979) Scand J Work Environ Health 5 (suppl 3) : 205-210

Occupational Epidemiology. H. Sakurai et al., editors

MUSCULOSKELETAL DISORDERS AND ERGONOMIC STRESS IN THE RETAIL MEAT INDUSTRY

LAURA PUNNETT

Department of Work Environment, University of Lowell, One University Avenue, Lowell, MA 01854 (USA)

INTRODUCTION

Previous analyses of injuries reported by meat cutters and wrappers to retail food store managers suggested that musculoskeletal disorders occurred frequently among this population. The objectives of this study were: 1) to estimate the prevalence of upper limb and back disorders among workers in the retail meat industry in the New York City area; 2) to determine the prevalence of ergonomic stressors in this industry; 3) to evaluate any associations between ergonomic stressors and musculoskeletal disorders in the study population; and 4) to recommend intervention measures for reducing the exposure to occupational ergonomic stressors and thus the risk of musculoskeletal disorders.

METHODS

Questionnaires were completed by workers who attended a health and safety training class voluntarily and on work time. Questionnaire items included demographics, work and medical history, symptoms of musculoskeletal disorders and description of working conditions, including specific ergonomic factors (lifting demands, postural stresses) and general aspects of the work environment (cold, work pace). Several "psychophysical" scales were used to rate the intensity of ergonomic stressors. In addition, exposures were evaluated by the investigator during visits to three retail food stores.

The key health questions pertained to soft tissue pain during the year prior to the date of the survey. "Cases" were defined as those workers with pain that met four criteria: (a) at least 20 episodes in the previous year or usual duration of at least one week; (b) reported date of onset of pain after date of first employment in the retail meat industry; (c) no history of systemic disease that might cause soft tissue pain; and (d) no history of acute injury to the same part of the body. Cases were defined separately for the back, neck/shoulder, elbow/forearm, wrist/hand, and leg/foot regions.

In external comparisons, the prevalence of each case group was compared with the prevalence of musculoskeletal cases defined with the same criteria in a recent study sponsored by the U.S. National Institute of Occupational Safety and Health (NIOSH) (1). This study included 650 workers, in seven different industries, categorized as to the manual force requirements and repetitiveness of their jobs. For shoulder and elbow/arm disorders, the reference rates from the "NIOSH study" were those observed in the entire population; for wrist/hand disorders, the reference group consisted of workers with jobs ranked "low" on scales of both manual repetitiveness and manual force. Gender- and age-stratified prevalence odds ratios (OR) and 95% confidence intervals (CI) were calculated to estimate the risk associated with work in the retail food industry.

In internal comparisons, cases and non-cases within the current study population were compared with respect to specific ergonomic stressors. For discrete exposure variables, ORs and 95% CIs were calculated; continuous variables were compared with non-parametric (Wilcoxon) tests and Mantel tests for linear trend. These analyses explored the extent to which exposure to specific ergonomic factors increased the risk of musculo-skeletal disorders, beyond employment in the industry *per se*.

RESULTS

Descriptive

A total of 254 workers, or 92% of the 275 who attended the classes, completed the questionnaire. The average age of the respondents was 42 (±12) years; their average height and weight were close to those of the general U.S. population (2). The average length of employment was 13 (±10) years in the current job title and 19 (±12) years in the retail food industry. The four job categories represented were cutter, wrapper, manager and other (delicatessen or fish department) (Table I).

TABLE I

JOB ASSIGNMENTS AND GENDER OF 254 RETAIL MEAT DEPARTMENT WORKERS

Job Title	Men (%)	Women (%)	Total
Cutter	122 (100)	0	122
Wrapper	0	89 (100)	89
Manager	33 (100)	0	33
Deli, Fish	6 (60)	4 (40)	10
TOTAL	161 (63)	93 (36)	254

The specific tasks that cutters performed most often were cutting meat by hand or with a band saw, and "boating," or packaging portioned meat into small styrofoam trays for sale. Handling boxes, cutting by hand and by band saw were judged by the cutters to be the most difficult tasks to perform. Wrappers' most frequent tasks were wrapping the "boats" of portioned meat with clear plastic wrap, weighing or "scaling" the packages and attaching price labels, and stocking the cases. Stocking the display cases, handling boxes, and wrapping were judged to be the most difficult tasks by a majority of wrappers.

Exposures. These workers' jobs were both repetitive and strenuous. Cutters daily cut an average of 121 ($\pm$ 278) large pieces of fabricated meat and filled 701 ($\pm$ 830) boats. Wrappers filled 374 ($\pm$ 602) boats, wrapped 1299 ($\pm$ 1365) boats, and scaled 1347 ($\pm$ 1339) boats per day. Among all respondents, the rating of work pace intensity was 5.6 ($\pm$ 1.3) on a psychophysical scale from 1 to 7; 89 workers (33%) rated the pace as 7.

Virtually all (251) of the respondents performed lifting tasks at work. On average, respondents judged that the load lifted most often on a typical day was 41 ($\pm$ 23) lb, lifted 33 times per day and carried 9 feet. The heaviest load was 71 ($\pm$ 31) pounds (lb), on average, lifted 11 times per day and carried 9 feet per lift.

In exposure to environmental cold, the cutters spent an average of 4.3 hours per day and the wrappers 3.2 hours per day in the refrigerated cutting room or other refrigerated areas. Forty-five (37%) cutters spent the entire work day in the refrigerator; 17 (19%) wrappers spent 8 hours per day there. Twenty-one (17%) cutters worked in the freezer room between 0.5 and 8 hours per day (median one hour). Fourteen (16%) wrappers worked in the freezer between 1 and 4 hours (median one hour).

Health outcomes. A total of 242 (95%) workers reported pain at one or more joints in the year preceding the survey. Of these, 180 had pain that improved if they were away from work for one week or more. The body regions where pain was most frequent were the back (59%), neck/shoulder (53%), and wrist/hand (86%). Both female and male workers reported high rates of pain overall (99% and 94%, respectively). Back and neck/shoulder pain varied little among the four job categories; elbow/arm and wrist/hand pain were more frequent among wrappers than among cutters.

External Comparisons

Among male retail food workers, the age-stratified risk of upper limb disorders was about twice the expected rate among men in the NIOSH study (Table II). Among female retail food workers, only the elbow/arm age-stratified OR was elevated.

Internal Comparisons

Back and neck/shoulder cases lifted both the "typical" and the "heaviest" loads with greater frequency than non-cases. Back, neck/shoulder, arm/elbow, and wrist/hand pain were associated with workers' ratings of their jobs' lifting demands.

With respect to postural stresses of the back, trunk flexion was more common among back cases than non-cases. For both forward flexion and lateral flexion/twisting of the spine, the risk was particularly high for workers who reported having to remain in the posture at least 5 seconds or having to lift at least 5 lb in the posture. Similar associations with neck/shoulder disorders were found for extended duration of, and lifting weight in, abduction/flexion and extension of the shoulder.

The risk of wrist/hand disorders was associated with flexion, extension, radial and ulnar deviation of the wrist. In addition, cases were more likely to hold at least 5 lb in each of these postures than non-cases. Wrist/hand cases were also six times more likely to have to work with a pinch grip, especially exerting force in that grasp.

TABLE II
RISK OF MUSCULOSKELETAL DISORDERS AMONG RETAIL MEAT WORKERS
Compared with U.S. Industrial Population (Age-stratified)

Body Region	Gender	OR	(95% CI)
Shoulder	Men	1.8	(1.0, 3.2)
	Women	0.9	(0.5, 1.9)
Elbow/Arm	Men	1.7	(0.8, 3.8)
	Women	1.5	(0.7, 3.1)
Wrist/Hand *	Men	2.2	(1.3, 3.7)
	Women	0.9	(0.6, 1.6)

* Reference group = jobs with low repetition, low force demands.

ACKNOWLEDGEMENTS
Funded in part by a grant from the NY State Dept of Labor to the Safety, Education and Cultural Fund of Local 342, United Food and Commercial Workers, AFL-CIO. Grateful acknowledgement to Barbara Silverstein, especially for reference data (study funded in part by NIOSH, CDC #200-82-2507). The author also thanks the members of Local 342-50, John Ziv and Thelma King (questionnaire administration), Deborah Woodland (coding), and Diane St. Onge (data analysis).

REFERENCES

1. Silverstein BA, Fine LJ, Armstrong TJ (1986) Brit J Industr Med 43:779-784.
2. U.S. DHEW (1979) Weight and Height of Adults, Series 11 (211), National Center for Health Statistics, Hyattsville, MD (USA).

Occupational Epidemiology. H. Sakurai et al., editors

AN EPIDEMIOLOGIC COMPARISON OF DIFFERENT STANDARDIZED INSTRUMENTS FOR MUSCULO-SKELETAL DISORDERS OF THE NECK AND LOWER BACK

BEATE RITZ, WILFRIED KARMAUS

Institute of Medical Sociology, University Hospital Eppendorf,
University of Hamburg, FRG

INTRODUCTION

Despite the grand old history of musculo-skeletal epidemiology there is still a need for standardized instruments to identify and classify musculo-skeletal disorders [1,2]. An intuitive and ambiguous classification hinders comparability between populations and over a period of time. Therefore the objective of this paper is to analyze (a) the validity of different approaches for gathering information, such as interviews and medical examinations; and (b) the validity of different methods of assessment with regard to the time period taken into consideration.

Regarding musculo-skeletal disorders, a clear-cut deviding line between diseased and non-diseased is not available. A dichotomization of a continuous measure is therefore arbitrary and can lead to an important loss of information. These are the reasons why we do not apply the classical measures of validity such as specificity and sensitivity but concentrate on a comparison based on correlation coefficients [3].

METHODS

The study population consists of female office workers (N=217) in governmental offices in Hamburg, FRG, who took part in all medical investigations in the years 1980 and 1985. Some of them retired (N=24) or changed jobs (N=16) between the two waves of collecting data. All female office workers who agreed to participate became part of the sample, irrespective of the status of their disorder. The data was collected in 1980 and 1985 in a standardized way. The clinical check-ups were performed by two different physicians in 1980 and in 1985. The study is described in more detail elsewhere [4]. Considering the issues at hand we collected data using different standardized methods:

(I) **medical examination** (examination / clinical data) and

(II) **personal medical interviews** (expert rated interview data) on pain, i.e. on different symptoms of the neck and lower back which represent the occurrence and limitations brought about by "pain in the course of the day".

(III) We also gathered **information on pain frequency** during the previous week in a personal interview and additionally in two

telephone interviews (frequency data), each after a period of four to six weeks (Proportion of episodes with pain (PROTEP), [5]).
For the neck and lower back we are therefore able to compare:
1) **period prevalence data** (12 months) from the medical interviews in 1980 and in 1985,
2) **point prevalence data** derived from the medical check-ups in 1980 and in 1985, and
3) the **proportion of time with complaints in three episodes**, each of seven days' duration.

RESULTS
Regarding table 1 it is obvious that no single Spearman correlation exceeds the value of 0.7. Thus the maximum of mutually explained variance (r^2) of two indices is lower than 50 percent. Some of the correlations are quite low.

Table 1: Spearman correlation coefficients between different signs/symptoms in the years 1980 and 1985

NECK DISORDERS (upper row) and LOW BACK DISORDERS (lower row) , (N=217)

VARIABLES	Restriction in move-ments 1980	Nerves, mus-cles, tendons 1980	Pain during check-up ma-noeuvres 1980	Pain-scale 1985	Restriction in move-ments 1985	Nerves, mus-cles, tendons 1985	Pain during check-up ma-noeuvres 1985
	Inter- Indices- Correlations 1980			Inter- Year- Correlations 1980/ 1985			
Pain-scale 1980	0.169	0.254	0.492	0.370	0.208	0.240	0.388
	0.013	0.286	0.463	0.497	0.182	0.384	0.376
Restriction in movements 1980		0.088	0.335	0.005	0.479	0.005	0.082
		0.205	0.159	0.075	0.451	0.239	0.109
Nerves, mus-cles, tendons 1980			0.403	0.030	0.095	0.172	0.162
			0.500	0.229	0.212	0.271	0.310
Pain during check-up ma-noeuvres 1980				0.284	0.264	0.245	0.457
				0.330	0.284	0.421	0.520
				Inter- Indices- Correlation 1985			
Pain-scale 1985					0.108	0.315	0.490
					0.116	0.468	0.449
Restriction in movements 1985						0.159	0.340
						0.187	0.184
Nerves, mus-cles, tendons 1985							0.645
							0.600
Days with pain in three epi-sodes				0.551	0.171	0.451	0.619
				0.598	0.137	0.475	0.537

Comparing the inter-indices-correlations (correlations of different indices) in 1980 with those of 1985 (upper left with lower right square except the last row), the pattern is similiar for both years.

Regarding the inter-year-correlations between 1980 and 1985 for the same indices (the diagonal in the upper right square of table 1 "signs in nerves, muscles, tendons" correlates low (0.172 and 0.271), and seems to be the least stable index, while all other indices correlate moderately. Regarding the inter-year-correlations between 1980 and 1985 for **different** indices (the upper right square of table 1 except the diagonal) "restriction in movement" and "signs in nerves, muscles, tendons" in 1980 do not correlate with other indices in 1985, anamnestic pain (pain-scale) and "pain during check-up manoeuvres" in 1980 have moderate correlations with other signs in 1985.

The last row of the lower right square shows that the indices "pain-scale", "pain during check-up manoeuvres" and "signs in nerves, muscles, tendons" correlate high with "days with pain .." ($0.451 \leq r \leq 0.619$).

3. DISCUSSION

Assuming either no change in the extent of a disorder (irreversibility or absence of any symptoms) or changes in one direction for all participants in a given period of time, one would expect high inter-year-correlations 1980/ 1985 for the same indices. However, assuming changes (acute and reversible chronic conditions), one would expect low correlations over time. In the last case investigation into predictors of the variablity over time, such as ageing, therapeutic interventions, and working or living conditions, seem to be relevant [6]. Inter-year-correlations for the same indices 1980/ 1985 are moderate for 'pain-scale', 'restriction in movements' and 'pain during check-up manoeuvres' ($0.37 \leq r \leq 0.52$), thus seem to incorporate stability over time. A lack of stability in case of the index 'signs in nerves, muscles, tendons' is correspondingly either an indicator of variablity/ changes over time or of measurement errors 1. The pattern of the inter-indices-correlations in 1980 and 1985 is similiar. In other words, we find that the indices which correlate best in 1980 also correlate best in 1985. This indicates that there are reproducible relationships between different indices in 1980 and 1985.

'Pain during check-up manoeuvres' in 1980 as well as in 1985, a point prevalence measure, is strongly related to another point prevalence measure (signs in nerves, muscles, tendons) in the same year and to two period prevalence measures of pain (pain-scale and days with pain..). Furthermore the period prevalence measure 'days with pain..' is highly correlated to the other pain indices and 'signs

1 The assessment of repeatability of measurements is not justified for the data at hand since a period of five years elapsed between the two investigations.

in nerves, muscles, tendons' but weakly to 'restriction in movements'. The main distinction therefore must be made between 'restriction in movements' on one hand and the indices of pain and 'signs in nerves, muscles, tendons' on the other. We suggest that this distinction indicates the restricted nature of information gained from approaches which rely only on restriction in movements data. It is further interesting that 'restriction in movements' in 1980 does not or only weakly predict other indices in 1985, whereas 'pain-scale' and 'pain during check-up manoeuvres' in 1980 do predict 'restriction in movements' in 1985. This suggests that the pain indices function as precursors of later restriction in movements.

Alltogether the results show the same correlation patterns in two different anatomical regions as well as in two points of time. This indicates an internal validity of the findings. Different approaches in gathering information such as interviews and medical examinations do not contradict each other. Both approaches provide valid information. The validity of different assessments with regard to the period taken into consideration also seems to be satisfactory for all pain indices. The sufficient correlation of the pain-scale with medical check-up findings also indicates that information provided through interviews can be used as a substitute for ascertaining clinical findings. Overall no single index serves as an optimal indicator for the extent of musculo-skeletal disorder of the neck and lower back.

4. REFERENCES

[1] WHO Expert Committee: Identification and Control of Work-Re lated Diseases. Word Health Organisation (Ed.). Technical Report Series 714. Geneva, 1985

[2] KUORINKA I, JONSSON B, KILBOM A, VINTERBERG H, BIERING-SORENSEN, ANDERSSON G, JORGENSEN K: Standardised Nordic Questionnaire for the Analysis of Musculo-Skeletal Symptoms. Applied Ergonomics 18:233-237, 1987

[3] MACLURE M, WILLET W C: Misinterpretation and Misuse of the Kappa Statistic. Am J Epid 126:161-169, 1987

[4] KARMAUS W, GLASER-MÖLLER N, HULLMANN B, RITZ B, SCHÄFER K-H, SONN E: Arbeitsbedingte rheumatische Erkrankungen. Ergebnisse einer Längsschnittsstudie von weiblichen Angestellten. Report for the Federal Minister of Research and Technology. Hamburg, 1987

[5] COBB S: A Method for the Epidemiologic Study of Remittent Disease. A.J.P.H. 52:1119-1125, 1962

[6] RITZ B, KARMAUS W, GLASER-MÖLLER N, SCHÄFER K-H: Risks of Musculoskeletal Disorders in Female Office Workers. Results of a Longitudinal Study. Scand J Work Environ Health. (to be published)

© 1990 Elsevier Science Publishers B.V. (Biomedical Division)
Occupational Epidemiology. H. Sakurai et al., editors

ANALYSIS OF SKIN TEMPERATURE, VIBRATION SENSE THRESHOLD, RECOVERY OF NAIL BLOOD FLOW, PAIN THRESHOLD, BLOOD PRESSURE, PINCHING POWER, TAPPING COUNTS AND HEARING LOSS OF RETIRED CHAIN SAW AND BUSH CUTTER WORKERS IN THE NATIONAL FORESTS OF JAPAN

KAZUO SAITO, TOSHIYUKI HOSOKAWA, MAMI KOBAYASHI, KOZO NIIZUMA, SONOYO WATANABE, TAKESHI SAITO, AKIO KOYAMA
Department of Hygiene and Preventive Medicine, Hokkaido University School of Medicine, Sapporo, JAPAN

SUMMARY

Twenty-five chain saw operators and fifty-five bush cutter operators were studied in order to make clear the effects of hand-arm vibration at the time when they retired from forestry work at 55 years of age. Skin temperature, vibration sense threshold, recovery time of nail blood color by the nail press test, pain sense threshold, blood pressure, pinching power, tapping counts and hearing loss were compared between two groups, those who had less than 5,000 and those who had 5,000 to 10,000 operation hours at the time of their retirement.

Only the vibration sense threshold of chain saw workers was significantly different between the group whose operation time was less than 5,000 hours and the group whose operation time was between 5,000 and 10,000 hours. That is, the threshold of vibratory sense of the latter group increased more than that of the former group in the left index and middle fingers and the right index, middle and ring fingers with 125 Hz, and left and right index, middle and ring fingers with 250 Hz.

INTRODUCTION

More than 30 years have passed since vibration syndrome of lumberjacks caused by using chain saws began to be widely observed in Japan. The authors reported the prevalent condition of vibration syndrome in the Hokkaido area of northern Japan in 1978 (1), the propriety of diagnostic items currently being used (2,3) and aging effects on recoveries of finger skin temperature, vibration sense threshold and nail blood flow by the nail press test after a 10-min immersion test in cold water at 10 ℃ (2,4). The main characteristic findings of vibration syndrome are disturbances of blood vessels, nerves, bones and joints of the hand and arm, but the mechanisms of white finger, polyneuritis, bone and joint disturbances have not been clarified. An analysis of the relationship between the age of workers and their operation time using vibrating tools will give important information to help understand the vibrating tool-oriented effect on the hand and arm.

This study was performed to make clear the real status of physiological functions at the age of 55 years when chain saw and bush cutter workers retired from forestry work.

SUBJECTS AND METHODS

Twenty-five chain saw operators and fifty-five bush cutter operators in the national forest in northern Hokkaido whose age was 55 years were engaged in this study. They were divided into groups A and B by the number of chain saw or bush cutter operation hours. Group A had worked less than 5,000 hours, and group B from 5,001 to 10,000 hours at the time of retirement. There were 18 chain saw operators and 18 bush cutter operators, in group A, and in group B there were 7 chain saw workers and 35 bush cutter workers. Skin temperature, vibration sense threshold, recovery time of nail blood color by the nail press test (5), pain sense threshold, blood pressure, pinching power, tapping counts and hearing loss were measured and also examined by the 10-min immersion test in cold water at 10°C. The data obtained were compared between the two groups.

RESULTS

Figure 1 shows the distribution of chain saw and bush cutter operation time at the age of 55 years when forestry workers retired. The mean operation time and its standard deviation for 25 chain saw works and 55 bush cutter workers were 5,108.6 ± 4,734.3 and 5,436.2 ± 1,969.5 hours, respectively. Operation times of group A and group B for chain saw workers were 2,527.6 ± 1,406.5 and 11,745.4 ± 3,560.2 hours, respectively, and those of group A and group B for bush cutter workers were 3,529.0 ± 987.5 and 6,364.0 ± 1,629.3, respectively.

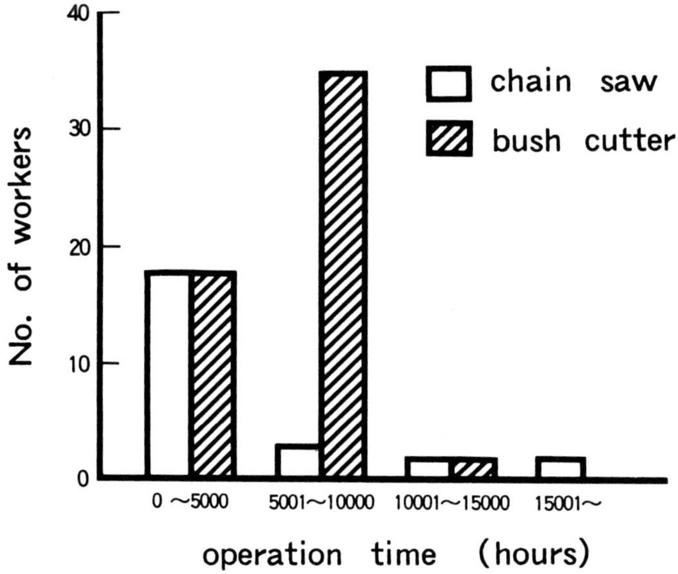

Fig. 1 Distribution of chain saw and bush cutter operation time at the time of retirement from forestry work at the age of 55.

Table I shows the finger skin temperature, vibration sense threshold, recovery time of blood flow after the nail press test, pain sense threshold, blood pressure, hand grip power, pinching power, tapping counts and hearing loss of chain saw and bush cutter workers. A statistically significant difference between two groups was observed only in the vibratory sense thresholds of chain saw workers in the left index and middle fingers and right index, middle and ring fingers at 125 Hz, and in the left and right index, middle and ring fingers at 250 Hz. The finger skin temperature, recovery time of nail blood flow by the nail press test, pain sense, blood pressure, hand grip power, pinch power, tapping counts and hearing loss in both chain saw and bush cutter workers did not show any significant differences between groups A and B.

Table I
Skin temperature, vibration sense threshold, recovery time of nail blood color after the nail press test, pain sense threshold, blood pressure, hand grip power, pinching power, tapping counts and hearing loss of chain saw and brush cutter workers.
Values present mean and standard deviation. # and ## show significant changes at 5 and 1 % levels respectively.

Items	Chain saw		Bush cutter	
	Group A (0-5,000)	Group B (5,000-10,000)	Group A (0-5,000)	Group B (5,000-10,000)
		Finger skin temperature		
Left finger				
2nd	31.2 ± 1.8	31.5 ± 1.5	30.2 ± 2.0	30.7 ± 1.9
3rd	31.4 ± 1.9	32.3 ± 0.8	30.2 ± 2.1	30.9 ± 2.2
4th	31.5 ± 2.1	32.5 ± 0.5	30.1 ± 2.3	30.7 ± 2.3
5th	31.4 ± 2.1	32.3 ± 0.3	29.8 ± 2.3	30.5 ± 2.4
Right finger				
2nd	31.9 ± 1.7	32.1 ± 0.3	30.4 ± 2.3	31.0 ± 2.3
3rd	31.9 ± 1.6	32.3 ± 0.3	30.8 ± 2.1	31.1 ± 2.2
4th	31.9 ± 2.0	32.5 ± 0.0	30.3 ± 2.5	31.0 ± 2.4
5th	31.8 ± 1.8	32.7 ± 0.3	30.1 ± 2.6	30.7 ± 2.5
		Vibration sense threshold		
125Hz				
Left finger				
2nd	4.9 ± 4.0	-1.7 ± 1.4#	2.1 ± 5.4	2.2 ± 4.2
3rd	4.2 ± 3.3	-5.0 ± 2.9##	1.9 ± 5.0	2.1 ± 5.3
4th	5.7 ± 5.8	-0.8 ± 2.9	2.5 ± 5.8	4.3 ± 5.7
Right finger				
2nd	4.9 ± 4.3	-1.7 ± 1.4#	1.9 ± 5.8	3.0 ± 4.7
3rd	4.9 ± 5.1	-2.5 ± 2.5#	1.8 ± 3.9	2.7 ± 5.5
4th	7.2 ± 6.0	-3.3 ± 6.3#	4.6 ± 5.2	5.4 ± 5.9
250Hz				
Left finger				
2nd	11.1 ± 5.7	2.5 ± 2.5#	9.4 ± 6.5	8.8 ± 7.7
3rd	11.5 ± 6.0	1.7 ± 2.9#	9.1 ± 6.6	9.6 ± 7.1
4th	11.9 ± 6.6	2.5 ± 2.5#	9.6 ± 7.0	10.4 ± 6.9
Right finger				
2nd	11.1 ± 5.2	3.3 ± 2.9#	9.9 ± 5.7	8.7 ± 7.6
3rd	11.4 ± 6.3	3.3 ± 2.9#	10.0 ± 5.3	9.6 ± 7.5
4th	12.2 ± 6.7	2.5 ± 2.5#	11.4 ± 6.7	11.9 ± 8.3
		Recovery time of blood flow after the nail press test		
Left finger				
2nd	1.3 ± 0.5	1.3 ± 0.2	1.3 ± 0.4	1.4 ± 0.3
3rd	1.3 ± 0.6	1.3 ± 0.0	1.4 ± 0.4	1.3 ± 0.3
4th	1.2 ± 0.4	1.2 ± 0.2	1.3 ± 0.4	1.3 ± 0.3
Right finger				
2nd	1.2 ± 0.3	1.6 ± 0.3	1.4 ± 0.4	1.3 ± 0.3
3rd	1.2 ± 0.4	1.4 ± 0.3	1.3 ± 0.3	1.3 ± 0.4
4th	1.2 ± 0.5	1.3 ± 0.4	1.3 ± 0.3	1.3 ± 0.3

		Pain sense threshold		
Left finger				
2nd	1.0 ± 0.0	1.0 ± 0.0	1.0 ± 0.0	1.0 ± 0.0
3rd	1.0 ± 0.0	1.0 ± 0.0	1.0 ± 0.0	1.0 ± 0.0
4th	1.0 ± 0.0	1.0 ± 0.0	1.0 ± 0.0	1.0 ± 0.0
5th	1.0 ± 0.0	1.0 ± 0.0	1.0 ± 0.0	1.0 ± 0.0
Right finger				
2nd	1.0 ± 0.0	1.0 ± 0.0	1.0 ± 0.0	1.0 ± 0.0
3rd	1.0 ± 0.0	1.0 ± 0.0	1.0 ± 0.0	1.0 ± 0.0
4th	1.0 ± 0.0	1.0 ± 0.0	1.0 ± 0.0	1.0 ± 0.0
5th	1.0 ± 0.0	1.0 ± 0.0	1.0 ± 0.0	1.0 ± 0.0
		Blood pressure		
	132.2 ± 19.6	116.7 ± 18.1	122.9 ± 14.4	127.4 ± 18.9
	85.0 ± 12.9	74.0 ± 6.0	78.3 ± 6.3	79.1 ± 8.9
		Hand grip power		
Left hand				
1st	42.9 ± 6.6	45.3 ± 8.6	44.3 ± 5.0	42.6 ± 4.9
2nd	41.8 ± 5.1	46.3 ± 8.0	43.4 ± 5.5	41.8 ± 5.7
3rd	43.3 ± 6.7	47.3 ± 8.5	42.9 ± 5.6	41.9 ± 5.3
4th	42.0 ± 6.3	45.3 ± 9.1	41.9 ± 5.5	41.7 ± 5.3
5th	41.8 ± 5.8	45.3 ±10.6	42.2 ± 4.9	41.5 ± 5.2
Right hand				
1st	42.9 ± 3.8	47.0 ± 6.6	42.1 ± 6.8	42.2 ± 4.9
2nd	42.3 ± 4.1	44.7 ± 5.5	41.6 ± 7.5	42.3 ± 5.4
3rd	42.7 ± 5.6	47.0 ± 4.6	41.5 ± 7.0	42.4 ± 5.8
4th	43.5 ± 4.9	47.3 ± 2.3	41.0 ± 7.1	42.2 ± 6.1
5th	43.0 ± 4.7	46.3 ± 3.1	41.4 ± 6.9	42.4 ± 5.4

Table II shows recovery of skin temperature, vibration sense threshold, recovery time of blood flow by the nail press test and pain sense threshold after the 10-min immersion test in cold water at 10 ℃.

These findings did not show any significant difference between the two groups for either chain saw or bush cutter workers.

DISCUSSION

In general, it is known that physiological functions deteriorate gradually with aging. It is an important problem whether or not certain types of work enhance aging effects. If a difference of physiological functions is observed among the persons of the same age, it may be caused by their occupation and by their life styles. From the standpoints of occupational health it should be clarified what kinds of occupations provoke such a difference. It is epidemiologically proved that the amount of operation time of chain saws correlates to the prevalence rate of hand-arm vibration syndrome in workers. However, the relationship between operation time and aging effects in the workers has not always been clear, so it is necessary to separate the aging effects from these.

Table II
Recovery of skin temperature, vibratory sense threshold, recovery time of blood flow by the nail press test and pain sense threshold after a 10-min immersion test in cold water at 10 °C.
Values present mean and standard deviation. # shows a significant change at 5 % level.

Items	Chain saw Group A (0-5,000)	Chain saw Group B (5,000-10,000)	Bush cutter Group A (0-5,000)	Bush cutter Group B (5,000-10,000)
Finger skin temperature				
Before immersion	33.3 ± 1.5	32.8 ± 1.2	31.0 ± 2.7	31.2 ± 2.4
During immersion				
6th min	11.5 ± 0.6	11.2 ± 0.6	11.1 ± 0.5	11.0 ± 0.7
7th min	11.3 ± 0.7	11.0 ± 0.5	10.9 ± 0.4	10.9 ± 1.1
8th min	11.2 ± 0.7	10.9 ± 0.4	10.8 ± 0.3	10.7 ± 0.8
9th min	11.1 ± 0.6	10.8 ± 0.4	10.7 ± 0.3	10.6 ± 0.5
10th min	11.1 ± 0.9	10.8 ± 0.5	10.6 ± 0.4	10.5 ± 0.5
After immersion				
5th min	21.5 ± 5.8	17.3 ± 1.7	17.1 ± 3.7	17.4 ± 3.5
10th min	27.3 ± 6.3	22.3 ± 4.3	22.1 ± 5.6	23.3 ± 5.4
Vibration sense threshold				
Before immersion	3.9 ± 4.1	-3.3 ± 2.9#	0.5 ± 8.5	1.4 ± 4.3
During immersion				
10th min	20.8 ± 5.3	25.0 ± 6.6	22.2 ± 10.1	24.6 ± 7.1
After immersion				
5th min	5.9 ± 7.8	10.8 ± 2.9	10.1 ± 9.3	11.1 ± 8.5
10th min	2.3 ± 6.3	2.5 ± 5.0	5.4 ±11.0	5.2 ± 9.4
Recovery time of blood flow after the nail press test				
Before immersion	1.3 ± 0.7	1.3 ± 0.3	1.4 ± 0.4	1.3 ± 0.3
During immersion				
10th min	2.8 ± 1.9	3.1 ± 0.4	3.2 ± 1.3	3.1 ± 1.6
After immersion				
5th min	1.8 ± 0.9	1.9 ± 1.0	2.7 ± 2.1	2.1 ± 0.8
10th min	1.5 ± 0.7	1.2 ± 0.2	1.9 ± 1.6	1.7 ± 1.4
Pain sense threshold				
Before immersion	1.0 ± 0.0	1.0 ± 0.0	1.0 ± 0.0	1.3 ± 0.8
During immersion				
10th min	1.0 ± 0.0	1.0 ± 0.0	1.4 ± 0.7	1.0 ± 0.0
After immersion				
5th min	1.0 ± 0.0	1.0 ± 0.0	1.2 ± 0.5	1.1 ± 0.3
10th min	1.0 ± 0.0	1.0 ± 0.0	1.1 ± 0.3	1.0 ± 0.0

It is thought that aging effects were excluded by this epidemiological analysis, and that only effects due not to aging but to the amount of operation time were observed in the chain saw workers who showed about a 9,000 hour difference between group A and B.

ACKNOWLEDGMENTS
We gratefully acknowledge Mr. Saburo Ishimura who made the excellent photos.

REFERENCES
1. Saito K, Kumashiro M, Niioka T, Fujimoto S, Shibano N (1980) Jap J Ind Health 22:348-354

2. Saito K, Niioka T, Fujimoto S, Kumashiro M (1980) Jap J Ind Health 22:355-367

3. Niioka T, Kojima Y, Kaji H, Saito K (1986) Scand J Work Environ Health 12:251-253

4. Saito K, Satoh H, Hosokawa T, Kobayashi M, Saito T, Niizuma K (1989) Proceeding of the 5th International Conference on Hand-Arm Vibration, Kanazawa (in press)

5. Yamada S (1972) Jap J Ind health 14:529-541

REPRODUCTIVE EFFECTS

Occupational Epidemiology. H. Sakurai et al., editors 549436

ASSESSMENT OF REPRODUCTIVE EVENTS IN ITALY IN RELATION TO THE CHERNOBYL ACCIDENT

I. Figà-Talamanca* E. Medda* A. Spinelli**
* Univ. of Roma "La Sapienza", Rome Italy; ** Ist. Super. di Sanità, Rome Italy

INTRODUCTION

The radioactive material released from the Chernobyl accident arrived in Italy over the Alps on Aprile 30, 1986. From May 2-5 northern Italy experienced a wet I-131 deposition of about 100 KBq/m^2. On May 5, a wet I-131 deposition of 96 KBq/m^2 was reported in central Italy (WHO, 1987). The committed effective dose equivalent was estimated to be about 1 mSv for children and 0.25 for adults in northern Italy. In central Italy exposure on the average was lower and the doses were estimated to be 0,40 mSv for children and 0,10 for adults. In the south the corresponding estimated doses were 0,35 and 0,09 (Annali Istituto Superiore di Sanità 1987). These doses are not considered teratogenic, and present knowledge does not exclude the possibility of a threshold in the range of 1 mSv (UNSCEAR, 1986). At higher doses, exposure has differential effects according to the developmental stage of the fetus (Karkinen - Jaaskelainen 1985). Human data on this subject however are sparse, and most statements are extrapolations from animal studies. In the present study we attempt to assess some reproductive effects of the exposure to eccess radiation in Italy by studying the frequency of selected reproductive events prior to, and after the Chernobyl accident.

METHODOLOGY

The reproductive events considered in the present study, comprise the monthly numbers of births, still births, voluntary interruptions of pregnancy and spontaneous abortions that occurred in the three main geographic areas of the country (north, central and south) in the period prior to Aprile 1986 and in one subsequent year. All above events are subject to compulsory registration, which is considered nearly complete.

The numbers of events observed in the months following the Chernobyl accident were compared with the number expected on the basis of the experience of the previous five years by a linear regression curve. Confidence limits around the expected values were set at the 95 per cent level.

RESULTS

1. <u>Live births</u>. Considering the births of conceptions occuring in the three months immediately following the Chernobyl accident we observe in table 1 that

in almost all cases the number of births expected was higher than those observed.

The reduction is evident in all regions mostly in February 1987, and for the North and the Center it is still apparent in March. All the observed values are within the 95% confidence limits of the expected numbers.

TABLE 1

OBSERVED AND EXPECTED NUMBER OF LIVEBIRTHS JAN-MARCH 1987 IN ITALY

	North			Center			South		
	observed	expected	% difference	observed	expected	% difference	observed	expected	% difference
JAN	15530	16089	- 3,5	7406	7439	- 0,4	20969	20911	+ 0,2
FEB	13106	14189	- 7,6	6300	6700	- 6,0	18306	18848	- 2,9
MAR	14798	15865	- 6,7	7094	7444	- 4,7	22008	22005	+ 0,01

2. Stillbirths. The numbers of stillbirths observed and expected in the three months of interest after the Chernobyl accident (Jan-March 87) corresponding to conceptions occurring in May-July 86, are shown on table 2. In the North, the observed stillbirths were fewer than the expected, while in the other areas the pattern is mixed. In the south we observed an excess of 30 stillbirths in the month of December corresponding to an increase of 21,3% which is statistically significant (C.L. 112-170).

TABLE 2
OBSERVED AND EXPECTED NUMBER OF STILLBIRTHS DEC. 1986 - FEB. 1987 IN ITALY

	North			Center			South		
	observed	expected	% difference	observed	expected	% difference	observed	expected	% difference
DEC	70	71	- 1,4	36	36	0	171	141	+ 21,3*
JAN	81	95	-14,6	42	15	+180	195	205	- 4,8
FEB	71	81	-12,3	38	37	+ 2,7	141	135	+ 4,4

* $P \leq 0.05$

3. Voluntary Interruptions of Pregnancy. Table 3 shows the numbers of induced abortions observed and expected during this period in the three areas of the

country in the three months following the Chernobyl accident. All of the differences between observed and expected are within the confidence limits.

TABLE 3

OBSERVED AND EXPECTED NUMBER OF INDUCED ABORTIONS MAY-JULY 1986 IN ITALY

	North			Center			South		
	observed	expected	% difference	observed	expected	% difference	observed	expected	% difference
MAY	7163	8192	-12,6	4003	4414	- 9,3	6533	6527	+ 0,09
JUN	6658	6836	- 2,6	3813	3540	+ 7,7	6074	5427	+11,9
JUL	6967	8088	-13,8	3982	4099	- 2,8	6230	5120	+21,6

4. Spontaneous Abortion. The data on this variable are available for only some regions of the country, and they are reported on table 4. The observed numbers of spontaneous abortions, as reported routinely in the local health authorities, are compared with those expected on the basis of the experience of the previous years (since 1980). Of the three geographic areas, the Northeastern was the most exposed to the radiactive contamination. It is interesting that a statistically significant excess in the number of spontaneous abortions was observed in June 1987, the expected number was 261 (upper 95% confidence limit 284), against 319 observed.

With the exception of an analogous excess in May in the Northwestern regions, all other monthly numbers of spontaneous abortions observed are either very close or smaller than those expected.

TABLE 4

OBSERVED AND EXPECTED NUMBER OF SPONTANEOUS ABORTIONS IN THE MONTHS PRIOR AND AFTER THE CHERNOBYL ACCIDENT IN SELECTED GEOGRAPHICAL REGIONS OF ITALY

	Northeastern			Northwest			Center		
	observed	expected	% difference	observed	expected	% difference	observed	expected	% difference
MAY	337	334	+ 0,89	883	825	∓ 7,0	167	228	-26,7
JUN	319	261	+22,2*	796	823	- 3,3	161	173	- 6,9
JUL	330	302	+ 9,3	746	784	- 4,8	162	186	-12,9
AUG	288	322	-10,5	573	707	-18,9	169	188	-10,1
SEPT	302	307	- 1,6	781	768	+ 1,7	154	182	-15,3

* $P \leq 0.05$

DISCUSSION

The results indicate that the Chernobyl accident might have caused a reduction in the births in the months immediately following its occurance. Such reduction, although not statistically significant is evident in all regions of the country and especially in the North. In some areas the reduction of births in the month of February 1987, corresponding to conceptions occuring in May 86 was particularly evident. In Trento for example, a region in Northeastern Italy the reduction was of the order of 15% in the urban areas. Since the reduction of births however does not correspond to an analogous increase in the number of stillbirths and abortions (spontaneous or induced), it may be hypothesized that this is to be attributed to an intentional prevention of conceptions on the part of the population in the areas more exposed to radiation. Analogous responses to the anxiety were observed in other countries (Trichopoulos 1987, Baum et al. 1983).

The data on stillbirths did not suggest any variations in their numbers that could be associated temporally or specially with the Chernobyl event. We are not in a position to interpret the excess observed in December 1986 in the sourthern region, but it seems unlikely that it is related to the Chernobyl accident, especially since the exposure there was negligiable, and the effect is evident for the sole month of december.

The data on spontaneous abortions on the other hand, do suggest an excess in the month of June in one of the more heavily contamined areas of Italy: the Northeastern region. The excess might correspond to conceptions that had occured prior to the accident or immediately after. Although the exposure level in the area was below what is considered embryotoxic, we cannot exclude the possibility that the excess observed might be related to the Chernobyl accident.

REFERENCES

1. Annali dell'Istituto Superiore di Sanità "Distribuzione della contaminazione in Italia" ISS vol. 23, n. 2 341-360 (1987).
2. Baum A., Gatchel R.J. e Schaeffer M.A. Emotional behavioral, and physiological effects of chronic stress at three Mile Island. Journ. of Consult and Clinical Psychology vol. 51, n. 4, 565-572 (1983).
3. Karkinen - Jaaskelainen M. "Maldevelopment abortion malformation and functional defects". Occupational Hazards and reproduction by Hemminki K., Sorsa M., Vainio H. Hemisphere publishing corporation; 81-85 (1983).
4. Trichopulos D. (Letter) Lancet Oct. 31, p. 1100 (1987).
5. UNSCEAR "Genetic and somatic effects of ionizing radiation". New York, United Nations Scientific Committee on the Effects of Atmoic Radiation (1986).

NOISE AT WORK AND THE OUTCOME OF PREGNANCY

ALISON MCDONALD, MARGARET SLOAN, BEN ARMSTRONG

School of Occupational Health, McGill University, 1130 Pine Avenue West, Montreal, H3A 1A3, Canada.

INTRODUCTION

Loud environmental noise has been shown to reach the fetus in utero[1], and to depress human lactogen levels late in pregnancy[2]. Delay in human fetal growth has been reported[3], as has an increased frequency of low birth weight close to a noisy airport[4]. On the other hand, a well designed study of noise exposure and congenital defects was negative[5].

Occupational factors and the outcome of pregnancy were investigated in current and previous pregnancies of 56,000 women interviewed while in 11 Montreal hospitals for delivery or treatment for a spontaneous abortion. Publications to date include reports on the main pregnancy outcomes[6] fetal death[7], prematurity[8] and congenital defect[9]. The findings on work demands and environmental factors in relation to spontaneous abortion and prematurity were reported at the 22nd International Conference on Occupational Health, Sydney, 1987. The relationships between occupational noise exposure and spontaneous abortion, preterm birth and low birth weight are presented in further detail here.

METHODS

The methods of data collection, processing, and analysis have been previously described[6]. Nurse-interviewers employed and trained for the purpose administered a standard questionnaire on personal social and occupational factors in recently completed (current) and all previous pregnancies. Questions on employment enabled occupations to be classified as in the Canadian Census. Among the questions on work environment was one on noise - whether the mother considered it absent, moderate or great. In six main occupational sectors the higher level of noise was reported by the following percentages of women: managerial and professional 4%, health 17%, clerical 16%, sales 14%, services 27%, manufacture 50%.

In current pregnancies information on outcome was obtained from obstetric and pediatric records. In previous pregnancies it was obtained from the mother and when uncertain by further enquiries from doctors and hospitals.

Current spontaneous abortions were those in which the women were hospitalized and successfully interviewed. Previous spontaneous abortions were less subject to selection and were probably well remembered (see 6). For prematurity current pregnancies only were studied because detailed information was available including ultra-sound findings in a high proportion. Single pregnancies of women who were employed 30 or more hours a week at the time of conception were used for the present analysis.

Statistical methods

1. Main analysis. Allowing by logistic regression for eight potentially confounding variables (age, parity, previous spontaneous abortion, ethnic group, educational level, height, cigarette smoking and alcohol consumption) expected (E) numbers of spontaneous abortions, preterm births (<37 weeks) and low birth weight births ($\leq$2500 g) were calculated for comparison with observed (O) numbers as a ratio O/E. 90 % confidence intervals for O/E ratios, one sided significance levels for excess adverse outcomes, and tests for heterogeneity or trend in O/E ratios were calculated on the assumption that observed numbers approximated to a Poisson sampling distribution.[6]

2. Grouped analysis. A grouped analysis was also undertaken for spontaneous abortions to minimise opportunities for recall bias in the reporting of a potentially damaging environmental factor when the outcome was known to be adverse. Sixty occupational groups were classified into eight groups according to the percentage of all pregnancies for which women reported a high level of noise. Regression (Poisson) of O/E ratios for spontaneous abortion in the eight groups on the percentage exposed to a high level of noise was carried out.

3. Birth weight for gestational age. In order to explore the possibility of an effect on the rate of fetal growth the lowest 5% of birth weights in each week of gestation after accounting for the same 8 confounding variables were classified as low weight for gestational age (see 10).

FINDINGS

Spontaneous abortion

Table 1 shows the O/E ratios for spontaneous abortion in 22,613 previous pregnancies of women who were employed for 30 or more hours a week at the time of conception and reported exposure to a high level of noise. The overall O/E ratio was 1.08 ($p < 0.01$). O/E ratios were significantly raised in three of the six occupational sectors: clerical 1.13 ($p < 0.01$), services 1.25 ($p < 0.01$), sales 1.41 ($p = 0.03$); ratios for the six sectors were not significantly heterogeneous. The O/E ratios differed according to length of gestation at time of abortion. At less than 10 weeks the O/E ratio was 1.00, at 10 < 16 weeks 1.12 and at 16 < 28 weeks 1.19 ($p = 0.02$). A trend was observed in O/E ratios with increasing noise exposure: none 0.96, moderate 0.99 and high 1.08 (p for trend < 0.01) - prima facie evidence of exposure-response. In the grouped analysis however the estimated relative risk for spontaneous abortion in women exposed to a high level of noise was 1.06 (90% CI 0.9-1.3, $p > 0.20$).

TABLE 1. SPONTANEOUS ABORTIONS OBSERVED (O) AND RATIO OF OBSERVED TO EXPECTED (O/E) IN PREGNANCIES WITH A HIGH LEVEL OF NOISE EXPOSURE

Occupational Sector	Spontaneous abortions		
	O	O/E	(90% CI)
Managerial	128	1.07	(0.92-1.23)
Health	78	1.05	(0.86-1.25)
Clerical	320	1.13	(1.03-1.24)
Sales	36	1.41	(1.05-1.82)
Services	138	1.25	(1.08-1.43)
Manufacturing	447	1.00	(0.92-1.08)
Total	1,147	1.08	(1.03-1.13)

Preterm and low birth weight

Table 2 shows O/E ratios for these two outcomes with a high level of noise exposure in 22,761 current pregnancies. For preterm birth the total O/E ratio was 1.03 and in none of the six occupational sectors was there a raised ratio significant at a 5% level. The total O/E ratio for low birth weight was 1.11 (p = 0.02). A significantly increased ratio was found in two of the six occupational sectors: health (O/E 1.49 p = 0.02) and manufacturing (O/E 1.20 p = 0.02). The association between high noise exposure and low birth weight was unaffected by adjustment for work demands, for example, lifting heavy weights and a long working week both of which increased the risk of low birth weight[8]. The O/E ratio for low birth weight for gestational age with high noise exposure was 0.97 (95% CI 0.84-1.11).

TABLE 2. RATIOS OF OBSERVED (O) TO EXPECTED (E) PRETERM AND LOW BIRTH WEIGHT BIRTHS IN PREGNANCIES WITH A HIGH LEVEL OF NOISE EXPOSURE

Occupational	Preterm			Low birth weight		
	O	O/E	(90% CI)	O	O/E	(90% CI)
Managerial	35	0.86	(0.64-1.12)	37	1.07	(0.80-1.38)
Health	33	1.17	(0.86-1.53)	36	1.49	(1.11-1.92)
Clerical	111	0.96	(0.81-1.11)	110	1.00	(0.85-1.17)
Sales	16	1.28	(0.80-1.94)	12	0.96	(0.55-1.56)
Services	41	1.07	(0.81-1.36)	40	1.03	(0.78-1.31)
Manufacturing	138	1.08	(0.94-1.24)	141	1.20	(1.04-1.37)
Total	375	1.03	(0.94-1.12)	376	1.11	(1.02-1.21)

COMMENT

The hypothesis that a high level of noise at work increases the risk of spontaneous abortion, presumably either by affecting directly the fetus or implantation site, or by causing stress is biologically conceivable. The association found between loud noise and spontaneous abortion and the trend of an increase in risk with increasing noise level suggest a causal relationship. On the other hand the negative result of the grouped analysis is against such a relationship and in particular raises the suspicion that the association was due to recall bias, an at least equally plausible explanation.

The finding of an association between loud noise and low birth weight without evidence of shortening of the period of gestation is consistent with the hypothesis that loud noise affects the rate of fetal growth. However no excess risk was found in birth weight after allowance for gestational age. These findings are not easy to interpret in conjunction, but do not present coherent evidence for an effect of noise on fetal growth.

The O/E ratios for both spontaneous abortion and low birth weight were only increased by about 10%. Confounding variables other than those allowed for in the analyses might be responsible for such marginal risks. Pregnancy outcome is affected by maternal (and paternal) characteristics, and by life style variables, environmental conditions and medical services. There is much variation in both choice of employment by individuals and choice of employees by employers. Inclusion of confounding variables known to be associated with occupation and with pregnancy outcome is likely to reduce the effect of selective factors but unlikely to eliminate them.

We conclude that occupational noise as reported by women in the Montreal survey was associated with a small increase in the frequency of spontaneous abortion and low birth weight, but that these associations were unlikely to be causal. There was no evidence of an association of noise with short gestations, or with fetal growth rate.

REFERENCES

1. Ando Y, Hattori H (1973) J Sound Vib 27: 101-103
2. Ando Y, Hattori H (1977) Br J Obstet Gynecol 84:115-118
3. Schell LM (1981) Am J Phys Anthropol 56:63-70
4. Knipschild P, Meijer H, Sallé H (1981) Int Arch Occup Environ Health 48:131-136
5. Kurppa K, Rantala K, Nurminen T, Holmberg PC, Starck J (1989) Scand J Work Environ Health 15:111-116
6. McDonald AD, McDonald JC, Nolin AD, Armstrong B, Cherry NM, Delorme C, Robert D (1987) Br J Ind Med 44:521-526
7. McDonald AD, McDonald JC, Armstrong B, Cherry NM, Côté R, Lavoie J, Nolin AD, Robert D (1988) Br J Ind Med 45:148-157
8. McDonald AD, McDonald JC, Armstrong B, Cherry NM, Nolin AD, Robert D (1988) Br J Ind Med 45:56-62
9. McDonald AD, McDonald JC, Armstrong B, Cherry NM, Côté R, Lavoie J, Nolin AD, Robert D (1988) Br J Ind Med 45:577-580
10. Armstrong B, Nolin AD, McDonald AD (1989) Br J Ind Med 46:196-199

WORK-RELATED DISEASES AND MEDICAL SURVEILLANCE

Occupational Epidemiology. H. Sakurai et al., editors

A CONSIDERATION ON HEALTHY WORKER EFFECT OBSERVED IN MORTALITY RECORDS OF WORKERS OF LARGE JAPANESE INDUSTRIES

TOSHIAKI HIGASHI(*), YASUHIKO BABA(*), HARUHIKO SAKURAI(**), KAZUYUKI OMAE(**), TOSHIO TOYAMA(**)

(*) Department of Health Policy and Management, Institute of Industrial Ecological Sciences, University of Occupational Environmental Health, Japan, 1-1 Iseigaoka, Yahatanishi-ku, Kitakyushu 807, JAPAN

(**) Department of Preventive Medicine and Public Health, School of Medicine, Keio University, 35 Shinanomachi, Shinjuku-ku, Tokyo 160, JAPAN

INTRODUCTION

Healthy worker effect (HWE), which can be described as a lower death rate within a work force when compared with the general population, has been observed in many epidemiological mortality studies of industrial work populations free of significant life-shortening hazards. The purpose of this report is to evaluate this effect in active work populations of large manufacturing companies in Japan, and to suggest possible factors which can be attributed to this phenomenon.

MATERIALS AND METHODS

Materials

A surveillance system of diseases that caused absence and caused death of workers has been established in member companies of The Japan Iron and Steel Federation (JISF) and The Japan Chemical Fibers and Textile Association (JCFTA). The diagnosis of disease, differentiation of new and old cases, sex, age and type of work were ascertained and recorded by the labor management or health department of each plant. The diseases were classified according to a simplified version of the 8th or 9th International Classification of Diseases. The present study was performed using these records registered in central file in JCFTA (1969-1981) and the reports on health statistics edited by JISF (1973-1981)(1).

Methods

The person-years, or numbers of subjects in each year were calculated from the number of workers recorded monthly by each company. The standardized mortality ratios (SMRs) were calculated for each year in JISF, which had large number of employee. In order to have enough number of subjects, SMRs in JCFTA were calculated for 1969-1971 and 1976-1981. Analysis for each industry was restricted to male employees. The expected number of deaths were calculated using the national age-specific death rate of Japan. Deviation of an SMR was tested according to the method of Monson, using a two-sided test of significance(2).

RESULTS

The average age of workers in JISF and JCFTA had been increasing due to the attrition of workforce caused by the change of industrial structure and progress of manufacturing process. The average of age in workers in JCFTA was increased from 36.7 in 1969 to 40.5 in 1981.

SMRs for all causes of death were within the range of 50 to 65 in JISF, and the tendency of decline was observed (Table I). From 1976 to 1981, 710 cases of death for cancer were observed in JISF and the SMR was 78 (95%CI: 72-84). In JCFTA, SMRs for all causes were 34 (1969-1981) and 41 (1976-1981), and the SMRs for cancer in each duration was 47 and 45, respectively (Table II). These results showed the significant HWE in terms of all causes of death and specific causes including cancer.

Table III shows the mortality of steel workers by age group in 1976-1981. The comparison of mortality between the steel workers and the general population in each age group suggests that the strength of HWE was significant even in the aged groups and that differences among age groups were not significant during the employment term.

TABLE I
SMR for all causes in steel workers in Japan, 1973-1981

	Number of Workers	Number of Death	SMR[a]	99%CI#
1973	263,076	421	65	56-75
1974	269,941	402	56	48-66
1975	267,610	413	63	54-72
1976	256,570	421	61	52-70
1977	243,570	341	54	46-63
1978	237,358	333	53	45-62
1979	225,752	334	55	46-64
1980	219,172	355	58	34-49
1981	210,200	292	50	42-52

a: calculated using The Vital Statistics Japan 1973-1981, Ministry of Health and Welfare
#: Confidence interval

TABLE II

SMRs and specific proportional mortality ratio (sPMR) in chemical textile plants, 1969-1971 (125,866 person years) and 1976-1981 (204,795 person years)

	1969-1971				1976-1981			
Cause of Death	Obs	SMR[a]	95%CI#	sPMR	Obs	SMR[a]	95%CI#	sPMR
All causes	119	34**	28-40	100	234	41**	36-46	100
Total cancer	29	47**	31-66	138	65	45**	34-56	110
Ischemic heart disease	7	46	22-104	160	15	53**	30-83	130
Cerebro-vascular disease	14	33**	18-53	97	35	43**	30-58	105
Liver cirrhosis	7	41*	16-77	121	23	51**	32-74	126
Other causes	62	29**	22-36	84	96	36**	29-44	89

a: calculated using The Vital Statistics Japan 1969-1981, Ministry of Health and Welfare
#: confidence interval
***: significant at 0.05, 0.01 risk level

TABLE III

Mortality (/100,000) of steel workers (1,289,204 person years) by age group in 1976-1981

Age group	-19	20-24	25-29	30-34	35-39	40-44	45-49	50-59
Subject Number	21,901	118,647	188,630	195,800	262,655	196,242	155,913	149,416
Mortality (A)	45.7	40.5	51.4	72.0	91.3	139.6	264.2	412.3
General population (B)[a]	70.7	87.7	90.3	102.9	159.7	255.1	436.2	756.3
(A)/(B)	0.65	0.46	0.57	0.70	0.57	0.55	0.61	0.55

a: from The Vital Statistics Japan 1976, Ministry of Health and Welfare, Japan

DISCUSSION

HWE reported from US and European countries has been within the range of 10% to 40%. This study shows a strong HWE, equal to or lower than the reported values in the United States in comparable studies(3).

The current consensus on factors involved in HWE, is thought that it is the composite result of factors such as: (I) selection of the workforce, (II) changes in life style accompanying employment, and (III) methodological characteristics of the SMR(4). To evaluate the findings of the present study, we could exclude the effect of factor (III), which are dependent on the percentage of active workers, because the purpose of this study was to evaluate the HWE in active workers.

Factors (I) has been emphasized as the strongest cause of HWE as a "selection" or "survival" effect: however, this effect was not thought to be sufficient to explain our findings in the lifetime employment system of large Japanese companies, even though selection is made prior to employment. Furthermore, selection of workers who tended to be suffered cancer was difficult but the strong HWE was observed in JCFTA even for cancer.

Factor (II), which is related to the economical status and/or health management and promotion programs in Japanese industry, is considered to have a relatively strong influence on the findings, especially for the work population engaged at large companies such as members of JISF or JCFTA, and it should be important that the strong HWE was observed in the aged workforce due to the attrition related to changes of industrial structure. Although health care or education, which may have been an impact on the prevention of death due to cancer, cannot be ascertained, recent reports which suggest that the medical management of blood pressure may help in preventing various diseases including cancer(5) should be properly assessed, because that has been one of the major indicators for medical management in Japanese industries.

This study might be criticised in terms of follow up of retired or terminated workers and the selection effect of workers through the attrition. In terms of the latter problem, the study was limited up to 1981, due to the rationalization of workforce caused by international change of industrial structure.

REFERENCES

1. JISF Occupational Health Committee (1987) J Steel Occup Health 31:138-148
2. Monson RR (1974) Comput Biomed Res 7:325-332
3. Wen CP, Tsai SP, Gibson RL (1983) J Occup Med 25:283-288
4. Wen CP, Tsai SP, Gibson RL, McClellan WA (1984) J Occup Med 26:118-127
5. Khaw KT, Conner EB (1984) Am J Epid 120:550-558

Occupational Epidemiology. H. Sakurai et al., editors

SERUM CONCENTRATIONS OF TRACE ELEMENTS AND FAT-SOLUBLE VITAMINS AND RISK FACTORS OF CHRONIC DISEASES IN A GROUP OF MIDDLE AGED JAPANESE WORKERS

TETSURO HONGO[1), TSUGUYOSHI SUZUKI[1), HIROSHI KASHIWAZAKI[1), HIDEKI IMAI[1), JUN YOSHINAGA[1), AKIKO HADA[2), AND TOMIE OYAMA[3)

1) Department of Human Ecology, School of Health Sciences, Faculty of Medicine, University of Tokyo, Hongo, Bunkyo-ku, Tokyo 113 (Japan)
2) Department of Food Service Management, Faculty of Home Economics, Tokyo Kasei Gakuin University, Aihara-machi, Machida-shi, Tokyo 194-02 (Japan)
3) Nippon Kokumin-shoku Co., Ltd., Ohte-machi, Chiyoda-ku, Tokyo 100 (Japan)

INTRODUCTION

Recent epidemiological studies have suggested that the low serum level of fat-soluble vitamins (retinol, α-tocopherol and β-carotene) and selenium (Se) were attributable to the subsequent risk of cancer (1-5). The imbalance in trace elements nutrition, such as those between sodium (Na) and potassium (K), magnesium (Mg) and calcium (Ca), and copper (Cu) and zinc (Zn), has also been related to occurrence of chronic diseases including cancer and heart disease (6-8). In this report, it is evaluated if the serum level of trace elements and fat-soluble vitamins are related to smoking and alcohol consumption, which are dominant risk factors of chronic diseases, in a group of middle aged Japanese working population. In the process of multiple regression analysis, other factors such as age, gender, obesity, and hypertension are simultaneously evaluated.

SUBJECTS AND METHODS

Subjects

Subjects were 180 (124 males and 56 females) employees in a stock trading company (79 males and 2 females) and a food service industry (45 males and 54 females) in Tokyo. Age of subjects ranged from 50 to 59 years old. They volunteered for participation after the objective and methodologies of the study were explained. In a stock trading company, 90% were office workers. In a food service industry, skilled laborers (cooks and dietitians) were 51% and office workers were 24% of the subjects.

Analytical Methods

Serum samples were collected in the afternoon without lunch. Sodium (Na), K, Mg, Ca, Cu, and Zn concentrations were measured by atomic absorption spectrometry after dilution with distilled deionized water, and Se was measured by Watkinson's fluorometric method after nitric acid digestion. Retinol, α-carotene, β-carotene, and α-tocopherol concentrations were measured using high performance liquid chromatography after extraction with ethanol and n-hexane.

Statistical Methods

Variables, distribution of which deviated from the normal distribution (α- and β-carotenes, α-tocopherol, and α-tocopherol/cholesterol), were converted to logarithmic values. Gender-related difference was tested by Student's t-test. Stepwise regression analysis was conducted to clarify the factors affected serum trace elements and fat-soluble vitamins levels. Independent variables were amount of weekly alcohol consumption, daily cigarettes consumption (0 piece/day = 0, 1-10 = 1, 11-20 = 2, 21-30 = 3, 31-40 = 4, 41 or over = 5), type of job (stock trading company = 0, food service industry = 1), age, gender (males = 0, females = 1), Body Mass Index (BMI), systolic (SBP) and diastolic blood pressure (DBP). The probability of F-values for selection of variables was set at 0.05.

RESULTS AND DISCUSSION

Table I shows mean (SD) value of trace elements and fat-soluble vitamins concentrations and molar ratio of Na/K, Ca/Mg, Zn/Cu, and α-tocopherol/cholesterol. All of the levels in our subjects fell into the ranges of reported values in literature on Japanese. Gender-related difference was significant in Na, Se, Zn/Cu, and retinol (males>females) and in α- and β-carotenes (males<females).

Table II shows the significant explanatory factors for serum trace elements and fat-soluble vitamins levels in the result of stepwise regression analysis. Smoking inversely influenced the levels of α- and β-carotenes. This negative effect of smoking was consistent with the result reported on Japanese (9), though they reported that the alcohol consumption was more effective than smoking.

Alcohol consumption was selected as a significant positive factor on serum retinol level. Toyoshima *et al.* (10) also reported retinol level was positively dependent on alcohol consumption in Japanese adults.

BMI was selected as a significant independent variable for serum α-tocopherol level. This relationship reflected that α-tocopherol level was significantly correlated with serum total cholesterol level ($r = 0.58$, $p<0.001$). When α-tocopherol level was adjusted for

TABLE I

MEAN (SD) VALUE OF TRACE ELEMENTS AND FAT-SOLUBLE VITAMINS CONCENTRATIONS AND MOLAR RATIO OF Na/K, Ca/Mg, Zn/Cu, AND α-TOCOPHEROL/CHOLESTEROL

Variable	Males (N=124)	Females (N=56)	Total (N=180)
Na(μg/ml)	3180(123)**	3130(127)	3170(126)
K(μg/ml)	172(15)	169(13)	171(14)
Na/K(mol/mol)	31.6(2.5)	31.6(2.2)	31.6(2.4)
Mg(μg/ml)	20.0(1.5)	19.9(1.6)	20.0(1.5)
Ca(μg/ml)	93.7(4.2)	93.3(6.5)	93.6(5.0)
Ca/Mg(mol/mol)	2.86(0.23)	2.85(0.22)	2.85(0.23)
Cu(μg/ml)	0.962(0.166)	1.004(0.164)	0.975(0.166)
Zn(μg/ml)	0.694(0.121)	0.670(0.120)	0.686(0.121)
Zn/Cu(mol/mol)	0.718(0.172)*	0.661(0.148)	0.701(0.167)
Se(μg/ml)	0.134(0.019)***	0.121(0.016)	0.130(0.019)
retinol(μg/ml)	0.612(0.158)***	0.425(0.106)	0.554(0.168)
α-carotene(μg/ml) #	0.051(1.9)***	0.073(1.4)	0.057(1.8)
β-carotene(μg/ml) #	0.120(2.6)***	0.318(1.7)	0.162(2.6)
α-tocopherol(μg/ml) #	9.71(1.4)	9.30(1.3)	9.58(1.4)
α-tocopherol/cholesterol(μmol/mmol) #	4.19(1.3)	3.91(1.2)	4.10(1.3)

Converted to the logarithmic values.
*,**,*** Significantly different from females, $p<0.05$, 0.01, and 0.001 respectively (Student's t-test).

cholesterol level (α-tocopherol/cholesterol molar ratio), DBP was selected as a explanatory factor.

For serum trace elements levels and molar ratio of Na/K, Ca/Mg, and Zn/Cu, neither smoking nor alcohol consumption was selected as a explanatory factor. Type of job influenced the levels of Na, K, and Ca — all were lower in food service industry workers —. This may be resulted from dietary or working conditions.

From these results, the effect of smoking on serum carotenes levels was noteworthy since it was suggested that serum carotene level was the remarkable predictor of increased cancer risk (4,5).

TABLE II

SIGNIFICANT EXPLANATORY FACTORS FOR SERUM TRACE ELEMENTS AND FAT-SOLUBLE VITAMINS LEVELS IN THE RESULT OF STEPWISE REGRESSION ANALYSIS

Dependent variable	Significant independent variables (β)	R^2
Na	type of job(-.474)***	0.225
K	type of job(-.349)***	0.122
Ca	type of job(-.249)**, age(.193)*	0.108
Se	gender(-.313)**	0.098
retinol	gender(-.438)***, alcohol consumption(.229)**	0.313
α-carotene	smoking(-.353)***, DBP(-.271)**	0.186
β-carotene	smoking(-.334)***, gender(.305)***, DBP(-.245)**	0.356
α-tocopherol	BMI(.330)***	0.109
α-tocopherol/ cholesterol	DBP(.192)*	0.037
Mg, Cu, Zn, Na/K, Ca/Mg, Zn/Cu	none	

β Standardized partial regression coefficient.
R^2 Multiple coefficient of determination.
*,**,*** Probability of F-values, $p<0.05$, 0.01, and 0.001 respectively.

REFERENCES

1. Willett WC, Polk BF, Morris JS, Stampfer MJ, Pressel S, Rosner B, Taylor JO, Schneider K, Hanes CG (1983) Lancet 2:130-134
2. Salonen JT, Salonen R, Lappetelainen R, Maenpaa PH, Alfthan G, Puska P (1985) Br Med J 290:417-420
3. Wald N, Idle M, Boreham J, Bailey A (1980) Lancet 2:813-815
4. Menkes MS, Comstock GW, Vuilleumier JP, Helsing KJ, Rider AA, Brookmeyer R (1986) New Eng J Med 315:1250-1254
5. Nomura AMY, Stemmermann GN, Heilbrun LK, Salkeld RM, Vuilleumier JP (1985) Cancer Res 45:2369-2372
6. Meneely GR, Battarbee HD (1976) Nutr Rev 34:225-235
7. Karppanen H (1981) Artery 9:190-199
8. Klevay LM (1975) Am J Clin Nutr 28:764-774
9. Ito Y, Minohara M, Otani M, Sarai S, Niiya Y (1989) Jpn J Hyg 44: 607-614
10. Toyoshima H, Hayashi S, Miyanishi K, Wakai S, Enoki S (1989) Jpn J Hyg 44:659-666

Occupational Epidemiology. H. Sakurai et al., editors

JOB MOBILITY DURING WORKING LIFE AND HEALTH AFTER RETIREMENT

Yuriko IWATSUBO, Francis DERRIENNIC :

INSERM U 170, 16 avenue P. Vaillant COUTURIER 94807 VILLEJUIF CEDEX FRANCE.

Bernard CASSOU : Consultations de Gérontologie, 49 rue Mirabeau, 75016 PARIS, FRANCE.

INDRODUCTION

Job mobility is a complex phenomenon which concerns an important part of the working population. So in most epidemiological studies on occupational exposures and working conditions in relation to health, the mobility of subjects in the studied population is raised. It may constitute a bias in the measure of the relation between occupational factors and condition of health in the observed sample (1-3).

The most frequently retained hypothesis supposes that health disorders are the factors influencing entering a job and leaving it. So it is interesting to examine among survivors of selection by health criteria and when working life is ended whether job mobility can be considered as a risk factor.

The aim of this study is to examine the relation between job mobility during working life and health disorders after retirement in a longitudinal study.

MATERIAL AND METHODS

A five year follow-up study among retired people was conducted in the Paris area between the period 1982-83 and 1987-1988 (4,5). A sample of 1000 subjects from the file of an inter-professional supplementary fund and who lived in the Paris area was randomly selected. The survey was carried out by home interviews using a standardised questionnaire. At the first stage 627 subjects participated in the study and at the second stage 464 of those 627 subjects were reinterviewed.

PARAMETERS OF HEALTH

Disorders of five major functions are defined as impairments (6) by grouping signs and symptoms which are covered systematically in the questionnaire.

Four impairments concern organic disorders : musculo-skeletal impairment (presence of pain in joints or spine since at least six months before the date of interview), cardiorespiratory impairment (presence of coughing or expectoration since two years before interview and for three consecutive months or breathlessness or palpitation), sight or hearing impairment (difficulties during daily activities), digestive impairment (presence of stomach pains every day). The fifth impairment concerns mental health defined by presence of at least five positive responses in a list of nine questions.

Elderly people's health is evaluated by the number of impairments that they reported at the moment of the survey.

In the present study, we will consider the number of impairments at both stages and any change in the number of impairments between those two stages.

JOB MOBILITY

Job mobility was defined by a dichotomic variable using the number of companies and the number of branches of economic activity. Those data were provided by the pension fund which has retraced the occupational history of each person by building up a list of companies that have hired the subjects. For most of the companies the branch of economic activity is known thanks to the INSEE code.

A subject was considered to have had high mobility when both numbers of changes were higher than the average values observed in the sample.

RESULTS

Men and women are considered separately in the analysis.

At the first stage, 320 men and 307 women participated in the study (response rate 62.7). They were on average 69 years old at the moment of the study. 65 male subjects (20.5 %) and 83 female subjects (27.4 %) belonged to the group with high mobility. The mean number of impairments was 1.4 (sd = 1.1) among men and 1.8 (sd = 1.2) among women.

In both sexes, subjects belonging to the group with high mobility had significantly higher mean number of impairments compared to those belonging to the group with low mobility : 1.3 in the group with low mobility and 1.7 in that with high mobility for men, 1.7 and 2.1 respectively for women (table I).

Adjustments of this relationship on potential confounding factors (age at the moment of the interview, previous health condition, socio-economic categories, physical or chemical occupational exposures during working life and physiological constraints) did not seem to modify the observed result.

At the second stage : 219 men and 245 women were reinterviewed (overall response rate of 74 %). Their mean age was 73 years for both sexes. 42 men (19.4 %) and 66 women (27.3 %) belonged to the group with high mobility.

The mean number of impairments was 1.4 (sd = 1.1) for men and 1.9 (SD = 1.1) for women.

TABLE I

JOB MOBILITY AND NUMBER OF IMPAIRMENTS AT THE TWO STAGES OF THE STUDY : CROSS-SECTIONAL RESULTS

		STAGE 1 mobility low		STAGE 1 mobility high	STAGE 2 mobility low		STAGE 2 mobility high
males	nb	252		65	175		42
	mean	1.3	*	1.7	1.4	a	1.7
	s	1.0		1.2	1.1		1.0
females	nb	220		83	176		66
	mean	1.7	*	2.1	1.8	*	2.2
	s	1.2		1.0	1.2		1.0

nb : number of subjects; mean : mean number of impairments; s : standard deviation; * : $p < 0.05$; a : $p < 0.10$; NS : no significant

Again at this stage, the subjects in the group of high mobility had on average a higher number of impairments (table I). Among men, subjects belonging to the group with low mobility reported 1.4 impairments on average and those belonging to the group with high mobility reported 1.7 impairments. Among women those averages were respectively 1.8 and 2.2.
However this difference was statistically significant only among women. And this relation was independent of the same potential confounding factors considered above.

CHANGE IN NUMBER OF IMPAIRMENTS DURING FOLLOW-UP PERIOD

The change in number of impairments was examined among those who participated in the two stages of the study (table II).
An increase in number of impairments was observed in both mobility groups and in both sexes. But these increases were not statistically significant.

DISCUSSION

Apart from men at stage 2, in both sexes and both stages of the study, the subjects with high mobility had on average, statistically, a significantly greater number of impairments. And those cross-sectional results seemed independent of the considered confounding factors.

A slight increase in number of impairments was observed on average during the follow-up period in both sexes and both mobility groups. But the difference was not statistically significant. The follow-up interval might be too short to observe a greater difference.

These results agree with the hypothesis on selections that account for the healthy worker effect. Nevertheless it is possible to argue that a great job mobility during working life could be a risk factor for health after retirement.

In this case what are the factors concealed behind the mobility considered here : stress effect due to the effort involved in adaptation to successive job environments, cumulative

TABLE II

JOB MOBILITY AND NUMBER OF IMPAIRMENTS AT THE TWO STAGES OF THE STUDY AMONG SUBJECTS FOLLOWED LONGITUDINALLY

	low mobility stage 1	stage 2	p	p paired	high mobility stage 1	stage 2	p	p paired
males nb	175	175			42	42		
mean	1.3	1.4	NS	NS	1.5	1.7	NS	NS
s	1.0	1.1			1.0	1.0		
females nb	176	176			66	66		
mean	1.7	1.8	NS	NS	2.0	2.2	NS	NS
s	1.2	1.2			1.0	1.0		

nb : number of subjets; mean : mean number of impairments; s : standard deviation; * : $p < 0.05$; a : $p < 0.10$; NS : no significant.

effects of several job exposures in one working life ? This question seems interesting because it suggests that health condition after retirement should be considered not only with regard to occupational exposures but also to factors associated with the pattern of working life before retirement.

REFERENCES

1. MONSON R.R Observations on the healthy worker effect. J. Occup Med 1986; 28: 425-433.
2. FOX A. J., COLLIER P. F. Low mortality rates in industrial cohort studies due to selection for work and survival in the industry. Br J Prev Soc Med 1976; 30: 225-230.
3. VINNI K., HAKAMA M. Healthy worker effect in the total finnish population. Br J Ind Med 1980; 37: 180-184.
4. CASSOU B., DERRIENNIC F., LECUYER G., AMPHOUX M. Déficience, incapacité et handicap dans un groupe de retraités de la région parisienne et relation avec la catégorie socio-professionnelle. Rev Epidem et Santé Publ 1986; 34: 332-340.
5. DERRIENNIC F., CASSOU B., LECUYER G., AMPHOUX M. Déficiences locomotrice et cardiorespiratoire après la retraite en relation avec certaines expositions professionnelles durant la vie active. Rev Epidem et santé Publ 1987; 35: 263-273.
6. International Classification of Impairments, Disabilities, and Handicaps . World Health Organization, Géneva, 1980

Occupational Epidemiology. H. Sakurai et al., editors

EFFECTS OF PERCEIVED JOB-STRESS ON GLYCOSYLATED HEMOGLOBIN

NORITO KAWAKAMI,* SHUNICHI ARAKI,* TAKESHI HAYASHI,** TAKESHI MASUMOTO**

* Department of Public Health, Faculty of Medicine, University of Tokyo, 7-3-1 Hongo, Bunkyo-ku, Tokyo 113 (Japan)

** Hitachi Health Care Center, 4-3-16 Ohse-cho, Hitachi, Ibaraki 317 (Japan)

INTRODUCTION

Proportion of glycosylated hemoglobin (HbA_{1c}) in total hemoglobin is an integrated measure of the changes in glucose metabolism in diabetic patients (1); this is used for a screening of diabetic mellitus (2). Recently, Cesana et al. (3) reported that the level of HbA_{1c} is higher in blue collar workers than in clerical workers; whereas no significant difference is observed in the level of fasting blood sugar between the two groups. The blue collar workers engaged in stressful conditions, such as shift work, noisy environment and low job-satisfaction; therefore it was explained that the findings resulted from frequent elevation in the blood glucose level due to job-stress mediated by sympathetic nervous system and cathecolamine secretion. Then Cesana et al. proposed HbA_{1c} as a stable and inexpensive measure of chronic job-stress. In this study, to study the finding by Cesana and his colleagues further, the relationships between HbA_{1c} and selected sources of psychosocial job-stress, i.e. job-overload and job-dissatisfaction, are examined where the major health-related behaviors, such as smoking and alcohol drinking, were adjusted for.

SUBJECTS AND METHODS

Subjects

307 male employees of an electric corporation, aged 30 or more years, came to a multiphasic health examination from July 2 to August 11 in 1987. They were surveyed with questionnaires concerning job-stress and health related behaviors. Blood analysis including HbA_{1c} and fasting plasma glucose (FPG) was made for these subjects. 275 or 90% of these workers responded the questionnaire survey. 146 blue collar workers were excluded because their physical activities during working hours were greatly different each other and might be confounding. The following analysis was made in 129 white collar workers. 10 subjects were omitted because they had been diagnosed as diabetes mellitus or they received medical treatment for diabetes mellitus or other disorders. Another 17 were excluded because they had 110 mg/dl or higher FPG concentration. Mean age±standard deviation (SD) of the 102 subjects was 38.0±5.1.

Methods

After fasting overnight, the subjects came to the examination center at about 8:00 am. The questionnaires concerning background data, job-stress variables and health-related behaviors were handed to the subjects and blood sample was taken. Health examination included blood pressure measurement, blood analysis and physical examination.

The job-stress items, which are 4-choice response scales, were subjected to a principal components factor analysis with varimax rotation; two factors with eigen values more than 1.0 were extracted; these items were classified into either of two factors in which their factor loadings were greater. A total score of each group of items was used as a measure of the correspondent factor of job-stress. Job-dissatisfaction (4 items) assesses how much the subject personally dissatisfied with content of his work and human relations at the workplace; the score was ranged from 0 to 12. Job-overload (3 items) refers to the amount of quantitative and qualitative pressure perceived by workers; the score was ranged from 0 to 9. Alpha coefficients of internal consistencies were 0.65 for job-dissatisfaction and 0.56 for job-overload. Overtime per month was also assessed in the questionnaires. Health-related behaviors consisted of smoking habit, alcohol consumption per week and obesity (body mass index).

HbA_{1c} was measured by an automatic analyzer (Kyoto Daiichi Kagaku HA-8121) by means of high performance liquid chromatography (2). Laboratory blood tests provided measures of FPG, hemoglobin, total cholesterol, triglyceride, GOT, GPT, LDH, gamma-GTP, uric acid and creatine. Relations of age, job-stress variables, health-related behaviors and health examination data to HbA_{1c} and FPG were examined using Pearson's correlation coefficients (rs). Student's t-test was used to examine difference in HbA_{1c} and FPG between groups classified on the basis of the variables.

RESULTS

Job-dissatisfaction score was positively correlated with HbA_{1c} in 40 non-smokers (figure 1). No significant correlation between job-dissatisfaction and HbA_{1c} was found in 55 smokers and 7 ex-smokers (r=0.019 and 0.112, respectively, $p>0.05$). Job-dissatisfaction score was significantly correlated with FPG in none of smokers, ex-smokers and non-smokers ($p>0.05$). The following variables were significantly correlated with HbA_{1c} in none of these three groups ($p>0.05$): job-overload score, overtime and possible confounders, i.e., age, alcohol consumption, obesity, sleeping time, blood pressures and results of blood tests other than FPG (hemoglobin, total cholesterol, triglyceride, GOT, GPT, LDH, gamma-GTP, uric acid, creatine).

Smokers had significantly higher HbA_{1c} levels than non-smokers in the subjects with lower job-dissatisfaction score (figure 2), where the subjects were stratified into two groups with higher and lower scores according to the median, i.e. 4 in the score. The mean values±SD in 20 smokers, 12 non-smokers and 2 ex-smokers in the group with higher job-dissatisfaction score were 5.33±0.30, 5.39 ±0.27 and 5.45±0.35, respectively; there were no significant differences among them ($p>0.05$). HbA_{1c} levels were not significantly different among smokers, non-smokers and ex-smokers in the subjects with high job-dissatisfaction score ($p>0.05$). FPG levels were significantly different among smokers, non-smokers and ex-smokers in the neither groups with higher nor lower job-dissatisfaction score ($p>0.05$). Job-overload score, overtime and the possible confounders described above were significantly correlated with HbA_{1c} in neither of these two groups ($p>0.05$).

DISCUSSION

In the present study, HbA_{1c} was significantly correlated with job-dissatisfaction score in non-smokers, but was significantly correlated in neither the smokers nor the ex-smokers. The results suggest that HbA_{1c} is a possible indicator of job-dissatisfaction in non-smokers.

Since job-dissatisfaction score

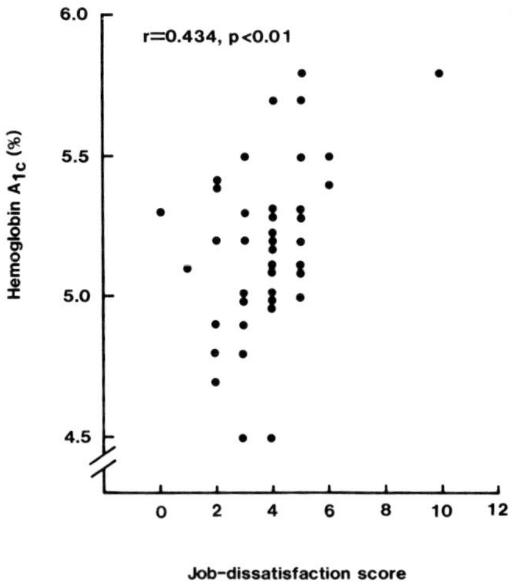

Figure 1. Relationship between job-dissatisfaction score and hemoglobin A_{1c} in 40 non-smokers.

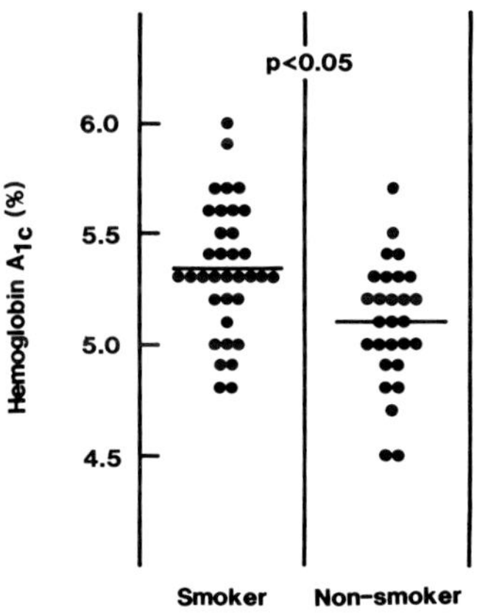

Figure 2. Difference in hemoglobin A_{1c} between 35 smokers and 28 non-smokers in the group with lower job-dissatisfaction score (t-test). Transeverse lines indicate mean values. The mean value±standard deviation in 5 ex-smokers in this group is 5.42±0.37 and significantly different from that in neither the smokers nor the non-smokers ($p>0.05$).

was not significantly correlated with FPG, higher HbA_{1c} levels in the subjects with higher job-dissatisfaction in non-smokers are mainly attributable to non-diabetic mechanisms. 1) Emotional reactions due to job-dissatisfaction may cause frequent release of counterregulatory hormones such as cortisol, growth hormone and cathecolamines (5) and a subsequent rise in blood glucose (6). 2) Changes in dietary habits under stressful conditions might cause elevated HbA_{1c} levels.

Smokers had significantly higher levels of HbA_{1c} than non-smokers in the subjects with lower score of job-dissatisfaction. Smoking itself or stress in smokers may stimulate release of the counterregulatory hormones and consequently cause temporal elevation in blood glucose (7,8).

Job-dissatisfaction was not correlated with HbA_{1c} in smokers and no difference by smoking habit was observed under higher job-dissatisfaction. The following explanations are possible: 1) Smoking itself (or stress in smokers) and the job-dissatisfaction act to increase HbA_{1c} levels through a common intermediatry, such as counterregulatory hormones, and this intermediatry might be limited in the degree to which it can respond to both characteristics. 2) There might be a difference in emotional or behavioral response to stress between between non-smokers and smokers. Further investigations are needed to explain psychophysiological mechanisms for the effects of job-dissatisfaction on the HbA_{1c} level in non-smokers as well as in smokers.

ACKNOWLEDGMENTS

The authors wish to thank Dr. Y. Arakawa and Mrs. S. Shoji at Hitachi Health Care Center. Part of this study was supported by a grant-in-aid for scientific research from the Ministry of Education, Science and Culture, Japan.

REFERENCES

1. Koenig RJ, Peterson CM, Jones RL, Saudek C, Lehrman M, Cerami A (1976) New Engl J Med 295: 417-420
2. Dunn PJ, Cole RA, Soeldner JS, Gleason RE (1979) Ann Int Med 91: 390-396
3. Cesana G, Panza G, Ferrario M, Zanettini R, Arnoldi M, Grieco A (1985) JOM 27: 357-360
4. Schneck AG, Schroeder WA (1961) J Am Chem Soc 83: 1472-1478
5. Rose RM, Sachar E (1981) In: Williams RH (ed) Textbook of endocrinology. 6th ed. WB Saunders, Philadelphia, pp 646-671
6. Eigler N, Sacca L, Sherwin R (1979) J Clin Invest 63: 114-123
7. Cryer PE, Hoymond MW, Santiago JV, Shah SD (1976) N Engl J Med 295: 573-577
8. Sandberg H, Roman L, Zavodnick J, Kupers N (1973) J Pharmacol Experiment Therapeutics 184: 787-791

Occupational Epidemiology. H. Sakurai et al., editors

CORONARY HEART DISEASE RISK FACTOR CHANGE IN RELATION TO OCCUPATIONAL CHANGE

JOHN A. MANDRYK, MICHAEL S. FROMMER, BERYL V. EDYE, GREG CURRY, DAVID A. FERGUSON

National Institute of Occupational Health and Safety, Worksafe Australia, GPO Box 58, Sydney, NSW, 2001, Australia

INTRODUCTION

As one aspect of a larger study of the possible influence of occupation on coronary heart disease [CHD] risk (1-4), this paper examines occupational change over five years in a large cohort of Australian government employees, and its possible association with CHD risk. Previous studies have suggested associations between occupational change and job dissatisfaction and stress, between occupational change and blood pressure, serum cholesterol and smoking, and between occupational change and CHD occurrence (5-9). However, other studies have not supported the existence of a relationship between occupational mobility and CHD occurrence (10), or between job change, line-of-work change and number of promotions over 10 years and CHD occurrence (11).

METHODS

The study population and methods have been described in detail elsewhere (1-4). A total of 4607 men and women employed by Australian government authorities in Sydney were enrolled on a voluntary basis between 1977 and 1980. On enrolment each subject had an initial contact with a study nurse, and a subsequent contact with a study physician two weeks later. Information on demographic, personal and occupational variables was obtained by questionnaire. Anthropometric and blood pressure measurements were made by the nurse, who also collected a random venous blood sample for chemical analysis. In the course of a general cardiovascular assessment the physician repeated the blood pressure measurement, and estimated fitness on a five point scale using a modification of Master's step test (2,12). The data collection process was repeated either annually for five years, or three and five years after enrolment, depending on initial risk factor levels.

The occupational change variables considered were upward mobility (promotions), lateral mobility (transfers), change in occupation, change in work-style and change in employer. Upward and lateral mobility and change in employer were expressed as the number of changes which occurred during the five year period. Change in occupation and change in work-style were binary variables with either no change (the majority of subjects) or some change. A change in work-style was recorded if the change was marked, such as from a clerical to a technical job.

The CHD risk variables considered were systolic and diastolic blood pressures, serum cholesterol, body mass index [BMI], smoking, alcohol consumption and fitness. Blood pressure measurement followed the method proposed by the World Health Organization for cardiovascular surveys (13), using Hawksley random-zero sphygmomanometers. Two successive measurements were made by the nurse, who recorded the average systolic and average diastolic pressures. The physician did the same, two weeks later. The mean of these readings was used in all calculations. Serum cholesterol was estimated in a hospital biochemistry laboratory using the Liebermann-Burchard reaction without precipitation (14). Weight and height were measured using balance scales and an Holtain anthropometer respectively, the subject being clothed but without shoes or jacket. Alcohol consumption (10-gram drinks/week) and smoking (cigarettes/day) were determined from the self-administered questionnaires.

Outcome variables comprised change in risk factors over five years, expressed as the difference between the final and initial values. Covariates in the analysis were the initial risk factor levels and age. Separate models were used to assess the effects of sex and initial occupation. Males were classified into eight occupational groups (administrators, professionals, technicians, clerks, skilled tradesmen, blue collar workers, tax investigators and tax assessors) and females into two occupational groups (office workers and technical or manual workers) (2). The SAS package was used for analysis (15). Multivariate analysis of covariance was used to examine the seven risk factors considered together as an outcome vector, while analyses of covariance were used to interpret the contribution of each of the seven risk factors to the more complex multivariate results.

Analysis was confined to subjects remaining in the employed workforce (though not necessarily still employed by the government authorities) five years after enrolment. Of the 4607 subjects who enrolled, 39 did not complete the enrolment procedure, 53 died and a further 874 were lost to follow-up. Fifth-year data were thus available for 3641 (79%). Of these, 455 had retired from the workforce. A further 329 persons were excluded because they were taking anti-hypertensive or other medications likely to affect blood pressure (122 of these had commenced taking anti-hypertensives during the five years of the study), and 30 females were excluded because they were pregnant either on enrolment or at the fifth-year follow-up. Relevant follow-up data were incomplete for 171 subjects. Thus the analysis was based on 58% of enrolled subjects (2125 males and 531 females). These subjects' ages were in the range 16 to 65 years, with the mean age of the males (± standard deviation) being 34 (±10) years and that of the females 31 (±11) years.

RESULTS

Changes in work-style, occupation and employer did not contribute significantly to the models tested. Upward and lateral mobility were also not significant when analysed as main effects. However, for males, the interaction of upward and lateral mobilities was significant ($p<0.01$) in the multivariate analysis of covariance, and this effect appeared to be associated with increases in serum cholesterol and BMI. The greatest increase in cholesterol (Table 1) and BMI (Table 2) occurred in association with three or more lateral moves but no upward moves, with no simple pattern for other combinations. This interaction effect did not appear to be restricted to any particular occupation(s). For females, no main effects or interaction terms were significant.

TABLE 1. MEAN INCREASE [a] IN SERUM CHOLESTEROL (mmol/l ± SE [b]) OVER FIVE YEARS (MALES, N=2125)

Number of upward moves	Number of lateral moves: 0	1	2	3+
0	0.43±0.04	0.45±0.06	0.65±0.10	0.90±0.11
1	0.57±0.04	0.57±0.05	0.45±0.07	0.45±0.09
2	0.51±0.06	0.57±0.07	0.49±0.09	0.64±0.09
3+	0.38±0.11	0.62±0.10	0.60±0.11	0.56±0.11

Significance of upward by lateral interaction: $p=0.008$

a. adjusted for initial values of: systolic and diastolic blood pressures, BMI, cholesterol, age, cigarettes smoked, alcoholic drinks and exercise response

b. pooled estimate of standard deviation = 0.79 mmol/l

TABLE 2. MEAN INCREASE [a] IN BODY MASS INDEX (kg/m^2 ± SE [b]) OVER FIVE YEARS (MALES, N=2125)

Number of upward moves	Number of lateral moves 0	1	2	3+
0	0.69±0.07	0.38±0.12	0.61±0.19	1.01±0.21
1	0.80±0.08	0.81±0.10	0.60±0.14	0.37±0.16
2	0.36±0.12	0.73±0.13	0.69±0.17	0.37±0.17
3+	0.55±0.21	0.40±0.19	0.42±0.21	0.47±0.20

Significance of upward by lateral interaction: p=0.013

a. *adjusted for initial values of: systolic and diastolic blood pressures, BMI, cholesterol, age, cigarettes smoked, alcoholic drinks and exercise response*

b. *pooled estimate of standard deviation = 1.47 kg/m^2*

DISCUSSION

Kaplan *et al* (6) suggest that upward mobility within a working lifetime has a more favourable outcome (less CHD) amongst upper social classes. Haynes *et al* (9) present weak evidence which implies that lack of occupational mobility amongst men is related to cholesterol level. Kirjonen and Hanninen (8) found that, within a five-year period, job and life dissatisfaction and stress symptoms decreased for their job-change group. The present longitudinal study of the effect of occupational change on change in CHD risk also suggests that there might be some association between occupational change and CHD risk. A statistically significant effect of the interaction of upward and lateral mobility on increases in serum cholesterol and body mass index in males was detected. Our inability to demonstrate any association of the interaction with one or more specific occupations may in part be due to small cell sizes which result when the data are stratified by occupation and cross-classified by numbers of upward and lateral moves. A further complication is that 122 subjects who commenced treatment for hypertension during the study were excluded (blood pressure was analysed as a continuous variable and so it was necessary to exclude subjects whose blood pressure was pharmacologically modified).

The present results invite consideration of the problems of studying health effects of occupational change in an epidemiological context. Occupational change is a complex phenomenon, and there is no standard approach to its measurement. While the approach adopted here was based on objective measures, it did not take account of the nature of the change or subjects' perceptions. Not all promotions (or transfers) are the same. Theorell *et al* (16) make a distinction between promotion and the perception of increased responsibility (they found that increased perceived responsibility amongst blue collar workers in the previous year was associated with increased myocardial infarction). Kasl (17) also emphasises that any link between objective measures of work and subjective perceptions is tenuous, and that the association with disease is usually stronger for the subjective perceptions.

The study of occupational change is complicated as well by the fact that the various occupational change variables may be interrelated in complex ways; for example, upward mobility might involve change of occupation and lateral mobility might lead to upward mobility. And although change of employer was found to be non-significant in the present study, this variable is associated with lateral mobility, as is change in work-style. Change of employer is also associated with change in work-style. These interrelationships were not explored in this paper.

Some other potentially relevant variables available in this data-set have also not been considered, namely: perceived work stress (the subject of another paper), education (although associated with occupation), work variables previously found to be associated with hypertension in a cross-sectional study of this population (contact with public, shift-work and overtime choice) (4), supervisory content, number of hours worked, work change prior to entry into the study and physical activity at work.

The present findings support the need to explore beyond the objective notion of job change, and to examine the possible contribution of components of work, and subjects' reactions to stress.

ACKNOWLEDGEMENTS

We thank the management, unions and employees of Telecom Australia and the Australian Taxation Office; the User Services Group, ADP Branch, Commonwealth Department of Community Services and Health; Dr Geoffrey Berry, Professor in Epidemiology and Biostatistics, University of Sydney; Ms Annie Chapman and Ms Sandra Healey, Research Officers, National Institute of Occupational Health and Safety.

REFERENCES

1. Edye BV, Mandryk JA, Frommer MS, Healey S, Ferguson DA (1989) *Med J Aust* 150:574-581
2. Edye BV, Healey SH, Mandryk JA, Ferguson DA, Frommer MS (1987) National Institute of Occupational Health and Safety. Blood Pressure Study: handbook of tables. Australian Government Publishing Service, Canberra
3. Frommer MS, Edye BV, Mandryk JA, Grammeno GL, Berry G, Ferguson DA (1986) *Scand J Work Environ Health* 12:476-48
4. Frommer MS, Ferguson DA, Edye BV, Mandryk JA, Berry G, Long AA, Ng TK (1983) *J Occup Health Aust NZ* 5:7-19
5. Haynes SG, Feinleib M, Kannel WB (1980) *Am J Epidemiol* 111:37-58
6. Kaplan BH, Cassel JC, Tyroler HA, Cornoni JC, Kleinbaum DG, Hames CG (1971) *Arch Intern Med* 128:938-942
7. Haynes SG, Feinleib M (1980) *Am J Public Health* 70(2):133-141
8. Kirjonen J, Hanninen V (1984) *Scand J Work Environ Health* 10:514-519
9. Haynes SG, Levine S, Scotch N, Feinleib M, Kannel WB (1978) *Am J Epidem* 107(5):362-383
10. Lehman EW, Schulman J, Hinkle LE (1967) *Arch Environ Health* 15:455-461
11. Haynes SG, Feinleib M, Levine S, Scotch N, Kannel WB (1978) *Am J Epidem* 107(5):384-402
12. Moorehouse LE, Miller AT (1971) Physiology of Exercise. 6th edition. C.V. Mosby Company, St Louis, pp 281-283
13. Rose GA, Blackburn H (1968) Cardiovascular survey methods. World Health Organisation, Geneva (WHO monograph series no. 56)
14. Lipid Research Clinic Program (1974) Manual of Laboratory Operations. Vol 1. Lipid and Lipoprotein Analysis. DHEW Publications No (NIH) 75-628. National Institute of Health, Bethesda
15. SAS Institute (1985) SAS User's Guide: Statistics. Version 5 edition. Cary
16. Theorell T, Lind E, Floderus B (1975) *Int J Epid* 4:281-293
17. Kasl SV (1981) *Am J Public Health* 71(7):682-684

Occupational Epidemiology. H. Sakurai et al., editors

CORONARY HEART DISEASE AND RISK FACTORS AMONG URBAN BUS DRIVERS IN DENMARK

BO NETTERSTRØM[1), KNUD JUEL[2)]

1) Clinic of Occupational Medicine, University Hospital, Copenhagen, Denmark.
2) The Danish Institute for Clinical Epidemiology, Copenhagen, Denmark.

The incidence of coronary heart disease and occupationally related coronary risk factors among urban bus drivers were studied. Two cohorts consisting of all male bus drivers in Copenhagen were followed from 1972 to 1977 (1741 men) and from 1978 to 1985 (1848). All cases of death due to coronary heart disease and all causes of myocardial infarction (MI) were registered from the Danish National Patient Register and the Register of Causes of Death. A subsample of the 1978-cohort underwent clinical examination including measurement of blood pressure and blood lipid levels. 2045 (83%) bus drivers in the three major cities in Denmark answered a questionnaire in 1978. The questions regarding work-related and psychosocial factors were later used as independent variables in the analysis of predictive factors for subsequent MI during the period 1978-1984.

The incidence of MI decreased among the Copenhagen bus drivers during the whole observation period 1972-85. During the period 1972-77 SMR for MI was 139 compared to other employed men, while no differences was found during the period 1978-85. The Copenhagen bus drivers had higher blood pressure and total serum cholesterol levels than the reference groups used. HDL-cholesterol was lower. Sixty-two cases of MI were registered during the period 1978-84.

The strongest work-related predictive factor for subsequent MI was high work load, defined as driving in the city traffic. The relative risk ratio was 4-6 among the city drivers compared to suburban drivers. The following factors too were correlated to subsequent MI: Smoking, feeling of increased work pace, and having no social contact with colleagues in spare time. Subjective stress symptoms and job dissatisfaction were however not associated with MI.

Occupational Epidemiology. H. Sakurai et al., editors

STATISTICAL ANALYSIS OF THE EFFECTS OF LIFESTYLE ON LIVER FUNCTION TESTS AMONG WORKERS

ISAO OKAZAKI, SUNAO ADACHI* and KATSUYA MARUYAMA**
Department of Preventive Medicine and Public Health, and *Laboratory of Biostatistics and Bioinformation Science, School of Medicine, Keio University, Tokyo 160, Japan, and **Clinical Research Unit, National Institute on Alcoholism, Kurihama National Hospital, Kanagawa 239, Japan

INTRODUCTION

In 1972 the Occupational Safety and Health Law was established in Japan for the purpose of systematic regulation and organization of the workplace and occupational health services in general. In order to pave the way for the already-encroaching era of high-technology, the law and its regulations were partially changed this year to include the implementation of a system of more extensive health checks. Before these modifications, the main purpose of health services was the early detection of occupational and general diseases, especially tuberculosis. However, recent health services provided by an occupational physician have come to include the prevention of occupational diseases as well as the education of health promotion.

The health examination required under this law can be divided into two major categories of tests, the general and special health examinations. A major facet of the general health examination is liver function blood chemistry, because abnormal liver function tests are observed in approximately 30% of those between the ages of 40-50 in the population of our country. Among the Japanese population ten years ago the incidence of HBs carrier was about 2.5%, but at the present time less than 1.8%. Due to the establishment of good sanitation conditions as well as education concerning sound hygiene practices, there are also few cases of hepatitis A in Japan. However, about 17% of males and 6% of females between the ages of 20 to 65 present with abnormal liver function tests[1,2].

The question then arises as to what factors influence liver function tests. I have therefore conducted an investigation into the effects of lifestyle on liver function tests to determine factors and causes that may lead to liver disease.

METHODS

The present study was conducted at a shipbuilding factory located in Kawasaki City which lies between Tokyo and Yokohama. The size of this company is typical of a large company in Japan with approximately 4,000 workers (3,800 males and 200 females) in its factory. At this company, in addition to the annual health examination, workers at the ages of 20, 25, 30, 35, 40, 45, 50 and 55 were given a more detailed health check. In this manner, a fifth of the employees, approximately 800 workers, would undergo a detailed health check every year. From this pool, 434 males actually received health examinations between May to October of 1985, the period of this present study. For this study, a questionnaire survey as well as this detailed health check were conducted on the workers in the 7 age groups. This study was limited to only male workers as there were too few females workers to conduct a proper study. The number of cases investigated in each age category is shown in Table 1.

Table 1. Number of Subjects

Age	Numbers
20 y.o.	22
25	34
30	43
35	100
40	53
45	66
50	68
55	48
total	434 males

To give a simple background picture of these workers, very few had been exposed to organic solvents or other hepatotoxic agents. The percentage of HB_s Ag carriers in this population was not considered to differ from the national average. Those with definite liver, cardiovascular, or other diseases were excluded from this study.

Table 2. Items in the Detailed Health Check Program

Questionaire	Age, Sex, Type of job, hours of sleep, commuting time, marriage status, smoking and alcohol drinking habits
Physical Exa.	height, weight, systolic and diastolic blood pressure,etc.
Chemical Analysis of Blood	AST(GOT), ALT(GPT), GGTP(gammaglutamyl transpeptidase),total cholesterol, triglyceride, HDL-cholesterol, total protein, ZTT, uric acid

Examination items conducted in this study are shown in Table 2. Subjects were asked to fill in a questionnaire and the answers were confirmed by oral interview by an industrial physician or an industrial health nurse. This information was input into a FACOM M-380R. In order to investigate the incidence and causes of abnormal liver function tests, statistical analysis was conducted in both workers with and without abnormal liver function tests. A person with abnormal liver function tests was defined to have GOT $\geqq$ 40K.U., GPT $\geqq$ 40K.U.,and /or GGTP $\geqq$ 50U/1.

RESULTS

314 workers presented with normal liver function tests and 119 workers presented with abnormal liver function tests. The incidence of abnormal tests was highest in the age groups between 40-55 y.o.(Table 3).

Table 3. Numbers of Cases with Abnormal Liver Function tests

Age	n	Numbers of workers with abnormal liver function tests
20+25	56	11 (19.6 %)
30+35	143	36 (25.2 %)
40+45	119	31 (26.1 %)
50+55	116	44 (37.9 %)

T-test of variance for each lifestyle variable was performed for both the groups with and without abnormal liver function tests. Among the various life style factors surveyed, statistically significant differences($P < 0.001$) were observed for each variable for: daily alcohol consumption for habitual drinkers(DAC), weekly alcohol consumption (WAC), systolic and diastolic blood pressure, body weight and obesity indices (Broca and BMI) (Table 4).

On the other hand, significant coefficients ($|r|>0.3$, $p< 0.0001$) for GOT were WAC, GPT and GGTP; for GPT, Broca BMI, triglyceride (TG) and GOT; GGTP, WAC, TG, body weight, GOT and GPT using Spearman's.

The multivariate relations of these variables were then examined by regression analysis, discriminant analysis and quantification analysis. Stepwise regression for each of the dependent variables for GOT, GPT and GGTP revealed the following formula.

Table 4. T-test for Each Variable Between Both Groups With and Without Abnormal Liver Function Tests

Each Variables	Without Abnormal Tests					With Abnormal Tests					T	Signi-
	Mean	SD	SE	Min	Max	Mean	SD	SE	Min	Max	value	ficance
Age	38.8	10.0	0.57	20	55	41.8	9.4	0.83	20	55	-2.86	.0045
hours of sleep	7.03	0.73	0.04	4.0	9.0	7.18	0.68	0.06	5.5	9.0	-1.98	.0483
alc.cons.daily*	23.7	23.3	1.31	0	206	35.9	25.0	2.24	0	110	-4.87	.0001
alc.cons.some+	50.1	41.1	2.33	0	202	63.0	46.5	4.20	0	300	-2.65	.0084
alc.cons.party	75.9	56.8	3.22	0	430	86.8	48.2	4.34	0	300	-2.02	.0443
alc.cons. week	121	133	7.54	0	700	219	176	15.8	0	732	-5.24	.0001
cum.alc.cons.**	99.6	119	6.83	0	717	185	164	14.9	0	732	-5.24	.0001
body weight	61.9	7.54	0.43	44	90	65.9	9.48	0.85	48	99	-4.20	.0001
systolic b.p.	119	13.6	0.77	90	172	125	14.0	1.25	98	192	-4.37	.0001
diastolic b.p.	73.6	10.7	0.60	50	110	78.5	11.4	1.01	50	114	-4.28	.0001
total cholest.	180	34.1	1.94	99	329	192	40.5	3.60	22	278	-2.84	.0049
triglyceride	131	82.8	4.69	15	567	217	160	14.4	31	998	-3.22	.0014
uric acid	5.10	1.16	0.07	2.0	9.8	5.42	1.28	0.11	2.0	9.5	-2.50	.0127
obesity(Broca)	102	10.3	0.59	72.6	134	110	12.1	1.08	83.3	143	-6.45	.0001
obesity(BMI)	22.0	2.16	0.12	16.0	29	23.7	2.60	0.23	18.1	31.6	-6.26	.0001

*daily alcohol consumption volume (gram);+alcohol consumption volume sometimes; **cumulative alcohol consumption volume (Kg)

Table 5. Close Relations Between Obesity (BMI) and Abnormal Liver Tests

BMI	Abnormal GOT	Abnormal GPT	Abnormal GGTP
16 ～ 18	0/6 (0%)	0/6 (0%)	0/6 (0%)
18 ～ 20	3/56(5.4%)	2/56(3.6%)	3/56 (5.4%)
20 ～ 22	11/126(8.7%)	19/126(13.5%)	23/126(18.3%)
22 ～ 24	8/138(5.8%)	24/138(17.4%)	25/138(18.1%)
24 ～ 26	13/73(17.8%)	29/73 (39.7%)	27/73 (37.0%)
26 ～ 28	3/31(9.7%)	17/31 (54.8%)	10/31 (32.3%)
28 ～ 30	2/ 4(50.0%)	3/ 4 (75.0%)	2/ 4 (50.0%)
30 ～	0/3	2/ 3 (66.7%)	3/ 3 (100 %)

$GOT=-3.938 + 0.215X_1^{**} + 0.012X_2^{**} + 0.149X_3^{*}$ (X_1: obesity (Broca index), X_2: cumulative alcohol consumption volume, X_3: Age) ; $R^2=0.105^{**}$ $(R=0.3240)$

$GPT=-31.672 + 0.628X_1^{**} + 0.021X_2 - 1.223X_4 - 0.768X_5$; $R^2=0.1127^{**}$ $(R=0.3357)$

$GGTP=-89.218 + 0.142X_6^{**} + 1.1330X_1^{*} + 0.047X_2 - 0.359X_7$ (X_6: weekly alcohol consumption volume, X_7: alcohol consumption per day); $R^2=0.1366^{**}$ $(R=0.3696)$;
** $Prob\{>F_i\}<0.01$, * $Prob\{>F_i\}<0.05$; all $Prob\{>F_i\}<0.15$.

Discriminant analysis for abnormal liver function tests revealed the contribution of obesity to be about 12% and that of WAC to be about 8%. A close correlations between alcohol intake and abnormal liver function tests (not shown), and also between Broca Index or BMI and abnormal tests were observed (Table 5). Although "obesity" and "drinking" did not show statistical correlation, these two variables independently affected liver function tests as shown statistically.

DISCUSSION

Alcoholic consumption in Japan has rapidly increased in the past decade[3]. A trend observed among the younger generation, especially, has been the consumption of strong alcohol and heavy calory intake. The result of the present study points to the fact that obesity and alcohol independently affected liver function. Both influence the other and these two factors are considered the causes of abnormal liver function tests in present-day Japan.

REFERENCES

1)Okazaki, I., Kobayashi, Y. and Kondo, H.:Worker education and health promotion-Prevention and management of liver diseases. XXII ICOH, Sydney, 1987.
2)Akiyama, M., IIda, M., Konishi, M., et al.:The analysis of mass screening survey for liver diseases in Osaka district. Jap.J.Pub.Health, 33:59,1986.
3)Ishii, H., Okazaki, I. and Tsuchiya, M.:Pathology of alcoholic liver disease. In:Alcohol Related Disease(Seitz,H.K., ed), Springer, 1985, pp.282-303.

Occupational Epidemiology. H. Sakurai et al., editors

THE NEUROBEHAVIOR CHANGES OF FERROMANGANESE SMELTING WORKERS

QING HUANG*, WEIQUN LIU*, CHUANXU PAN**.
* Occupational Disease Hospital, School of Public Health, West China University of Medical Sciences, CHINA.
** Department of Health Statistics, School of Public Health, West China University of Medical Sciences, CHINA.

INTRODUCTION

Manganese is a known neurotoxin. In the early stage of chronic manganese poisoning manganese may cause functional disturbance of central nervous system, but in the later period it may lead to irreversible pathological changes in human nervous system. From recent twenty years, a variety of neurobehavioral tests are available for evaluating nervous effects in working population exposed to neurotoxin agents. In order to make some exploration in early diagnosis and quantitative evaluation of chronic manganese poisoning. We examined the neurobehavior function of 61 ferromanganese smelting workers and 61 manganese-nonexposed workers using the neurobehavioral core test battery recomed by WHO (1) .

SUBJECTS AND METHODS

Subjects

61 ferromanganese smelting workers of a large steel factory in Chongqing of China were tested. A control group of manganese-nonexposed workers from the same factory were matched with the manganese-exposed subjects according to sex, age and level of education which showed with the number of school years completed.

Neurobehavioral Test

The WHO Neurobehavioral Core Test Battery (NCTB) consisted of a pre-test interview, a administration of the tests and a post-test interview. The examination was performed individually and last about one hour. The examiner always give the instructions in the standard wording according to Operational Guide for the WHO Neurobehavioral Core Test Battery.

Administration of the tests (the test methods is elided) :

1. Profile of Mood States (POMS): The POMS test give a description of the moods and feelings of the subject.

2. Simple Reaction Time: It measures how fast a person react. It requires sustained attention by the subject.

3. Digit Span: The Digit Span Test is a test of immediate (short-term) auditory memory which requires focused attention. The test

include Digit-Forward and Digit-Backward.

4. Santa Ana Manual Dexterity Test: The Santa Ana-Helsinki verson is a test of manual dexterity which requires rapid eye-hand coordinated movements.

5. Digit Symbol Test: The Digit Symbol Test is a test of perceptual motor speed which also requires leaning of associations.

6. Benton Visual Retention Test: The Benton Recognition Test is a measure of the ability to organize geometrical patterns in space and memorize them.

7. Pursuit Aiming Test: THe test measure the ability to make quick and accurate movements with the hand.

Statistical Analysis

Computation of Standard Scores. We converted the raw score into standard score according to the method of standardize raw score recommded by WHO (1).

Statistical Methods. The statistical methods adopted were Chi Square Test, Straight Bar Graph, Point Graph, Multiple Linear Regression, Compare of Multivariate two Group's Mean Vector, Canonical Correlation Analysis, Simple Coorelation Analysis,etc. The data analysis was performed using microcomputer.

Results

The concentrat of manganese in the air of ferromanganese smelting shop where the 61 manganese-exposed workers worked is obviously exceed 0.2mg/m3 that is the highest allowable concentrat of manganese in occupational environment of China.The 61 ferromanganese smelting workers were normal in Clinical Physical Examination, Encephalogram, and the level of manganese in urine.

Subjective Symptoms

The manganese-exposed group's percent of subjective symptoms was significantly exceed the control group's ($p<0.05$) in 13 subjective symptoms, such as weak memory, less coordination in hands, somnolence, insomnia, often wake up at night, nightmares, often forget things, thought are incoherent, lost in his own thoughts, difficulty to concentrate, vertigo, feel numbness in fingers, hands tremble.

Neurobehavioral Function

Table 1 showed that the mean score of contral group was generally higher than the exposed group's in almost behavior indexes except Aiming-Wrong and POMS-Vigor. When we analysis these data use Multiple Linear Regression. The result showed that most behavior indexes had significant difference ($p<0.05$) in two group's scores except Aiming-Wrong, POMS-Vigor and Digit Span when eliminating the influance of age factor and education factor. Inthe meantime, the result showed that age factor have not significant affection to the scores of Digit Span, Benton, Aiming-Wrong, Standard Deviation of Reaction Time and the education factor have not significant affection to the scores of Sant Ana Nonpreferred Hand, Aiming-Wrong,Fastest Reaction Time and POMS(all six mood scales).

The result of Simple Correlation Analysis showed that there were significant positive correlation between almost single behavior indexes except Aiming-Wrong with all the other behavior indexes, POMS-Vigor with Digit Span, Benton, POMS-Tension-Anxiety, POMS-Hostility, level of education with POMS-Hostility, POMS-Fatigue, POMS-Depression, POMS-Confusion.

DISCUSSION

This study found that ferromanganese smelting workers had shown clear deficits in short term memory, manual dexterity and eye-hand coordination movements, perceptual motor speed and learning of associations, the ability to make quick movements with the hand, the speed of reaction and attention while eliminate the influence of age factor and education factor, although it is normal in their Clinical Physical Examination, EEG and the level of manganese in urine. Weak visual memory have been reported in the neuropsychology examination of 48 electric welders (2). In the meantime, the manganese-exposed group showed poorer mood states in tension-anxiety, hostility, fatigue, depression and comfusion besides vigor. This result coorespond to the report about having emotional lability in the early symptoms of manganese-exposed workers (2,3,4). But the immediate auditory memory and the ability to make accurate movements with the hand of ferromanganese smelting workers were not affected.

This study indicate that the subject's scores of perceptual motor speed, manual dexterity, the ability to make quick movements with the hand decrease with their age getting older. But the immediate auditory memory, short term visual memory, the ability to make accurate movements with the hand, attention of subjects did'nt be affected by their age. When the subject's level of education increase, their scores of immediate auditory memory, short term visual memory, perceptual motor speed, manual dexterity of preferred hand, the ability to make quick movements with hand, attention also increase. But the level of education of subjects didn't affect their manual dexterity of nonpreferred hand and the ability to make accurate movements with the hand.

There were some significant positive correlation between behavior indexes of subjects, such as short term visual memory and immediate auditory memory, short term visual memory and perceptual motor speed, manual dexterity and the ability to make quick movements with the hand, the speed of reaction and attention,etc. It showed the internal connection of behavior functions.

In the manganese-exposed group, the persons who complain of weak memory, somnolence, insomnia, difficulty to concentrate,etc.was significanty more than the persons of control group who had the same symptoms. This result correspondto the clinical symptoms of manganese-exposed workers reported in literature (3,4).

This study pointed out that the test of behavior function may provide quantitation evaluation index in the early diagnosis of chronic manganese poisoning.

TABLE 1

SOME STATISTICS OF EXPOSED GROUP AND CONTROL GROUP

Item	Exposed Group			Control Group		
	Number	Mean	Stand.Dev.	Number	Mean	Stand.Dev.
D-Symbol	61	48.84	10.28	61	51.25	9.60
D-Span	61	48.75	10.43	61	51.56	9.25
Benton	61	48.25	11.17	61	52.61	8.50
St-Ana-P	61	46.64	9.95	61	53.11	9.28
St-Ana-N	61	46.23	8.66	61	53.28	10.12
Aiming-W	61	50.77	11.69	61	49.67	7.85
Aiming-T	61	48.15	9.29	61	51.74	10.49
React-M	60	48.27	9.25	61	52.49	8.19
React-F	60	49.1	9.63	61	51.75	6.65
React-S	61	46.70	11.57	61	53.33	6.93
React-St	61	47.39	10.63	61	52.70	7.45
POMS-T	61	46.21	10.57	61	53.89	7.95
POMS-H	61	46.44	10.33	61	53.59	8.37
POMS-F	61	47.31	10.77	61	52.64	8.67
POMS-D	61	46.31	10.28	61	53.69	8.38
POMS-V	61	50.87	8.96	61	49.05	11.02
POMS-C	61	47.02	10.28	61	52.90	8.97

REFERENCES

1. WHO: Operational Guide for the WHO Neurobehavioral Core Test Battery. WHO, Office of Occupational Health, Draft-25.5.1986
2. Huang Shupei. The Behavior Toxicology of Heavy Metal (A Survey) The Hygiene Fascicle of Oversea Medicine. 1985 (6);321
3. Chandra S.V. Psychiatric Illness due to Manganese Poisoning. Acta Psychiat Scand. 1983 67 Suppl. 303:49
4. Feldman R.G. Central and Peripherel Nervous System Effects of Metals: A Survey Occupational Neurology. Acta Neurol Scand. 1982 (66) Suppl 92:143

Occupational Epidemiology. H. Sakurai et al., editors

APPLICATION OF THE METHOD OF "DISTRIBUTION OF NERVE CONDUCTION VELOCITIES" IN OCCUPATIONAL MEDICINE

KAZUHITO YOKOYAMA, SHUNICHI ARAKI, KATSUYUKI MURATA
Department of Public Health, Faculty of Medicine, University of Tokyo, Bunkyo-ku, Tokyo 113 (Japan)

INTRODUCTION

Peripheral nerve conduction velocity has been used for evaluating peripheral nerve disorders of occupational and environmental etiology. However, the conventional methods for measuring conduction velocities yield only two discrete values that reflect the maximal and slower conduction velocities of fibers in the nerve trunk; the function of the vast majority of fibers cannot be directly assessed. We have established a technique to derive the distribution of conduction velocities (DCV) of large myelinated fibers (alpha group) using computer analysis in our laboratory (1,2). In this paper, findings in four different groups of workers, i.e. those exposed to lead, thallium, styrene and local vibration, are reported.

MEASUREMENT OF DCV

The DCV was measured by the method reported by us (1,2). The study was conducted in a warm laboratory (28-32 °C) using a Medelec MS-92 electromyograph; skin temperature was in the range of 30-36 °C for all subjects. After electrical stimulation of the right median nerve at the second digit with a 70 to 100 V square wave pulse of 0.2 msec duration, the compound action potential (CAP) was picked up at the wrist and elbow. The DCV was calculated from the two CAPs by the double conduction distance method (3) between the velocities of 30.0 and 77.5 m/sec using a microcomputer. The calculated DCV was expressed by the the conduction velocities below which 10, 20, ..., 90% of active fibers lie (V10, V20, ..., V90 velocities).

DCVs IN FOUR GROUPS OF SUBJECTS

Workers exposed to lead, zinc and copper

Subjects were 20 male gun metal founders, aged 34-59 (mean 48) years, with blood lead (BPb) concentrations of 22-59 (mean 39) μg/dl. In nine of them (high lead group) the BPb was 40 μg/dl or above; in the remaining workers (low lead group) it was below 40 μg/dl. Control subjects were 20 healthy men whose age, skin temperature and alcohol consumption were not significantly different from those in the high and low lead groups (P>0.05).

Fig. 1 illustrates the DCVs in 20 gun metal founders. In the high lead group, the V10 velocity and the maximal sensory conduction velocity (SCV) were significantly slowed (Fig. 2); no significant reduction were observed in the V20-V90 velocities ($p>0.05$). The low lead group showed no significant slowing of the V10-V90 velocities and SCV ($p>0.05$). In 20 gun metal founders, the V10 velocity was inversely correlated with BPb (Fig. 3) and with 24 hr mobilization yield of lead in urine (MPb) by CaEDTA ($r = -0.595$, $P<0.01$); the V20 velocity was correlated with MPb ($r = -0.449$, $P<0.05$). On the other hand, the V90 velocity was positively correlated with the amount of zinc excreted in urine for 24 hrs (UZn) (Fig. 3); the V80 velocity and SCV were positively correlated with UZn ($r = 0.459$, 0.455, $P<0.05$).

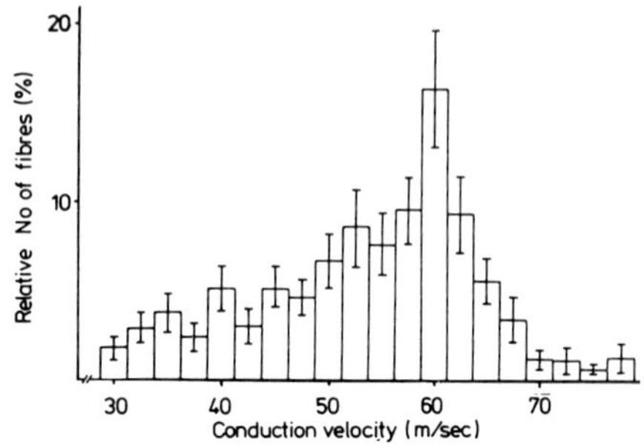

Fig. 1. DCV in 20 gun metal founders (means and standard errors) (ref. 1).

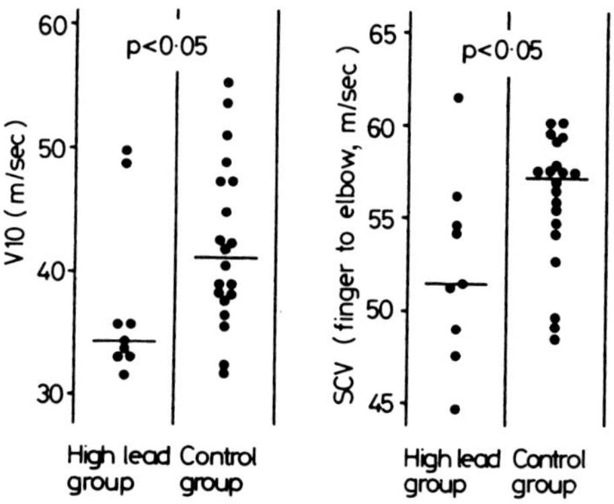

Fig. 2. Differences in DCV (V10 velocity) and SCV between the high lead group (nine subjects) and 20 controls (Wilcoxon's rank sum test). (ref. 1). Transverse line indicates median values.

It is suggested that conduction velocities of slower fibers are inversely affected by lead resulting in a significant reduction at the BPb level of 40-59 μg/dl; the effects of lead might be antagonized by zinc.

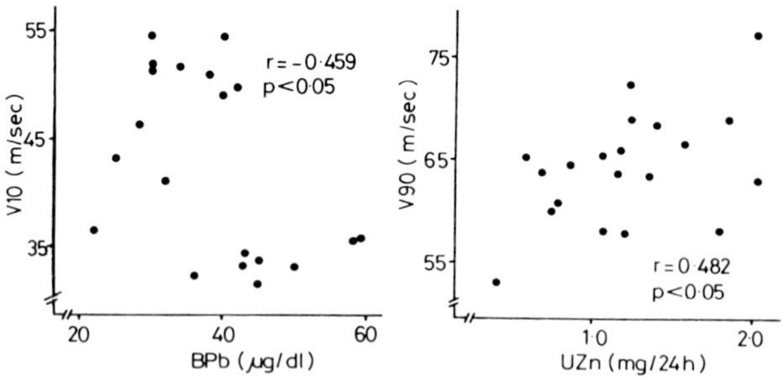

Fig. 3. Relations between DCV (V10 and V90 velocities) and blood lead (BPb) concentration and 24 hr urinary excretion of zinc (UZn) in 20 gun metal founders (ref. 1).

<u>Acute thallium poisoning patient</u>

The patient was a male building contractor aged 31 years; the DCV was measured two and 11 months after the onset of clinical symptoms. Control subjects were 16 healthy men aged 22-41 (mean

32) years. In the first examination, the patient showed elevated urinary thallium (3.5 mg/l) with sensorimotor neuropathy; the V70-V90 velocities and SCV were below the normal lower limit (mean - 2 SD in control subjects) (Fig. 4). In the second examination, the V70-V90 velocities and SCV returned to normal level; the V10-V60 velocities were higher than the initial levels (Fig. 4). These results indicate that the conduction velocities of all faster and slower fibers are affected in thallium poisoning and recover following recuperation from the poisoning; and faster fibers are more sensitive to thallium.

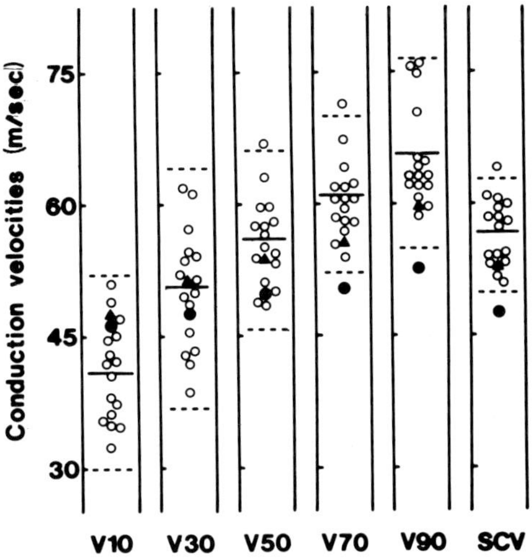

Fig. 4. DCV (V10, V30, V50, V70, V90 velocities) and SCV in thallium poisoning patient 2 (●) and 11 (▲) months after onset of symptoms and in 16 controls (○) (ref. 4). Transverse solid lines indicate mean values for controls; broken lines are mean ± 2 SD (upper and lower normal limits). The V20, V40, and V60 velocities were within normal limits for two examinations; the V80 velocity was below normal in the first examination and within normal limits in the second.

Workers exposed to styrene

Eleven male workers in a fiber-reinforced plastic (FRP) boat factory aged 22-61 (mean 40) years were examined. Their phenylglyoxylic acid concentrations in end-of-shift urine were 31-419 (mean 169) mg/g creatinine. Control subjects were 11 healthy men matched to each styrene worker by age; their skin temperature and alcohol consumption were not significantly different from those in styrene workers ($p>0.05$). It was observed that the V80 velocity and SCV were significantly slowed in styrene workers, suggesting that conduction velocities of faster fibers are more vulnerable to styrene (Fig. 5).

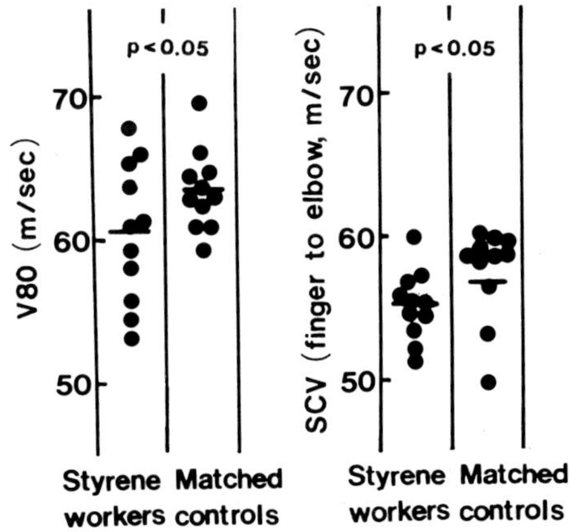

Fig. 5. Differences in DCV (V80 velocity) and SCV between 11 styrene workers and same number of matched controls (paired sample t-test). Transverse line shows mean values.

Chain saw operators (workers exposed to local vibration)

Subjects were 10 male forest workers, aged 41-59 (mean 53) years, who had engaged in chain saw operations for 16-26 (mean 22) years. Three had frequent attacks of white finger; the attacks were only occasional in four and negative in three). Control subjects were 10 healthy men matched to each worker by age; there were no significant differences in skin temperature and alcohol consumption between chain saw operators and controls. The V10-V90 velocities and SCV were significantly slowed in chain saw operators, indicating that local vibration affects all faster and slower fibers (Fig. 6). It is also suggested that chain saw operators with white finger attacks tended to have slower conduction velocities for all the V10-V90 velocities than those without; on the other hand, slowing of SCV was independent of the attacks (Fig. 6). The DCV, therefore, may be sensitive indicator of the vascular effects of local vibration.

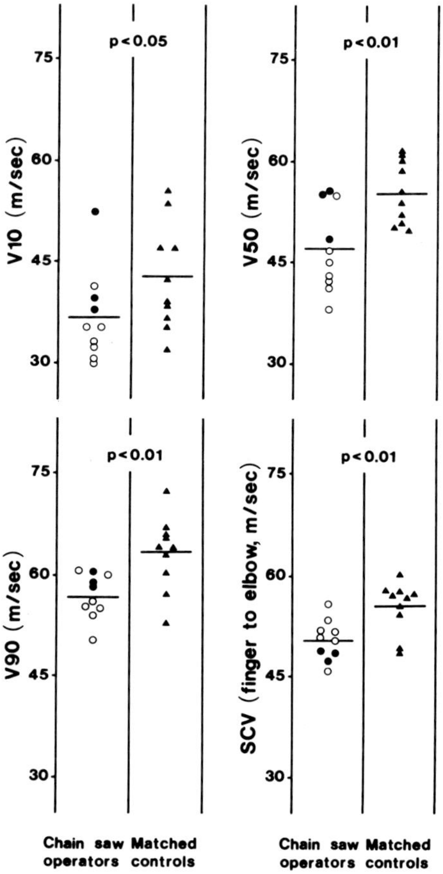

Fig. 6. Differences in DCV (V10, V50, V90 velocities) and SCV between 10 chain saw operators and same number of matched controls (paired sample t-test) (ref. 5). Open (○) and solid (●) circles indicate chain saw operators with and without a history of white finger attacks, respectively; black triangles (▲) are matched controls. Transverse lines are mean values.

CONCLUSION

Evidence has been given that there is a good correspondence between the DCV and the distribution of fiber diameter in large myelinated fibers (6). It is concluded that determination of the DCV is useful for assessing the effects of various occupational and environmental factors on all faster and slower large myelinated nerve fibers.

REFERENCES

1. Araki S, Yokoyama K, Murata K, Aono H (1986) Brit J Ind Med 43:321-326
2. Yokoyama K, Araki S, Murata K, Aono H (1987) Jpn J EEG EMG 15:282-290
3. Barker AT, Brown BH, Freeston IL (1979) IEEE Transac Biomed Eng BME-26:76-81
4. Yokoyama K, Araki S, Abe H (in press) Muscle & Nerve
5. Araki S, Yokoyama K, Aono H, Murata K (1988) Brit J Ind Med 44:341-344
6. Yokoyama K, Feldman RG, Sax DS, Salzsider BT, Kucera J (in press) Muscle & Nerve

Occupational Epidemiology. H. Sakurai et al., editors

A DOSE-RESPONSE RELATIONSHIP FOR NOISE-INDUCED HYPERTENSION

Zhao Yiming, Zhang Shuzhen*, Steve Selvin** and Robert C. Spear**

Cardiovascular Research Lab., Third Hospital; *Department of Occupational Medicine, School of Public Health, Beijing Medical University, Beijing 100083, China; **Northern California Occupational Health Center, School of Public Health, University of California, Berkeley, CA 94720, U.S.A

There have been many investigations of the relationship between noise exposure and hypertension in worker populations. Several researches indicated that industrial noise exposure was associated with increases in the prevalence of hypertension. But some other researches did not find the association. A principal objective of the present study was to explore further the association between noise exposure and hypertension in a setting in which exposure was well defined and in which there was a reasonable expectation of describing any dose-response relationship free from the influence of known confounding variables, albeit within the constrains of a cross-sectional design.

MATERIALS AND METHODS: The subjects were 1,101 female workers in a textile mill in Beijing. Each of these workers had worked in a single workshop in this mill for essentially their entire working life. All had been employed in the mill for at least five years. The subjects were drawn from six workshops and divided into 4 exposure groups by sound pressure level as shown in Table 1 which also contains the mean age and years worked in that environment for each group. As might be expected with such a stable population, there is a very high correlation between age and years worked in the mill (r = 0.966).

The sound pressure levels (SPL) of time-weighted average (TWA) were estimated to range from 75 to 104 dB(A). As far as can be determined, the SPLs have been essentially steady in each workshop since 1954. In those groups where noise exposure is classified by a single SPL, the levels at various locations in the workshops did not vary from this values by more than two dB(A) and the TWA exposure of all workers was very close to the value given. In cases where the exposure group contained a range of TWA exposures, the group mean, as well as the range, was estimated from measurements of the spatial distribution of SPLs and observations of the time spent at various stations within the workshop. The noise spectrum was typical of textile mills and broad band in nature.

Only second shift workers were studied (2:00 p.m. to 10:00 p.m.). the measurement of blood pressure and the administration of questionnaire were carried out between 1:30 p.m. and 4:30 p.m. and prior to the beginning of the day's work. All data were collected from July 8 to August 10, 1985. Blood pressure was measured twice in sitting subjects by mercury sphygmomanometer after 10 minutes rest. Hypertension was defined as systolic pressure greater than or equal to 160 mmHg and/or diastolic pressure greater than or equal to 95 mmHg. The subjects were also classified as hypertensive if they were currently using anti-hypertensive drugs.

RESULTS: The crude hypertensive prevalence in 4 SPL groups is shown in Table 2. Hypertensive prevalence increases markedly at the higher exposure levels. In order to explore this association in greater detail, a logistic regression was carried out using hypertension, as defined above, as the dependent binary outcome variable. The predictor variables were SPL, years worked, salt use (low, normal or high) and history of hypertension in either parent. No evidence was found of any substantial interactive influence and an additive logistic model was employed in the following analysis. Table 3 contains the summary estimates for this analysis. The coefficience of SPL, self-reported salt use and parental history of hypertension are all associated with the probability of hypertension as judged by significance values of less than 0.05. The signs of the coefficients indicated an increasing likelihood of hypertension with increasing noise exposure, increasing salt use and with a parental history of hypertension.

TABLE 1 Distribution of age and working years of female textile mill workers by SPL group

SPL	Age		Working Years		Cases
dB(A)	Mean	S.D.	Mean	S.D.	
104	38.51	8.07	19.76	9.59	164
96	37.20	8.64	18.23	9.87	294
86-90	33.93	7.99	14.18	8.99	428
75-80	33.90	8.20	14.59	9.34	215
Total	35.46	8.43	16.17	9.64	1101

TABLE 2 Sound pressure level and hypertension prevalence in female textile mill workers

SPL dB(A)	Number Hypertension	Total	Hypertensive Prevalence %
104	25	164	15.2
96	25	294	8.5
86-90	18	428	4.2
75-80	11	215	5.1
Total	79	1101	7.2

TABLE 3 Estimated parameters for logistic regression model for hypertension prevalence among 1011 female textile mill workers

Variable	Term	Coefficent	S.E.	P-Value	Odds Ratio
Constant	b0	-10.610	2.070	-----	-----
S P L	b1	0.0303	0.015	0.047	1.031
Age	b2	0.0959	0.063	0.126	1.101
Working Years	b3	0.0544	0.055	0.323	1.056
Salt (Normal)	b4	-0.827	0.408	0.043	0.437
Salt (High) More	b5	0.569	0.314	0.856	1.059
Family History	b6	0.748	0.260	0.004	2.113

The maximum likelihood estimates of the logistic model parameters (Table 3) produces an adjusted SPL odds ratio of 1.031. Therefore an increase of 30 dB(A) increases the odds of hypertension by $(1.031)^{30} = 2.479$ regardless of the values of the other predictor variables as long as they are held constant. In terms of probability, a 50 years old workers, employed

20 years, with normal salt intake and no family history of hypertension, and who is exposed to 70 dB(A) has a probability of being hypertensive of 0.089. In contrast, a worker with the same levels of the other predictor variables, but an exposure of 100 dB(A), has a probability of 0.195 of being hypertension.

TABLE 4 Relative influence of predictor variables on probability of hypertension: differences in likelihood values

Variable	Difference	P-Value
S P L	4.061	0.044
Age	2.234	0.135
Working Years	1.021	0.312
Salt Use	7.752	0.005
Family History	8.520	0.004

A set of commensurate values is achieved by the comparison of two likelihood values; one likelihood value measuring the influence of the entire set of variables (all five variables) and a reduced likelihood where one variable at a time is deleted from the model. The difference in the likelihood values measures the influence on hypertensive risk solely attributable to the deleted variable. Contrasting these two likelihood for the 1101 female workers (Table 4) shows that a family history of hypertension and high salt intake have about equal significant impact (8.52 and 7.75; $p < 0.001$) on the probability of hypertension, followed in order of importance by SPL at about half the magnitude (4.061; $p = 0.044$). Age and years worked have less influence and are not statistically significant (2.23 and 1.02; $p > 0.05$).

TABLE 5 Confounding influence on logistic regression: coefficients for a series of sequential analyses

S P L	Age	Working Years	Salt Normal	Salt Excess	Hypertension History
0.0523					
0.0297	0.148				
0.0287	0.0789	0.0639			
0.0279	0.0686	0.0722	-0.784	0.130	
0.0303	0.0959	0.0544	-0.827	0.0569	0.748

The influence on risk of hypertension associated with SPL is relatively unaffected by the other four predictor variables. Table 5 shows the logistic coefficient associated with SPL as other variables are added to the analysis. The SPL coefficients remain essentially constant when the other variables are included in the analysis, particularly after age of the worker if taken into account.

The ability of the logistic model to summarize the multivariable relationships under investigation can be judged by the "goodness-of-fit" of the values predicted by the logistic model to those observed as shown in Table 6. The 1101 workers were distributed into 24 categories using three variables, hypertension, SPL and age. The expected frequencies and observed frequencies show close agreement with the exception of one aberrant cell where five workers were observed and only 1.08 were expected. Formally, the chi-squared value for goodness-of-fit of the values predicted by

TABLE 6 Goodness-of-fit of values generated from the logistic regression model using hypertension, SPL and age categories

Hyper-tension	SPL	Age	Observed Number	Expected Number	Difference	Chi-square Contribution
Yes	104	45	19	12.878	6.122	2.910
Yes	104	35	5	2.589	2.411	2.245
Yes	104	25	1	0.508	0.492	0.477
Yes	96	45	20	15.942	4.058	1.033
Yes	96	35	5	3.731	1.269	0.432
Yes	96	25	0	0.898	-0.898	0.898
Yes	90	45	13	11.450	1.550	0.210
Yes	90	35	2	4.515	-2.515	1.401
Yes	90	25	3	1.615	1.385	1.188
Yes	77	45	6	4.860	1.140	0.267
Yes	77	35	5	1.081	3.919	14.208
Yes	77	25	0	0.620	-0.620	0.620
No	104	45	50	56.122	-6.122	0.668
No	104	35	47	49.411	-2.411	0.118
No	104	25	42	42.492	-0.492	0.006
No	96	45	84	88.058	-4.058	0.187
No	96	35	89	90.269	-1.269	0.018
No	96	25	96	95.102	0.898	0.008
No	90	45	74	75.550	-1.550	0.032
No	90	35	133	130.485	2.515	0.048
No	90	25	203	204.385	-1.385	0.009
No	77	45	46	47.140	-1.140	0.028
No	77	35	42	45.919	-3.919	0.334
No	77	25	116	115.380	0.620	0.003
Total			1101	1101.000	0.000	27.348

the logistic model to those observed as shown in Table 6. The 1101 workers were distributed into 24 categories using three variables, hypertension, SPL and age. The expected frequencies and the observed frequencies show close agreement with the exception of one aberrant cell where five workers were observed and only 1.08 were expected. The chi-square value for goodness-of-fit is 27.348 with 20 degree of freedom producing a p-value of 0.126.

DISCUSSION: The crude rates of hypertension as a function of noise exposure shown in Table 2 suggested a dose-response relationship which, accounting for the influence of other predictor variables, is now confirmed by logistic regression. An increase in noise level from 70 to 100 dB(A) approximately doubles the probability of hypertension for any combination of other variables. The overall risk of hypertension is strongly dependent on the present of other predictor variables, in particular, family history of hypertension, dietary salt intake and age. Cumulative exposure to noise, as measured by years worked in a particular noise environment, did not appear to be an important predictor of hypertension risk. This might be due to the manifestation of this effect within the first five years exposure, which we would not have detected, or to an inability to separate the effects of age and years worked because of the collinearilty between these factors in this population.

Index of authors